MUST WE SUFFER OUR WAY TO DEATH?

The Park Ridge Center exists to explore the relationships among health, faith, and ethics. In its programs of research, publishing, clinical consultation, and education, the Center gives special attention to the bearing of religious beliefs on questions that confront people as they search for health and encounter illness. It also seeks to contribute to ethical reflection on a wide range of health-related issues. In this work the Center collaborates with representatives from diverse cultures, religious communities, health care fields, and academic disciplines and disseminates its findings to people interested in health, religion, and ethics.

The Center is an independent, not-for-profit organization supported by Advocate Health Care, by subscribing members, and by grants and gifts from foundations, corporations, and individuals. Additional information may be obtained by writing to the Park Ridge Center, 211 E. Ontario, Suite 800, Chicago, IL 60611-3215.

MUST WE SUFFER OUR WAY TO DEATH?

CULTURAL AND THEOLOGICAL PERSPECTIVES
ON DEATH BY CHOICE

Edited by

Ronald P. Hamel
Edwin R. DuBose

*A book from the Park Ridge Center
for the Study of Health, Faith, and Ethics*

Southern Methodist University Press
Dallas, Texas

First edition, 1996

Requests for permission to reproduce material from this work should be sent to:

Permissions
Southern Methodist University Press
P.O. Box 750415
Dallas, TX 75275-0415

Cover art: Mark Rothko, American, 1903–1970, *Purple, White and Red*, oil on canvas, 1953, 197.5 x 207.6 cm, Bequest of Sigmund E. Edelstone, 1983.509, photograph © 1994 The Art Institute of Chicago. All rights reserved.

Library of Congress Cataloging-in-Publication Data
Must we suffer our way to death? : cultural and theological
    perspectives on death by choice / edited by Ronald P. Hamel, Edwin
    R. Dubose. — 1st ed.
        p.   cm.
    "A book from the Park Ridge Center for the Study of Health, Faith,
    and Ethics."—T.p.
    Includes bibliographical references and index.
    ISBN 0-87074-392-9 (cloth). — ISBN 0-87074-393-7 (pbk.)
    1. Assisted suicide—Moral and ethical aspects. 2. Euthanasia—
Moral and ethical aspects. I. Hamel, Ronald P., 1946–   .
II. DuBose, Edwin R. III. Park Ridge Center (Ill.)
R726.M87 1996
174' .24—dc20   96-13818

Printed in the United States of America on acid-free paper

10   9   8   7   6   5   4   3   2   1

CONTENTS

FOREWORD

In 1991 the Park Ridge Center published its first work on the topic of euthanasia, *Choosing Death: Active Euthanasia, Religion, and the Public Debate*. Contributors to that volume mapped the terrain of the emerging public discussion concerning assisted suicide and euthanasia, offering reasons for the surge of interest in euthanasia, defining frequently used terms, and sketching the dominant societal attitudes toward euthanasia. Writers presented arguments on the justifiability of euthanasia and the wisdom of creating public policies concerning the practice at this time in the United States. Because religious concerns are central to any discussion of the morality of performing or legalizing euthanasia, considerable attention was also given to the stances of various religious bodies.

Debate concerning assisted suicide and euthanasia has not subsided. The activities of Dr. Jack Kevorkian and his lawyer continue to sensationalize euthanasia, and public initiatives in the states of Washington and California evidenced substantial public support for the legalization of assisted death for the terminally ill. And more recently a narrowly worded referendum in Oregon addressing just physician-assisted suicide was passed, although it now faces court challenges. These indications of growing support should not be surprising since they reflect our national bias in favor of individual rights and our relatively meager sense of social consciousness.

The pervasive influence of religion in this public policy discussion must be acknowledged. Some religious traditions have endorsed euthanasia and assisted suicide, while others have opposed these practices as fundamentally immoral. Whether religious traditions endorse or reject specific positions, they offer rich resources that can be used to expand and deepen the ongoing debate. Failure to take religion seriously in these matters will in all probability lead to increased political polarization and less-informed conversations.

While it is not the intention at the Park Ridge Center to move the public debate about euthanasia and assisted suicide in a particular direction, it is our aim to raise and examine key issues in the discussion. In this volume theologians from various religious traditions answer a direct challenge: to theologize creatively and to offer concrete responses to the dilemmas associated with the acceptance of assisted suicide and euthanasia. What theological insights are relevant, and how do they influence a movement toward or away from the social acceptance of benignly administered death?

Against the backdrop of an interdisciplinary discussion of the current social context, the theologians have mined the rich deposits of their respective theological traditions. In doing so, they have illuminated yet another facet of the complex conversation that must be part of the development of public policies that will so intimately affect the lives of people in the United States.

Although public opinion may ultimately favor the legalization of certain actions taken to hasten death, such acceptance should come only after a full understanding of the ramifications of such a policy. Pondering the perspectives offered in this volume should keep us from rushing to premature closure and flawed social policy. The Swahili proverb captures the point: "Haste, haste has no blessing!"

Laurence J. O'Connell
President and CEO
The Park Ridge Center

ACKNOWLEDGMENTS

In addition to the contributors, several other people played a major role in bringing this volume into being: Elizabeth Casey, Barbara Hofmaier, and Sondra Pittman edited the manuscript; Stephen Hudson and Rose Luciano did text processing; Loretta Faber proofread the manuscript; and Larry Greenfield provided support and guidance throughout the project. To all of them, we are immensely grateful.

The Editors

CONTRIBUTORS

Christine K. Cassel, M.D., is professor and chairman of geriatrics and adult development, Mount Sinai Medical Center, New York.

James M. Childs, Jr., Ph.D., is academic dean and professor of ethics at Trinity Lutheran Seminary, Columbus, Ohio.

Nicholas A. Christakis, M.D., Ph.D., M.P.H., is assistant professor of medicine and sociology at the University of Chicago, Chicago, Illinois.

Elliot N. Dorff, Ph.D., is provost and professor of philosophy at the University of Judaism, Los Angeles, California.

Edwin R. DuBose, Ph.D., is clinical ethics consultant, Clinical Healthcare Ethics Support Services, Park Ridge Center for the Study of Health, Faith, and Ethics, Chicago, Illinois.

Arthur W. Frank, Ph.D., is professor of sociology at the University of Calgary, Calgary, Alberta, Canada.

Ann Dudley Goldblatt, J.D., L.L.M., is an assistant director of the MacLean Center for Clinical Medical Ethics at the University of Chicago, Chicago, Illinois.

Ronald P. Hamel, Ph.D., is director of the Department of Clinical Ethics at Lutheran General Hospital of Advocate Health Care, Park Ridge, Illinois.

Patricia Beattie Jung, Ph.D., is associate professor of theology at Loyola University, Chicago, Illinois.

Lonnie D. Kliever, Ph.D., is professor of religious studies at Southern Methodist University, Dallas, Texas.

Martin E. Marty, Ph.D., is senior scholar in residence at the Park Ridge Center for the Study of Health, Faith, and Ethics and is Fairfax M. Cone Distinguished Service Professor at the University of Chicago, Chicago, Illinois.

William F. May, Ph.D., is Cary M. Maguire Professor of Ethics at Southern Methodist University, Dallas, Texas.

Daniel B. McGee, Ph.D., is professor of religion at Baylor University, Waco, Texas.

Laurence J. O'Connell, Ph.D., S.T.D., is president and CEO of the Park Ridge Center for the Study of Health, Faith, and Ethics, Chicago, Illinois.

Carol A. Tauer, Ph.D., is professor of philosophy at the College of St. Catherine, St. Paul, Minnesota.

Allen Verhey, Ph.D., is Evert J. and Hattie E. Blekkink Professor of Religion at Hope College, Holland, Michigan.

MUST WE SUFFER OUR WAY TO DEATH?

INTRODUCTION

Ronald P. Hamel and Edwin R. DuBose

Among the basic goals of medicine are to restore patients' health and alleviate their suffering, as in the old adage: "To cure sometimes, to relieve often, to comfort always." Another aim that is often mentioned is to prolong life. At times these goals can be achieved simultaneously. At other times, however, as the adage suggests, even the formidable scientific and technological armamentarium of contemporary medicine cannot restore the patient's health. In many of these instances, medicine relieves and comforts. But in others, it sustains or prolongs lives accompanied by much pain and suffering. When living comes to be so painful or oppressive that some desire to die, or even to have their lives ended, then difficult questions must be faced by patients, families, and care providers.

For the past twenty years, society has struggled with the moral and legal justifiability of forgoing life-sustaining treatment in patients whose disease cannot be cured and for whom prolonging life is no longer reasonable. It was probably the Karen Ann Quinlan case in 1976 that galvanized the public's attention to the issue. But *Quinlan* was followed by a succession of other prominent cases, among them *Saikewicz* (1977), *Spring* (1980), *Eichner* (1981), *Barber* (1983), *Bartling* (1984), *Conroy* (1985), *Brophy* (1986), *Jobes* (1987), and *Cruzan* (1988). The numerous debates associated with these cases—in homes, in the media, among health professionals and medical ethicists—and a number of

1

court decisions have resulted today in widespread moral and legal agreement regarding the permissibility of withholding and withdrawing life-sustaining treatment. But no sooner had society achieved some consensus on this issue than another, perhaps much more difficult one, came to the fore. Attention has begun to shift in the past few years from forgoing life-sustaining treatment to intervening actively to bring about a patient's death either with the assistance of another (assisted suicide) or by the direct action of another (euthanasia).

For many, there is a qualitative moral difference between forgoing life-sustaining treatment and participating in assisted suicide or euthanasia. The former, sometimes referred to as withholding or withdrawing life-sustaining treatment, abating treatment, allowing to die, or passive euthanasia (an unfortunate, confusing term that should be avoided), permits the patient's terminal disease process to run its course by forgoing those interventions that are delaying death from occurring. This practice involves a judgment that continued medical intervention is really no longer of benefit to the patient or may even impose burdens on the patient that outweigh any benefits. Consequently, it is no longer reasonable to continue interfering with the dying process. With the removal of death-delaying interventions, it is the underlying disease that ends the patient's life.

Assisted suicide (also referred to as physician-assisted suicide when the assistance comes from a physician) and euthanasia, many believe, are another matter. Assisted suicide consists in a patient's deciding to end his or her life and doing so with the assistance of someone who provides the means for bringing death about. The patient, however, actually administers the means, whether it be an overdose of sleeping pills, Kevorkian's carbon monoxide gas, or something else. Assisted suicide is a form of self-inflicted death. Euthanasia is different in that death is brought about by a third party either with the consent of the patient (voluntary), without the consent of the patient (nonvoluntary), or against the will of the patient (involuntary). Many if not most would consider euthanasia to be homicide but for compassionate purposes. With both assisted suicide and euthanasia death is directly intended and is caused by something other than the disease process. Until recently, entertaining the possibility of either of these courses of action as a legitimate response to the burdens of chronic and terminal illness was virtually taboo. The ethos of the medical profession and the condemnation of both actions by virtually all religious traditions kept them out of the realm of serious consideration. Discussions that did occur (frequently in classrooms) tended to view these practices as interesting ethical issues that prompted animated debate, but not, generally, as real options. This is no longer the case.

The current debate about physician-assisted suicide and euthanasia, and any resulting change in public policy on these issues, poses an enormous challenge to the traditional bulwarks against the acceptance of these practices—the medical profession and religion, particularly the latter. For the medical profession these practices call into question fundamental tenets of the Hippocratic ethos: not taking life and not doing harm. For religion they call into question some of the most basic and long-standing convictions of the major religious traditions—that life is sacred and is a gift of the Creator; that human beings' lives do not belong to them to do with as they wish; that innocent human life should not be ended; that suffering can be meaningful and beneficial; that human autonomy is limited by one's status as creature; that human beings are social by nature. An acceptance of assisted suicide or euthanasia by mainstream religious believers would seem to require a reinterpretation of these beliefs or, in some cases, their rejection. Either way, mainline Christian and Jewish religious traditions find themselves and their beliefs severely challenged from both within and without. In the face of a growing societal shift in attitude toward these practices, these religious communities are confronted with the task of developing constructive responses to those who defend the practices and their possible legalization.

In the fall of 1991, the Park Ridge Center embarked on a project called "Choosing Death in America: The Challenge to Religious Beliefs and Practices." For this phase of the project, we chose to focus on the larger mainline Jewish and Christian traditions in the United States. Although the latter part of the twentieth century often is described as postmodern, perhaps even post-theistic, it is important to remember that much of what we understand to be human nature, of who and what we are as persons, is taken from the biblical doctrine of our creation in the *imago Dei* (Kilner, Cameron, and Schiedermayer 1995:ix). In spite of the challenges presented by the postmodern cultural ethos to a theistic understanding of the nature and purpose of humanity, generally the Jewish and Christian traditions have been slow in grappling with the implications of an increasing public interest in "choosing death." To be sure, there has been strong and active support of, as well as resistance to, the idea of assisted suicide and euthanasia over the last several decades. Yet as aid in dying moves into the legislative arena, within both this country and others, the pressure to move to legalization of these practices or to close off debate about them altogether may occur too precipitously. For the mainline Jewish and Christian traditions, it is time for a thoughtful review and analysis of the reasons that many people in this country are interested in aid in dying.

We therefore gathered a group of religious professionals—theologians, hospital chaplains, congregational clergy, and denominational public-policy analysts—representing six religious traditions: Baptist, Jewish, Lutheran, Methodist, Reformed, and Roman Catholic. Their charge was to respond creatively and constructively, out of the best of those traditions and their personal experience, to the challenge posed to them and to members of the traditions by the increasing openness to assisted suicide and euthanasia in this country. To facilitate a better understanding of the social situation, we invited an interdisciplinary faculty composed of physicians, an attorney, a medical sociologist, a theologian, and a philosopher to probe, from their respective disciplines, the factors contributing to shifting societal attitudes toward aid in dying. A significant shift such as this can take place only if the environment makes it possible. Particular beliefs, values, needs, experiences, structures, and events coalesce and become catalysts of change in social attitudes, practice, and even public policy. Recognition of these driving forces is crucial not only to an informed debate but also to a response to the shaping forces themselves. Quite simply, it is imprudent at best to debate a change in public policy without first uncovering, examining, and in some way addressing those factors that contribute to requests for physician-assisted suicide and euthanasia and for a public policy permitting them.

The essays in this volume contain the analyses of the interdisciplinary faculty and the responses to the social situation by one of the four groups of religious professionals, namely, the theologians. Reflections by members of the other groups will be published, we hope, in a future volume. This project was not our attempt to garner the forces of the religious traditions in order either to oppose or to support the practice or the legalization of assisted suicide and euthanasia. Rather, we meant to foster creative theological thinking and constructive practical proposals in response to this social reality. Throughout, it was our hope that theologizing be informed by experience, that experience be informed by theology, and that ultimately public-policy initiatives would be influenced by both.

The essays in Part 1 constitute an interdisciplinary examination of the cultural factors driving public interest in euthanasia and especially in assisted suicide. Not surprisingly, given the deep moral concerns of thoughtful people surrounding the issue, the contributors express a variety of views about the morality of actively, albeit compassionately, taking life or assisting in a suicide. At the same time, common concerns run through their essays.

First, the contributors detect in the public some fear and uneasiness about medicine's successes and limitations. Undoubtedly, medicine is capable of great things. With all that it has to offer, however, many people are becoming convinced that an unnatural death is one that befalls the patient who is removed from his or her family, surrounded in an institution by strangers, machines, procedures, tubes, and medications that at some point no longer enhance his or her well-being. Living, not dying, may be burdensome in modern medicine. Under these conditions, people fear losing control of their lives and their personal dignity in a dying process that is often medicalized, professionalized, and inhumane, needlessly prolonged, inordinately expensive, and filled with uncontrolled suffering. As this view of death comes to be held by both physicians and patients, assisted suicide and euthanasia gain greater acceptance, symbolically reasserting the patient's and the physician's control over machines, over suffering, and over dying.

A second concern in these essays is the desire of many people to control their dying as a way of finding meaning in their death. The desire for control over dying usually surfaces in talk about patient autonomy, professional power, or the appropriate balance between individual self-determination and society's responsibility to care for its members. To carry on the discussion through debates about principles such as autonomy and beneficence misses the point, however: for many people, how they die—organically and technically, as well as emotionally and spiritually—has come to represent a measure of life's final value. Too often, under the current institutionalization and medicalization of death in our culture, the perception reigns that death is a pretty meaningless affair. People want a good death; how to achieve such a death is, of course, the question.

The desire for control over dying raises a third issue: who is responsible for ensuring a good death—the individual or society? In part, this question exposes an underlying issue in the assisted suicide and euthanasia debate: what we understand human beings to be, particularly whether each person is an atomistic individual, or whether we all are essentially relational beings, formed by personal and historical communities of interdependence.[1] Given the individualistic orientation of our society, over the last thirty years the focus of medical ethics has shifted gradually from a paternalistic medical practice to an emphasis on patients' rights. Indeed, by 1996, much ethical and legal thinking in this country weights personal autonomy heavily, even in the case of a person no longer capable of self-determination. The right of a competent patient to refuse or withdraw life-sustaining treatment, either directly or through advance directives, is widely accepted ethically and legally. As a result, many people argue that if one has a right to refuse life-sustaining treatment, knowing that the refusal will result in death, why should one not have a similar right to request that euthanasia be caused directly or assistance in suicide be provided, thereby assuring a meaningful "death with dignity"?

Several of the contributors, however, argue that how we care for each other as persons and as a society is expressed through the ways in which we care for the vulnerable among us: the poor, the elderly, the chronically and terminally ill, and people with disabilities. Have the faith communities, in an effort to be positive, warm, welcoming places, neglected their traditional responsibility to help their members face the limits of life? Some among the contributors to Part 1 worry that people who are chronically or terminally ill may feel so strapped with present and anticipated suffering and loss of function, and feel so unsupported by the people around them, that they see a continuation of their lives as meaningless. What is our individual and social responsibility to provide for suffering people the care that would alleviate their desire for assisted suicide or euthanasia? In a push toward legalized assisted suicide or euthanasia, are we trying to control suffering by eliminating the sufferer?

Because the issues surrounding assisted suicide and euthanasia so affect the nature of the relationship between doctor and patient, a fourth concern that connects these essays is the appropriate role and duties of the physician in the dying process. After all, if painless and merciful death is a goal, anyone can be trained to provide it; nothing inherent in the process of assisting suicide or actively taking the life of another person requires the presence of a physician. Yet no matter how the debate swings between a right to life and a right to die, the public refuses to exclude physicians from any discussion of decision making at the end of life. While the public may limit through legislation physicians' authority in these matters, it seems to feel something about their presence to be valuable. An insistence that physicians be agents of assistance in dying raises questions about what it means to be a physician, about a doctor's duty to patients and to his or her profession. It forces physicians into conflict between the duty to heal and to prolong life, and the duty to serve patients' best interests and to relieve their suffering.

The assisted suicide and euthanasia debate—with its implications for our understanding of personal rights and policy limitations and for our understanding of the value of a human being and the goals and limits of medicine—offers an opportunity to reexamine the belief that death is a profound and meaningful part of life. If we try to deny or avoid death, we lose a central part of what it means to be human.

The challenge to religious communities of responding to the social and cultural factors driving public interest in assisted suicide and active euthanasia is taken up in Part 2. This section consists in reflections by six theologians. While working with the theologies of particular theistic traditions, they do not necessarily claim to speak *for* those traditions but rather *to* them and to anyone else who might want to listen. Some have come to conclusions about physician-assisted suicide and euthanasia consistent with the position of the tradition that they represent; others come to a conclusion at variance with their tradition yet, they claim, not inconsistent with its basic theological convictions.

The theologians chose to focus their discussions on four themes they themselves considered central to (though not exhaustive of) any theological treatment of assisted suicide and euthanasia: healing and caring, mercy and justice, freedom and responsibility, and suffering and dying. Within these themes, other pivotal issues emerged as central in the cultural analysis, such as the role and limits of autonomy and fundamental understandings of what it means to be human. While there are differences in the way these various themes and issues are articulated among traditions, there are also significant similarities.

Healing, or making whole, is viewed as central to God's work of salvation in the world, a mission in which physicians participate through their healing work. Although it can be difficult, the work of caring belongs primarily to families and communities who need to provide community for the suffering and dying. It is, however, the inadequacies in the way we currently care for the dying that propel many toward an interest in assisted death.

Mercy and justice are viewed as two defining aspects of the nature of God. Mercy is God's forgiving love or loving kindness expressed in compassion for the suffering and those in need. It consists in compassionate forgiveness and compassionate concern for the needs of the whole person. It is something concrete; it is prepared to sacrifice and is patient beyond reasonableness. God's justice consists in action that favors those whom life has neglected, responding to them on the basis of their need. It cries out against structures that harm human beings. Most contributors recognize the danger of minimalist notions of mercy and justice or of responding to one while neglecting the other. Mercy and justice must exist in tension with each other. One contributes to social order; the other responds to human need in the particular situation. We are left to wrestle with what the law requires and what love allows in the concrete case. Justice must be fueled by mercy; mercy alone, however, cannot be the basis of social order.

Freedom and responsibility, as one contributor notes, are Siamese twins in most religious traditions. One is inconceivable without the other. They are marks of personhood, of having been created in God's image and likeness. The common tendency is to emphasize the first and neglect the second, to insist on an autonomy that has no limits or no need of others. But freedom, understood in a religious context, is a gift of the Creator and consists not so much in a freedom from duty as in a freedom for love and service of God and neighbor. Biblical freedom is not individualistic, concerned with the pursuit of individual rights, but rather is relational, communal. It is limited by human finitude as well as responsibility to God and to others. Consequently, decisions about life and death are not simply one's own to make. Those decisions must take account of one's creaturehood and one's relationships.

Suffering and death are recognized as inevitable aspects of human existence, human tragedies assaulting the core of our being, threatening our identity and the meaning of our existence. There is nothing that can rescue the human condition from finitude and mortality or vulnerability to suffering. Both are tragedies, but neither is ultimate tragedy. Both are destructive enemies of human life, but they are not finally destructive of meaning and purpose because God has the power to triumph over both. Life and flourishing are not ultimate goods, and death and suffering are not ultimate evils. They are not as strong as the promise of God. The religious traditions represented here do not deny the destructive power of death and suffering, but most deny their claim to victory. While there is nothing inherently good in human suffering, most of these traditions hold that it can be educative and serve as occasion for deepening holiness if rightly borne.

At least one of the theologians contributing to this volume (Lonnie D. Kliever) believes that the tradition about which he speaks can justify aid in dying. The sanctity and solidarity of life, he believes, can provide crucial arguments for, rather than against, assisted death. To uphold the solidarity of human life is what the dying owe the living. The dying may choose to die to spare their loved ones torturous grief or extraordinary sacrifices in providing care. They may wish to avoid being a burden to others. And they may well be acting out of the deepest respect for life and out of a profound commitment to others. In this way, assisted death can be an act of moral sacrifice and moral heroism, a dying for the sake of others.

A few of the other theologians, while essentially reflecting the position of their respective traditions, do pose questions to those traditions. For example, while suffering may contribute to holiness and may be educative, how much suffering can people be expected to endure? Can everyone be expected to endure pain and suffering without limit, given varying capacities for pain and suffering? Do moral prescriptions to preserve life always take precedence over compassionate efforts to relieve suffering? Might the latter on occasion and in special circumstances need to triumph? Could good stewardship of life sometimes entail helping someone escape from a life worse than death?

The six theologians bring the resources of religious traditions to bear on the growing interest in and, in some cases, acceptance of physician-assisted suicide and voluntary euthanasia. Each provides an alternative interpretation to many of the basic beliefs that are fueling changing societal attitudes. Some of these interpretations are dependent upon underlying theological convictions; others are not necessarily so. All offer insights and valuable perspectives on the issues. These theologians do not provide the final word on assisted suicide and euthanasia, but they do provide an important word.

There can be no doubt that the discussions and debate about these issues will continue, as evidenced in part by several states' recent initiatives to legalize assisted suicide and by the acquittals of Jack Kevorkian in Michigan on charges of violating that state's ban on assisted suicide.

As this volume was going to press, the U.S. Court of Appeals for the Ninth Circuit handed down its decision that a mentally competent, terminally ill person, under the due-process clause of the Fourteenth Amendment, has a right to seek help to end his or her life. In striking down a Washington state law making it a criminal act for a doctor to assist in the suicide of a terminally ill and competent patient, the court held that such patients who wish to hasten their deaths in order to avoid protracted pain and suffering have a liberty interest in controlling the time and manner of their deaths, an interest "that must be weighed against the state's legitimate and countervailing interests, especially those that relate to the preservation of human life."[2]

The implications of this ruling are far-reaching and will be widely discussed. Almost certainly, the court's decision will be appealed to the U.S. Supreme Court. The ruling, however, demonstrates again the direction in which our society is moving with regard to aid in dying.

The essays in this book represent the kind of ongoing dialogue that must take place between those who hold religious convictions about aid in dying and those who suffer and are dying, and between those who share particular religious convictions and those who don't. In a sense, they model the kind of discussion that needs to take place as all segments of society struggle with these issues. In this process, it is critical that open and mutually respectful conversations occur between and among religious and nonreligious communities, and that religious communities and their individual members, as they formulate their responses to assisted suicide and euthanasia, continually engage both their own traditions and human experience in the most honest, sensitive, and truthful ways possible. This volume is meant to be a step in that direction.

NOTES

1. We are grateful to W. D. White, professor of social medicine, for this insight.
2. *Compassion in Dying v. Washington*, 1996 WL 94848 (9th Cir.).

REFERENCE

Kilner, John F., Nigel M. de S. Cameron, and David L. Schiedermayer, eds. 1995. *Bioethics and the Future of Medicine: A Christian Appraisal*. Grand Rapids, Mich.: Wm. B. Eerdmans.

PART ONE

Assisted Death in American Society:
A Cultural Analysis

CHAPTER 1

Managing Death: The Growing Acceptance of Euthanasia in Contemporary American Society

Nicholas A. Christakis

The great majority of Americans die within the confines of health care institutions (McMillan et al. 1990).[1] In the social group formed by the patient, physicians, nurses, other health professionals, and the patient's family and friends, decisions are made and sanctioned regarding how, precisely, the patient's death and dying optimally shall be handled (Prigerson 1992). The physician in particular has considerable control over the manner of death, determining the treatment instituted to forestall death, the degree of pain relief (Wilson et al. 1992), the medical interventions withheld or withdrawn (Smedira et al. 1992; Christakis and Asch 1993), and the facts patients have about their illness (Miyaji 1993). As a result of both the proliferation of medical technology and the sequestration of large numbers of dying patients in institutions, contemporary American physicians, more so than ever before, influence the timing, rapidity, and painlessness of patients' deaths. Nevertheless, they exercise this influence under pressure from patients and society.

Euthanasia can be seen as just one of several expressions of physicians' control over the manner of death; it is an almost logical extension of the physician's role in managing death. Recent events in American

15

society point to an increasing public awareness and acceptance of such a role for physicians. Nearly half of the voters in California and Washington voted to accept bills permitting physicians to practice euthanasia (Reinhold 1992; Steinfels 1993; Misbin 1991). Grand juries in Michigan have repeatedly refused to indict pathologist Jack Kevorkian for his very public practice of euthanasia (Margolick 1993). Editorials in the popular press call for a review of proscriptions against the practice (Caplan 1990; Engram 1990). Surveys show that the majority of the public favors both allowing patients to die (Harvey and Shubat 1989; Frampton and Mayewski 1987)[2] and euthanasia ("The Ethics of Choosing Death" 1990). In the context of considerable physician control over death in American society, euthanasia appears to have found increasing acceptability.

In this chapter I examine features of American society and medicine—both recent trends and timeless values—that militate for the acceptance of euthanasia. I focus on forms of aid in dying that involve physicians, including euthanasia and physician-assisted suicide, and on the way in which recent trends are vitiating the physician's role within society, particularly with respect to the management of death.

The change in attitudes regarding euthanasia has largely been forced upon the medical establishment by exogenous forces, most prominently by patient dissatisfaction with current ways of dying. Modern modes of death and dying have become so problematic that euthanasia is achieving new legitimacy. The most fundamental reason for this, as the examples below make clear, is that modern medicine—whatever else it does—seems often to increase suffering when it prolongs life. Moreover, this increase in suffering takes place in a setting wherein, for example, patients see front-page newspaper headlines asserting that "doctors are lax in easing pain" (Haney 1991) and "doctors admit ignoring dying patients' wishes" (Brody 1993).[3] Patients appear to want not just the right to die but also the right to be killed (Areen 1991).

People are dissatisfied with the technicalization, medicalization, professionalization, institutionalization, and sanitization of death in modern American society. Euthanasia stands in opposition—often paradoxically—to these developments. Euthanasia is finding acceptability both within American society and within institutionalized medicine because it is congruent with several large-scale social and medical trends and values, including naturalism, individualism, anti-authoritarianism, and secularism. These trends, directly or indirectly, tend to detechnicalize, demedicalize, deprofessionalize, and deinstitutionalize death.

Physicians and Death in American Society

Other people's deaths are part of physicians' workaday routines.[4] Physicians try to forestall our death, tend to us before death, and care for us at death. Indeed, in our society, one is not legally dead until a physician so pronounces.[5] Moreover, contact with death and dying plays an important role in how physicians are trained and socialized. For example, at the center of the socialization process of medical students is contact with death in the anatomy and pathology labs (Fox 1988:51–77, 78–101). And training time spent in intensive care units, wherein the patients are critically ill and mortality rates are high, is particularly valued by resident physicians as an opportunity to hone their skills "on the borderland between life and death."[6]

Nevertheless, physicians have generally reviled and avoided death, fearing it as a mark of failure. For example, the function of prognostication in clinical practice was, for a long time, to help physicians avoid contact with dying patients. The Hippocratic texts suggest that one function of prognosis is to protect physicians from assuming responsibility for unmanageable or terminal patients and to help absolve themselves of blame in cases with adverse outcomes (Lloyd 1983:170; Unschuld 1979).[7] Modern surgeons will sometimes refuse to operate on a critically ill patient for fear that they might be blamed for the patient's presumably inevitable demise or for fear that they might have poor mortality statistics. And many internists still neglect their patients once a terminal diagnosis is made, avoiding associating with them, if possible (see Mizrahi 1986:72).

Although this pattern began to change in the 1960s, for many years there was a pattern of institutional denial regarding death in American medicine. Physicians and patients did not directly discuss death. Physicians tended to reassure dying patients that everything was fine. Amongst themselves, physicians referred to dead patients as having merely been "transferred" to "Ward X" or to the "fifteenth floor" in a building with only fourteen floors. This reticence about death was not always self-serving. Many physicians avoided discussion of death out of a beneficent concern for the patient's well-being. One physician characterized the thinking as follows:

> When I started [in the 1940s], you didn't tell anybody that they were going to die, unless they really pushed you. And I think it is all wrong that [today] we operate in medicine the way we used to in the army, with a "standard operating procedure," and that standard operating procedure seems nowadays to be that you tell people when they have a malignancy, or if they have a problem [you tell] them just how big of a problem it is. And I don't think that all patients can tolerate this. Medicine is something that just can't operate with an s.o.p. It is something that should be thought about and something where you treat the patient as an individual, and that you involve the family as well as the patient. I don't think that every patient ought to know that they're going to die. That's just my feeling. But it's a whole new ethos that's developed during my time in medicine. . . .
>
> I think a physician always ought to let the *family* know [however]. Long ago, my wife's father had angina and he came to our city, and I went over him, and there was nothing you could really do in those days. His electrocardiogram was all right, his chest X ray was all right. It was clear that he had angina. And, uh, I guess I told him that he had a problem and so forth and that he did have

heart disease, but I told my wife and his wife that he was probably going to die one of those days and die suddenly. But I didn't tell him that.

And what really happened was that sometime a year later, he was digging in the garden—he had always wanted to know whether he should stop digging in his garden, given his heart problem, and what he should do if he got pain [while digging] and I said, "Well, stop when you get the pain"—but anyway, digging in the garden, which he loved to do, he collapsed and died. Now, you know, I guess people today express various things to patients that this or that would happen to them. But anyway, my wife was very understanding about it and so was his wife. . . . We just didn't tell patients in those days. (Christakis field notes, 10 April 1992)

This ethos of beneficent silence persists today among some physicians and in certain relatively traditional subcultures within American society (for example, the Hispanic community).[8]

In reaction to this avoidance of discussions about death—and consonant with then-contemporary societal trends toward "consciousness raising" and questioning of authority—a death-awareness movement emerged in the 1960s, led by books such as Herman Feifel's *Meaning of Death* (1959) and Elisabeth Kübler-Ross's *On Death and Dying* (1969). Kübler-Ross showed, among other things, that dying patients did not wish to be isolated, abandoned, or misled by their physicians. These books, both authored by psychiatrists, galvanized the public and spurred a rethinking of conventional medical practice. This pattern prefigured the way that popular ideas about euthanasia are currently leading the way to a change in professional ideas.[9]

The sentiment that patients and physicians should discuss death more openly eventually gave way, in the 1970s and 1980s, to the compulsion that they do so. The ethics of the profession changed, and what has since been criticized as "terminal candor" took hold (Lear 1993). By today's standards, physicians have the duty to inform their patients of their illness, and patients have a right to know. As we shall see, this represents a displacement of the locus of control over death from the physician to the patient, a displacement that has contributed to the greater acceptability of euthanasia.

A physician expressed his own uneasiness about the haste to tell patients the worst this way:

> I don't think if I were Dr. Smith, my son's doctor, that I would have expressed the whole thing—my son's prognosis—quite as early as he did. It was like out of the blue. I sat there when Dr. Smith told him, and I think that's what they do with everybody!
>
> Or I had a colleague who had a carcinoma of the breast. And someone told her, just after she had a breast removed, while she was still recovering from the anesthesia and had just got back to her room, that she had six nodes positive. And I thought, Hell, you don't need to discuss all those things that early. But there seems to be a real feeling on the part of physicians today that the more open they are the better, but I don't think that's always true. (Christakis field notes, 10 April 1992)

Despite the resurgent intellectual interest and the critique of the prevailing thinking about death that began in the late 1960s, there was nevertheless relatively little change initially in the clinical care of the dying or in doctor-patient communication. This lack of change in physician behavior had to do with the social roles assumed by physicians. In a differentiated, modern society, citizens and institutions acquire specific social roles with specific duties. Technical advances and discoveries in medicine have held such promise that, from the turn of the century, society has endowed physicians with the duty and the privilege to eradicate disease (see Starr 1982). From this triumphal perspective, death connotes failure—not just of the therapeutic armamentarium to achieve its objective, but also of the physician to fulfill his or her social role. When physicians speak of the death of their patients, they often use expressions that suggest a mistake that might be rectified, such as "we lost the patient," or a failing on the part of the patient, such as "that patient died on me." Physicians' rituals (for example, giving false reassurance to the dying) and institutional practices (for example, rapid sequestration of dead bodies in hospitals) served to protect the physicians from being identified with the failure to fulfill this role. It reflects both irony and arrogance that physicians feel guilt when their patients die—irony because they are not (ordinarily) truly responsible for the patient's death and arrogance because they believe that they are so powerful they might have prevented it.

Physicians have thus tended to regard their patients' deaths as personal failures (Mauksch 1975). Powerful emotional and intellectual strands within the professional culture of medicine also contribute to this perspective: optimism, activism, meliorism, and a hubristic, "against-the-odds" attitude are endemic in physicians. Sociologist Renée Fox has noted both the deeply held values underlying this thinking about death and the troubling questions raised by a medical technology capable of extraordinary life-support measures:

> The Judeo-Christian tradition emphasizes that, because human life is divinely given, it is inherently sacred and important, has absolute, inestimable worth and meaning, and should be protected and sustained. . . . [But] in recent years, the unqualified commandment to support and sustain life has become increasingly problematic in American society, particularly in the medical sector. The sanctity of life ethic has helped to push physicians, nurses, and other medical professionals into a pugilistic tendency to combat death at any cost, and to define its occurrence as a personal and professional defeat. This heroically aggressive, "courage to fail" stance has been reinforced by the development of more powerfully effective forms of medical technology that increase the medical team's ability to save and maintain life. However, some of the consequences of doing everything possible to keep all chronically afflicted and terminally ill patients alive have come to be questioned. (Fox 1988:429–30)

Over the last twenty years, the material and psychic costs of this institutional denial of death have come to light; patients and physicians are addressing the suffering that the prolongation of life may entail for the dying person, and, as the nation's health care system has come under public scrutiny, many question the squandering of resources in the care of the dying.

The emergence of euthanasia as a desirable option, though a departure from tradition in that it puts the doctor face-to-face with death and seems to represent surrender to death, is, as we shall see, in other (somewhat paradoxical) senses a return to the traditional roots of clinical medicine and an exertion of control over modern ways of dying. Within the context of modern medical practice, total control over life is achieved only through control over death. At the same time, the increasing acceptance of euthanasia represents another step—evolutionary more than revolutionary—in the development of the physician's relationship to death and dying: an increasing acceptance of the inevitability and, in some circumstances, desirability of death.

The Detechnicalization and Demedicalization of Death

Since the 1960s, there has been a resurgent current of naturalism in American society expressed in ways as diverse as the "natural look" in appearance, organic cuisine, environmental activism, natural childbirth, and the glorification of the traditional family. This trend runs counter to the rampant technological advances present in modern society, advances that many view as distancing human beings from nature itself.

Though some forms of dying might at first glance seem completely unnatural (such as physician-assisted suicide or euthanasia), they, like allowing to die and the withholding of life support, actually stand in contradistinction to that which, today, is regarded as truly unnatural: death in an institution, perhaps in an intensive care unit, removed from one's family, surrounded by strangers, invaded by machines and devices, and needlessly enduring iatrogenically prolonged pain and suffering. Ironically, it is artificially sustained living, not dying—even by euthanasia—that has become inhumane in modern medicine.

A fundamental shift is now occurring in our society with respect to perceptions of medical technology. After years of great confidence in the promise of modern medicine, people are becoming concerned with the unseemly side of technical advances. The technicalization of death finds its chief expression in the provision of intensive care to patients just before death in the ICU. Patients have expressed deep sadness, frustration, and anger with modern medical care of all patients, but especially of the extraordinary measures taken for the dying in ICUs. For example, the son of one patient opened an editorial in the *New York Times* by stating, "The hospital was a torture chamber. Doctors were the torturers." This man—whose ninety-four-year-old mother developed colon cancer and, after surgery, developed multiple organ system failure requiring admission to an ICU—wrote of his anger with the medical community:

> My mother's face was swollen beyond recognition. Her lips were raw from the respirator.
> . . . A young doctor called to say that my mother had died. Momentary relief overshadowed anger. Now anger will linger for a long time:
> Anger at a system that makes torture legal.
> Anger at the medical profession that fights hard to protect its own prerogatives but has shown little courage in fighting inhumane legal restrictions which make doctors accomplices in torture.
> Anger at doctors who are so wedded to charts and monitors that they seem oblivious of patients' pain.
> At the funeral parlor I was told that I would be required to identify my mother. A few minutes later the men who were dealing with the body reversed that. They wanted to spare me a final look at the havoc modern medicine had wreaked on her. ("They Tortured My Mother" 1991)

This same theme of torture appears in a physician's evocative description of ICU care, entitled "The Prisoner":

> The lights came on at exactly 5 am, revealing more clearly the gaunt elderly man lying naked amidst the disordered sheets on the bed. In response to the blinding light, the old man awoke, opened his eyes, then shut them just as quickly against the painful glare from above. Now awake, he struggled to resist the sound that had plagued him in the previous days (weeks? months?) of his imprisonment. The stiff gag in his mouth prevented him from talking and caused a constant pain in his throat. Alarms and other strange noises unceasingly assaulted him. His arms and legs throbbed from the multiple cuts they had inflicted upon him.
>
> Under the brilliance of the lights, he became aware of his nakedness. Ashamed by this newest form of torture, he tried frantically to cover himself, but found his arms and legs tied down. . . .
>
> Suddenly his captors surrounded the bed, each masked, each clamping down on his arms and legs. He tried desperately to tell them he had done nothing wrong, that they had imprisoned the wrong man, but the gag in his mouth prevented him from uttering a sound. Unable to talk or to free himself, he continued to resist. His captors kept him subdued and spoke loudly among themselves, seemingly unaware of the writhing, shriveled form beneath them. . . .
>
> To the masked figures rushing by the bed, only [the] constant movement of the old man's chest distinguished him from a bloodless corpse. (Eveloff 1992:313–14)

A similar description was offered by a son of a patient—here, both patient and child were physicians: "It has been more than a year since my father died, and I have come to believe that the circumstances of his death demonstrate much of what is wrong with our medical system. . . . [My father] held me and whispered that everything would be O.K. 'Norman, I have been a surgeon for almost fifty years,' he said. 'In that time, I have seen physicians torture dying patients in vain attempts to prolong life. I have taken care of you most of your life. Now I must

ask for your help. Don't let them abuse me. No surgery. No chemotherapy'" ("Making a Living" 1992). The parents of yet another patient,
a young man with AIDS, described their son's experience in an ICU thus:

> *Mother*: Well, you know, you could die from all those medi-
> cines [that they gave him]. . . . Every time they moved those IV's,
> and they had to move them all the time because there were too
> many things flowing through him. There was no skin left on him
> anyway. He was in excruciating pain [as a result].
>
> *Father*: There was one particular incident, and I think that
> was when he decided that he wanted out, that was when they put
> an IV in incorrectly, and he complained about the burning, and it
> stayed in for several hours, and they then discovered that it was
> infiltrated. And they took it out.
>
> *Mother*: Then they were going to do that subclavicle thing
> [place a central venous line, a type of intravenous catheter] on him
> and that's when he said "I want out of here."
>
> *Father*: I think it was that incident that was the end!
>
> *Mother*: I mean it hurts like hell. (Christakis field notes, 23
> April 1992)

Patients fear being victimized by a technology and a medical system run amok. One fifty-one-year-old woman, suffering from amyotrophic lateral sclerosis, paralyzed, and ventilator dependent, "used
her eyes to ask to die," a newspaper headline declared. Her
eighteen-year-old daughter told the judge in the case: "All I want is for
you to see her and see what she's going through. She could continue to
suffer for another week and another week and another week. [Please] do
something for her" ("She Uses Eyes to Ask to Die" 1990).

Another illustration of the horror felt by some physicians at this
needless prolongation of suffering is a tasteless joke that some physicians
at my hospital have expropriated in order to characterize what often happens to patients in an ICU. They characterize the torture they feel they
inflict on terminal patients as "mamba." The joke is as follows: Three

travelers are captured by vicious cannibals. The chief asks the first one whether he prefers death or mamba. Naturally presuming that nothing is worse than death, the first traveler picks mamba. He is subjected to unspeakable torture and then is killed. The same choice is posed to the second traveler. Uneasily, he picks mamba. He is also tortured and then killed. The chief then asks the third traveler to choose. Cognizant of the experience of his colleagues, the traveler says, "I choose death." "That is fine," the chief replies, "but first a little mamba." Many physicians feel that ICU care can be cruelly unnecessary, simply delaying an otherwise inevitable death. The implication, moreover, is that even when patients wish to die, the system refuses to let them.[10]

It is in this context, in a setting where medical care is equated with "excruciating pain," "imprisonment," and "torture," that euthanasia in all its forms finds increasing acceptability.[11] Such technical and invasive therapy is viewed as both violating the person (causing meaningless suffering) and violating the body (even making it unfit to be seen). These perceptions of modern medicine frame public desires and make euthanasia more acceptable.

Euthanasia, consequently and paradoxically, represents (1) the quintessential relief of suffering, (2) the firm repudiation of life-support technology, and (3) the paradigmatic exercise of physicianly restraint epitomized by the Hippocratic aphorism "First, do no harm" (Lloyd 1983:67).[12] The last point illustrates how traditional medical values are being recast: in the past, "do no harm" was used to limit medical practice and prevent death; now it may be used to limit medical practice and foster death. This paradoxical state of affairs has arisen because, compared to current, high-technology treatments, death is often perceived as less noxious. The practice of euthanasia, while ancient, assumes new meaning because it throws into relief the terrible bind of modern physicians: they can do more to treat their patients, but at a greater physical and psychic cost. The physician's increased power to heal is coupled with increased power to harm.

Euthanasia symbolically reasserts the patient's and the physician's control over suffering, over machines, and over dying. It symbolizes the fact that there are limits to technology. It is countertechnical: it involves the removal of machines and, if anything, the administration of a simple, lethal drug. Euthanasia is construed as facilitating the inevitable, as preserving the occurrence of what is natural. Just as society commends aggressive intervention to restore the otherwise healthy—but for disease—back to their natural health,[13] society commends aggressive intervention to restore the otherwise dead—but for modern medicine—back to their natural death. Modern medicine is construed as an unnatural impediment to a normal life event.[14]

If modern medicine, with its advanced life-support technologies, ranging from mechanical ventilation to hemodialysis to extracorporeal membrane oxygenation to cardiopulmonary resuscitation, medicalizes death, then euthanasia to a great extent demedicalizes it (see Fox 1988:465–83). The increasing acceptability of euthanasia reflects a societal response to and backlash against the increasing technicalization of medicine and death and the misery rather than the promise that technology is currently felt to offer.[15]

The Deprofessionalization and Deinstitutionalization of Death

The increasing acceptability of euthanasia is also part of a trend granting greater autonomy to patients in general and granting greater control to patients over their deaths in particular, reactions against both the paternalism of medicine and the professionalization of death. Elements of the trend against the professionalization of medicine over the last two decades include the emergence of the hospice movement (James and Field 1992), the increasing popularity of patient-controlled analgesia (Kerr 1988), the rise of the home care movement (Steel 1991; Sankar 1991), and legal and legislative developments such as advanced directives, living wills, and the Patient Self-Determination Act (Greco et al. 1991). Patients are being encouraged more and more to care for themselves rather than to rely so heavily on the services of physicians and medical institutions. These efforts are "not so much a change in [American] values as the initiation of action intended to modify certain structural features of American medicine, so that it will more fully realize long-standing societal values" (Fox 1988:482). These values include equality, independence, and self-reliance. Moreover, euthanasia is consonant with anti-authoritarian trends in American society, such as the consumer advocacy movement, the civil rights movement, and the women's movement. It returns control over death to patients.

Part of the demedicalization trend in American society has involved efforts to make the doctor-patient relationship less hierarchical and more egalitarian. Patients are being given a slew of rights—with corresponding duties being placed upon physicians: the right to treatment, the right to information, the right to informed consent, the right to privacy, and the right to die. Patient autonomy in terminal care may manifest itself in several ways: patients may choose not to initiate medical therapy (including lifesaving therapy), they may refuse lifesaving therapy, and, with ultimate self-determination, they may end their own lives. The last right to die is gradually being extended to include the right to euthanasia.

Such patient rights are emerging at a time when medicine as a profession is coming under attack. In a paper titled "When Self-Determination Runs Amok," philosopher Daniel Callahan is critical of euthanasia in part because it treats physicians as "hired hands" rather than as moral agents (Callahan 1992). Yet there is no arguing that this is happening. That is, to some extent, physicians are themselves being deprofessionalized in contemporary American society. Their role is being commercialized as it is coming to be construed as one of serving their clients as much as treating their patients. Physicians have voluntarily and involuntarily abrogated many of their fiduciary duties. They must answer to insurance companies, government agencies, quality assurance committees, professional review boards, malpractice attorneys, their employers, and their patients. Physicians are coming to be more *employees* than professionals (Friedson 1970). Indeed, the very term *physician-assisted suicide* places the physician in a secondary role of an assistant.

Thus, the issue is coming to be framed as a question of what role to allow physicians in helping patients to exercise their "rights." More generally, physicians are deprived of their authority over dying. Indeed, one of the remarkable things accomplished by the availability of books like Derek Humphry's *Final Exit*—which, in describing in specific detail how patients might end their own lives, achieved best-seller status—is to make it possible to remove physicians altogether from the social network responsible for euthanasia. Patients are empowered, with varying degrees of family assistance, to end their own lives, painlessly and with dignity. Euthanasia itself, in other words, while still involving a knowledge of toxicology and physiology, is largely deprofessionalized and deinstitutionalized; it takes place outside of a health care institution, with laypeople assuming functions such as pain relief and drug administration previously reserved for physicians, and with laypeople in decision-making roles. This development is analogous to patients' taking responsibility for their own health.

When physicians have proven to be unwilling or unable to forgo painful or unnecessary therapy or unwilling to practice euthanasia, patients have sometimes shown themselves willing and able to take matters into their own hands, either inside or outside the hospital. There has been a spate of stories in the popular press concerning family members insisting on the withdrawal of life support and assisting relatives with suicide. In a sense, people outside the medical profession, patients and their families, are leading the way, with the medical and bioethical communities following (Fox 1994).[16]

Recurrent themes in the cases of family-assisted suicide are frustration with an overly aggressive medical system and deep love and

almost ritualistic pacts between the family members. These cases sometimes wind up in court. One man was brought to trial for manslaughter
when he "kept his promise" to his seventy-nine-year-old mother by
handing her a pistol the day she was told by her doctors that she had terminal liver cancer. She killed herself minutes after he left the room
("Trial Begins" 1992).[17] In another case, a daughter desperately tried to
"free" her mother from the "trap" of inoperable ovarian cancer and
obtained pills for her to kill herself with ("I Helped" 1992). Sometimes
family members will volunteer to be of assistance; they prepare themselves to help a patient kill himself even when the patient says nothing
(Cranford 1989). In a particularly heartbreaking case, Rudolfo
Linares—in desperation over his profoundly brain-injured infant's prolonged stay in an ICU—swept into his son's room and, keeping hospital personnel at bay with a handgun, disconnected his son's respirator
and cradled him until he died thirty minutes later. His actions were supported by many, and a grand jury refused to indict him ("Armed Man
Pulls" 1989; "Father Speeds" 1989; "Father Who Pulled" 1989). It is a
sad commentary on modern medicine that such desperate action was
necessary to achieve an end that all participants regarded as desirable.
One has the sense that part of the reason this case was so newsworthy
was that Linares was acting as the public felt that physicians should
have. In a profoundly American way, he took matters into his own hands
so that justice might be served.

Sometimes doctors go so far as to suggest to families that they
commit euthanasia. On the one hand, this complies with physicians'
duty to do no harm in treating their patients, but, on the other, it is an
abrogation of their responsibility and shifts the burden to others.
Suggestions to families that they take matters into their own hands are
sometimes met with surprise and sometimes without resistance. In the
case of a young AIDS patient, a doctor suggested to the patient's parents that they themselves might wish to help their son to die. The parents described the situation as follows:

Mother: When I was questioning the doctor as we were leaving, I was really very concerned. My son was a wreck. And he was in awful pain, and all those medicines had just done this number on him. I said that I had to be able to keep him comfortable: "You're giving me this new prescription for Dilaudid [a powerful narcotic]; do I give him two, do I give him four, how much. . . . What's reasonable, how frequently?" And he looked me level in the eye and gave me a progression: "If one doesn't work give him two, if two don't work give him three, and if you can't make him comfortable and you want to, just give him the whole bottle." And I believe I understood him clearly. He didn't think there was anything good coming down the pike for my son.

Interviewer: Do you think that he was suggesting to you that you take your son's life or that you provide him the means to take his own life?

Mother: I think he was suggesting that if what it took . . . if he was so miserable and so uncomfortable . . . if what it took to put him out of his misery was an overdose, it was a good idea. I think that was exactly what he was saying.

Interviewer: This seems to trouble you.

Mother: It didn't trouble me. It surprised me . . . that somebody was giving me leave to go home and take this medication and do with it as I saw fit. That's not usually what you get from a doctor. But it was humane.

Father: It was just shocking to us because we have no experience and, you know, you hear something like that from a health professional—who is supposed to be there to save life no matter what. . . .

Interviewer: You said a minute ago that there may be a tension between the duty of health professionals to save life and this function [of ending life].

Father: I was just trying to explain where my wife is coming from. One grows up in our society with the expectation that doctors are somebody special. And why are they special? They are special because they help and [because] they save lives. And for them to now say that here it is okay for them to execute somebody, that goes against the grain of what we in our society are culturally accustomed to. Intellectually, I can agree with the doctor. On the other hand, it does go against the grain in some way. We may overlook it, or push it back, or ignore it, but I at least realize that there is a conflict in me thinking about that.

Mother: So, suddenly, here you are. You've got this person in front of you who is dying. And the physician says to you, "We've pretty much done all we can do." It's going to take its own course: he's going to die. On the other hand, acknowledging that you don't want him to suffer too much, there is a way maybe to speed that process, especially if he's very uncomfortable. It's taking the physician out of the role of—as my husband says—healer, and it's putting him in the position of saying, "I can't help you or protect you any more; the best I can do for you is to make this person's end . . . [be] with as little pain as possible." *You just don't expect it! It is admitting defeat!* (Christakis field notes, 23 April 1992)

Despite their ultimate willingness to facilitate their son's death, this couple did not refer to the action the doctor suggested as "euthanasia" but rather—demonstrating a distinction made in society-at-large— referred to it as "killing" or "executing" the patient. For them, when a doctor commits this action, it is euthanasia, but when they do, it is not. Similarly, Humphry refers to such patient actions as "self-deliverance," not as self-euthanasia.

Nevertheless, it is noteworthy that, in general, when practiced by nonphysicians outside of health care institutions, such deaths are not, in fact, referred to as euthanasia but rather as "suicide," whether or not the individual was assisted by a physician or relative. This suggests that the public still desires that physicians assume the serious responsibility of ending life, that only physicians can be socially sanctioned to bring about the death of another person by "euthanasia." However uncomfortable our society might be with euthanasia practiced by physicians, it is that much more uncomfortable when it is practiced by laypeople. This observation also suggests that, from a societal perspective, since physicians are assigned the task and honor of preventing death, only they can properly cause it; physicians, not laypeople, are still the only ones that society permits to practice euthanasia.

Sometimes doctors encourage euthanasia and encounter both surprise and resistance from families. When they do so, they often invoke an emerging theme in American bioethics: futility. A futile action is one that cannot achieve the goals desired of the action (Schneiderman et al. 1990). Thus, providing medical therapy in order to improve health in a case where such therapy *cannot* improve health is futile. Even when therapy is futile, however, doctors rarely seek to withdraw life support against the wishes of the family. The case of Helga Wanglie became famous in part because doctors are ordinarily so reluctant to advocate publicly the death of a patient, but also because the family was opposed to the doctors' intentions. In addition, the very public admission of impotence by the physicians was also cause for consternation in a society accustomed only to claims of heroic successes in modern medical care. In this case, the doctors argued that further life support for eighty-seven-year-old Mrs. Wanglie, who was in a persistent vegetative state, was futile. Her husband disagreed ("As Family Protests" 1991; see also "Atlanta Court" 1991). Mr. Wanglie contended that he and his wife felt that human life was sacred and God-given and that only God could take it. The director of the hospital replied that they did not feel obliged to provide inappropriate treatment that was not in the patient's medical interest.

The recent emergence of futility as an important theme in American medicine and bioethics reflects the moral desirability of acknowledging medical limitations and the practical necessity of allocating scarce resources (Jecker and Schneiderman 1992; see also Fox 1994). Futility and euthanasia may have the same roots. Although futility runs counter to the quintessential American ethos of limitless medical progress and virtually omnipotent physicians, it is nonetheless consonant with other important values within medicine, such as nonmaleficence and rationality.

One assumption underlying the increasing acceptance of euthanasia in American society is that dying is a private, individual, personal, intimate event. Dying in modern contexts connotes a fear of losing control, which loss is antithetical to a core American value. The option to be killed restores control. This is not necessarily so in other societies, where the death of one person may be viewed as the concern of the entire community. This American perception of death is contingent on a quintessentially individualistic view of the person (De Craemer 1983). To this view, however, some are opposed on moral grounds (Callahan 1992). Indeed, to insist that dying is a private act does, to some extent, eliminate public accountability and oversight.

Anti-authoritarianism, individualism, and autonomy are also manifest as anti-institutionalism—here, in particular, as a rejection of death at a hospital in favor of a more natural and autonomous death at home. Hospitals are increasingly viewed as singularly unsuited not only to a "natural" but also to a painless and dignified death. The juxtaposition in a hospital of high technology, bureaucracy, and professionalism on the one hand and the most fundamental and unchanging of human experiences—such as birth, death, and pain—on the other hand is increasingly viewed as inauspicious (see Rosenberg 1987:3). Studies have shown that terminally ill people would prefer to die at home rather than in a hospital (see McCormick et al. 1991), and home death is increasing (McMillan et al. 1990). People are rejecting both biomedical therapy and biomedical institutions.

Terminally ill patients think of hospitals as "buildings full of strangers" (Belkin 1992) and regard them as unwelcoming, uncaring, and alienating. Patients reject what they see as the meaninglessness and indignity of dying in a hospital and prefer death at home, removed from high technology. Hospitals are coming to be seen as a necessary evil for the curable but an unnecessary evil for the incurable.

One twenty-nine-year-old cancer patient who had been hospitalized eight times in the preceding two years refused to go back to the hospital, arguing: "I want to die at home. My doctor calls me stubborn. I'm not stubborn. I'm taking control" (Belkin 1992). The husband of another patient, a fifty-eight-year-old woman with breast cancer, observed of his wife: "In the hospital, they could have kept her alive for a few days, maybe a few weeks. For what? What kind of life is that? She cried whenever she had to go back to the hospital. All she would do there is stare at the ceiling" (Belkin 1992). Indeed, terminally ill patients often prefer to die rather than be aggressively treated in what they perceive to be the wrong fashion in the wrong setting. Euthanasia thus provides escape from the hospital, an institution which many regard as an impersonal monolith "little concerned with needs that [cannot] be measured, probed, or irradiated" (Rosenberg 1987:3). As care has become more and more impersonal, patients have lost confidence that their true needs will be met, and so euthanasia has become more appealing.

This observation may partly explain the hostility between the right-to-die, pro-euthanasia movement and the hospice movement. The hospice approach to the care of terminally ill patients emphasizes attention to patients' physical, emotional, and spiritual suffering; its primary goal is the palliation and relief of this suffering rather than treatment of the patient's underlying disease. Proponents of hospice feel that if patients were better cared for, they would not be demanding euthanasia. Indeed, one physician titled his book on hospice care *Euthanasia Is Not the Answer*, arguing that uncontrolled pain and suffering lead to a desire for euthanasia (Cundiff 1992).[18] In my field interviews, hospice personnel indicated that they are pleased with American Medical Association and American Bar Association opposition to pro-euthanasia laws. Hospice personnel regard death reverently; they feel that euthanasia is irreverent, meaningless, and undignified. From the hospice perspective, euthanasia is meaningless because it is the ending of a life without the relief of the suffering. It does not address the pain of the patient's family or the psychiatric and spiritual suffering of the patient. Proponents of hospice regard death as incidental to the relief of suffering. In contrast, proponents of euthanasia regard death as instrumental to the relief of suffering. Nevertheless, like the hospice movement, which rejects unnecessary medical technology and bureaucracies in favor of personal, simple, traditional, low-technology health care for the terminally ill, advocates of euthanasia also reject unnecessary medical technology (Mor et al. 1988).

Other Social Factors

Several other trends contribute to the increasing acceptability of euthanasia in American society. First, the post–World War II era has seen a trend toward the progressive secularization of our society, evidenced in the elimination of school prayer, falling church attendance, and the waning of religious influence over everyday life. With respect to euthanasia, this trend has found expression in the desacralization of death and healing. In a secular and humanistic society, euthanasia becomes more permissible. Second, over the last two decades, there has been a progressive societal obsession with physical fitness. At a minimum, this glorification of fitness may foster a general feeling that it is better to die than to become infirm. Physical and mental deterioration prompts patients and their families to opt for a way out—for example, through family-assisted suicide—rather than face a slow senescence, even when the senescence is not painful. Those that are mentally or physically infirm feel so socially deviant that euthanasia is legitimized. Third, public concern with cost containment and setting limits in health care also unavoidably makes euthanasia an attractive alternative to lengthy and costly terminal hospitalizations. Like the proverbial elderly Eskimo wandering onto the ice floes in self-sacrifice rather than burdening his or her clan, the practice of euthanasia is consonant with the husbanding of what are increasingly viewed as limited societal resources for health care. Finally, as the American population ages, greater attention is being given to the problems and needs of the aged in our society;

the growing numbers of aged patients may lead to increased pressures for euthanasia as an alternative to an extended, hopeless debilitation.

Eliminating Suffering

The increasing acceptability of euthanasia in American society is thus congruent with a number of values of American society, including especially naturalism, individualism, and anti-authoritarianism.

Paradoxically, physician-assisted suicide and the other forms of euthanasia we have been considering represent a retrenchment to the humanitarian ethos that used to guide medicine. Euthanasia, at its best, represents an atavistic phenomenon. When physicians do support euthanasia, they couch it in the best traditions of their profession, as a humanitarian act that represents an ultimate act of good doctoring (Quill 1991). It is a bedside practice. It is a relief from suffering. Typically, it is done in circumstances where the doctor has known the patient for a long time.[19] Euthanasia and its greater acceptability can thus be seen as part of an effort to rehumanize medicine and return it to its roots.

The public and professional debate about euthanasia revolves not just around its acceptability but also around its definition. If euthanasia is acceptable, under what terms is this so? Who may commit it? Who may succumb to it? When and why is it acceptable? Many physicians would say that their duties include both the prolongation of life and the relief of suffering. But American society is poorly equipped to handle situations where the two conflict. Which has precedence? Who decides?

The debate about the acceptability of euthanasia in our society unavoidably—if inexplicitly—raises important questions about the ideal relationship of a doctor to death. Much energy has gone into resisting any change in the physician's relationship to death—as evinced by opposition to physician-assisted suicide and active euthanasia, which are felt to be a perversion or inappropriate extension of the physician's social role—but less energy has been expended examining what the proper relationship to death should be. How should the physician usher us out of this world? How should the physician view death? In our society, we generally expect physicians to study and learn from dead bodies, certify death when it has occurred, attend the death of their patients, and relieve the suffering associated with it. Yet we expect our physicians, while doing all this death-related work, to be on the side of life, to preserve and extend it. Some of the triumphalism that used to characterize the relationship of the doctor and death is now giving way to a new realism, as contemporary physicians, emerging from an era of unbridled optimism and success, are finally reaching and recognizing their limits.

Euthanasia in many of its forms has come to be seen as salvation, not only as release from the suffering and pain of the underlying disease but also as relief from the suffering, pain, and alienation engendered specifically by modern medicine and modern health care institutions. It provides deliverance from both the disease and the therapy. In the past, euthanasia was often construed as a repudiation of a moral good, namely life itself, and was therefore unacceptable. Moreover, to commit it was to acknowledge incompetence on the part of the physician in curing disease and relieving human misery. Now, euthanasia may often represent the repudiation of an evil, namely iatrogenic suffering. The equation of hospitalization and medical care with suffering has to some extent made death less feared. Euthanasia does what therapy seemingly cannot: relieve the suffering. In so doing, it calls into question the status of suffering in contemporary American society (Kleinman 1988; Cassell 1991).

Relief of physical suffering is in principle relatively easy. Yet physicians, in practice, do as poor a job relieving physical suffering as they do relieving psychic and spiritual suffering. For many, euthanasia addresses—nay, eliminates—all three.

NOTES

This work was partially supported by the Robert Wood Johnson Foundation Clinical Scholars Program. I am grateful to Renée C. Fox for many helpful insights regarding this topic.

1. In 1986, the most recent year with available data, 83 percent of aged Americans who died did so in health care institutions (McMillan et al. 1990).

2. For example, in a 1988 survey, 78 percent of physicians and 73 percent of the public favored the withdrawal of life support for hopelessly ill patients (Harvey and Shubat 1989).

3. The original study was Solomon et al. 1993.

4. Sociologist Everett C. Hughes notes, in his discussion of professions and work, that "one man's routine of work is made of the emergencies of other people" (1971:316).

5. This function is particularly intriguing, but, even more intriguing, the performance of this function by physicians is generally assumed and unexamined. Even Ivan Illich does not criticize physicians for the arrogation of this priestly function (1976).

6. From my field notes for 10 April 1992. The research for which these field notes were obtained is an effort to understand the use of prognosis in modern clinical practice, particularly as it influences physician behavior at the end of a patient's life (Christakis 1995). Prognosis is a key element in a physician's decision to withdraw or withhold life support, administer lethal medicines, refer a patient to a hospice, or perform euthanasia. Among other methods, the research involves interviewing physicians, patients, and their families. Subsequent references to these field notes appear in the text.

7. This use of prognosis is not restricted to Western medical systems; similar themes appear in the texts of other literate medical traditions, such as Ayurveda and traditional Chinese medicine (Unschuld 1979).

8. Some patients and their families are calling for its return and criticizing contemporary practice (Lear 1993:17). This beneficent silence is widely practiced in Europe, China, Japan, Latin America, and other parts of the world (Freedman 1993).

9. This pattern appears to have been the case for quite some time, at least with respect to active euthanasia (Fye 1978).

10. Some doctors have described their agony and embarrassed complicity in participating in futile medical care. For a case described by one physician, see Hansen-Flaschen 1990.

11. I should add that proposals to reform the medical system's approach to the dying and to foster the hospice approach arise from similar sources.

12. The oath also contains the following statement: "I will not give a fatal draught to anyone if I am asked, nor will I suggest any such thing."

13. This "restoration" is nevertheless often felt to be unnatural in any case. For example, medical technology applied to such patients is spoken of as "artificial"—such as the artificial kidney or heart. Similarly, physicians euphemistically refer to "end-stage" rather than "terminal" renal disease (see Fox and Swazey 1978).

14. In a way, "natural death" is the counterpart of "natural childbirth." For an excellent consideration of "new metaphors" for birth, including "pure childbirth" and "home birth," see Martin 1987, chap. 9. Indeed, there are interesting parallels between the professionalization and deprofessionalization of death and birth in general.

15. See also Illich 1976:102–3: "The modern fear of unhygienic death makes life appear like a race towards a terminal scramble. . . . The patient's unwillingness to die on his own [without a physician nearby] makes him pathetically dependent. He has now lost his faith in his ability to die, the terminal shape that health can take, and has made the right to be professionally killed [i.e., euthanasia] into a major issue."

16. Regarding the pattern of reaction rather than proaction by the bioethics community see Fox 1994.

17. Ironically, in this case, the doctor's diagnosis was in error, and the patient might have survived ("Trial Begins" 1992).

18. For more on the antipathy of hospice proponents toward euthanasia, see Thompson 1984.

19. Indeed, the furor over the Debbie case was in large part motivated by the fact that the doctor in question did not know the patient. The furor over Dr. Kevorkian's practice has similar roots.

REFERENCES

Areen, Judith. 1991. "Advance Directives under State Law and Judicial Decisions." *Law, Medicine and Health Care* 19:91–100.

"Armed Man Pulls Plug on His Son." 1989. *Boston Globe*, 27 April, 1.

"As Family Protests, Hospital Seeks an End to Woman's Life Support." 1991. *New York Times*, 10 January, A1.

"Atlanta Court Bars Effort to End Life Support for Stricken Girl, 13." 1991. *New York Times*, 18 October, A10.

Belkin, Lisa. 1992. "Choosing Death at Home: Dignity with Its Own Toll." *New York Times*, 2 March, A1.

Brody, Jane E. 1993. "Doctors Admit Ignoring Dying Patients' Wishes." *New York Times*, 14 January, A18.

Callahan, Daniel. 1992. "When Self-Determination Runs Amok." *Hastings Center Report* 22 (March–April): 52–55.

Caplan, Arthur. 1990. "Suicide Machines and 'Obitoriums.'" *Baltimore Sun*, 17 June, D1.

Cassell, Eric J. 1991. *The Nature of Suffering and the Goals of Medicine*. New York: Oxford University Press.

Christakis, Nicholas A. 1995. *Prognostication and Death in Medical Thought and Practice*. Ann Arbor, Mich.: University Microfilms.

Christakis, Nicholas A., and David A. Asch. 1993. "Biases in How Physicians Choose to Withdraw Life Support." *Lancet* 324:642–46.

Cranford, Ronald E. 1989. "Going Out in Style, the American Way, 1987." *Law, Medicine and Health Care* 17:208–10.

Cundiff, David. 1992. *Euthanasia Is Not the Answer: A Hospice Physician's View*. Totowa, N.J.: Humana Press.

De Craemer, Willy. 1983. "A Crosscultural Perspective on Personhood." *Millbank Quarterly* 61:19–34.

Engram, Sara. 1990. "Medical Treatment and the Right to Die." *Baltimore Sun*, 17 June, D1.

"The Ethics of Choosing Death." 1990. *Baltimore Sun*, 17 June, D1.

Eveloff, Scott. 1992. "The Prisoner." *American Journal of Medicine* 93:313–14.

"Father Speeds Baby's Death as Questions of Law Linger." 1989. *New York Times*, 7 May, 26.

"Father Who Pulled Plug on Comatose Son Is Freed." 1989. *Boston Globe*, 19 May, 3.

Feifel, Herman, ed. 1959. *The Meaning of Death*. New York: McGraw-Hill.

Fox, Renée C. 1988. *Essays in Medical Sociology*. New Brunswick, N.J.: Transaction Books.

———. 1994. "The Entry of U.S. Bioethics into the 1990s: A Sociological Analysis." In *A Matter of Principles? Ferment in U.S. Bioethics*, ed. Edwin R. DuBose, Ronald P. Hamel, and Laurence J. O'Connell, 21–71. Philadelphia: Trinity Press International.

Fox, Renée C., and Judith P. Swazey. 1978. *The Courage to Fail*. 2d ed. Chicago: University of Chicago Press.

Frampton, M. W., and R. J. Mayewski. 1987. "Physicians' and Nurses' Attitudes toward Withholding Treatment in a Community Hospital." *Journal of General Internal Medicine* 2:394–99.

Freedman, Benjamin. 1993. "Offering Truth: One Ethical Approach to the Uninformed Cancer Patient." *Archives of Internal Medicine* 153:572–76.

Friedson, Elliot. 1970. *Profession of Medicine*. Chicago: University of Chicago Press.

Fye, W. Bruce. 1978. "Active Euthanasia: An Historical Survey of Its Conceptual Origins and Introduction into Medical Thought." *Bulletin of the History of Medicine* 52:492–502.

Greco, Peter J., Kevin A. Schulman, Risa Lavizzo-Mourey, and John Hansen-Flaschen. 1991. "The Patient Self-Determination Act and the Future of Advance Directives." *Annals of Internal Medicine* 115:639–43.

Hafferty, Frederic W. 1991. *Into the Valley: Death and the Socialization of Medical Students.* New Haven: Yale University Press.

Haney, Daniel Q. 1991. "Study: Doctors Lax in Easing Cancer Pain." *Philadelphia Inquirer,* 22 May, A1.

Hansen-Flaschen, John. 1990. "Choosing Death or 'Mamba' in the ICU: 'Where There's Life, There's Hope' Is Not Necessarily True." *Washington Post,* 8 May, "Health," 9.

Harvey, Lynn K., and Stephanie C. Shubat. 1989. *Physician and Public Attitudes on Health Care Issues.* Chicago: American Medical Association.

Hughes, Everett C. 1971. "Mistakes at Work." In *The Sociological Eye,* ed. E. C. Hughes, 316–25. Chicago: Aldine-Atherton.

Humphry, Derek. 1991. *Final Exit.* Eugene, Oreg.: Hemlock Society.

"I Helped My Mother Die." 1992. *People,* 20 January, 56.

Illich, Ivan. 1976. *Medical Nemesis: The Expropriation of Health.* New York: Pantheon.

James, Nick, and David Field. 1992. "The Routinization of Hospice: Charisma and Bureaucratization." *Social Science and Medicine* 34:1363–75.

Jecker, Nancy S., and Lawrence J. Schneiderman. 1992. "Futility and Rationing." *American Journal of Medicine* 92:189–96.

Kerr, I. G. 1988. "Continuous Narcotic Infusion with Patient Controlled Analgesia of Chronic Cancer Pain in Outpatients." *Annals of Internal Medicine* 108:554–57.

Kleinman, Arthur. 1988. *The Illness Narratives: Suffering, Healing, and the Human Condition.* New York: Basic Books.

Kübler-Ross, Elisabeth. 1969. *On Death and Dying.* New York: Macmillan.

Lear, Martha W. 1993. "Should Doctors Tell the Truth: The Case against Terminal Candor." *New York Times Magazine,* 24 January, 17.

Lloyd, Geoffrey Ernest Richard, ed. 1983. *Hippocratic Writings.* New York: Penguin Books.

McCormick, Wayne C., Thomas S. Inui, Richard A. Deyo, and Robert W. Wood. 1991. "Long-term Care Preferences of Hospitalized Persons with AIDS." *Journal of General Internal Medicine* 6:524–28.

McMillan, Alma, Renee M. Mentnech, James Lubitz, A. Marshall McBean, and Delores Russell. 1990. "Trends and Patterns in Place of Death for Medicare Enrollees." *Health Care Financing Review* 12:1–7.

"Making a Living Off the Dying." 1992. *New York Times,* 25 April, 23.

Margolick, David. 1993. "New Level of Debate Arising over Doctor-Assisted Suicide." *New York Times,* 22 February, A1.

Martin, Emily. 1987. *The Woman in the Body: A Cultural Analysis of Reproduction.* Boston: Beacon Press.

Mauksch, Hans O. 1975. "The Organizational Context of Dying." In *Death: The Final Stage of Growth,* ed. Elisabeth Kübler-Ross, 5–24. Englewood Cliffs, N.J.: Prentice-Hall.

Misbin, Robert I. 1991. "Physicians' Aid in Dying." *New England Journal of Medicine* 325:1307–11.

Miyaji, Naoko T. 1993. "The Power of Compassion: Truth-Telling among American Doctors in the Care of Dying Patients." *Social Science and Medicine* 36:249–64.

Mizrahi, Terry. 1986. *Getting Rid of Patients.* New Brunswick, N.J.: Rutgers University Press.

Mor, Vincent, David S. Greer, and Robert Kastenbaum. 1988. *The Hospice Experiment.* Baltimore: Johns Hopkins University Press.

Prigerson, Holly G. 1992. "Socialization to Dying: Social Determinants of Death Acknowledgement and Treatment among Terminally Ill Geriatric Patients." *Journal of Health and Social Behavior* 33:378–95.

Quill, Timothy E. 1991. "Death and Dignity—A Case of Individualized Decision Making." *New England Journal of Medicine* 324:691–94.

Reinhold, Robert. 1992. "California to Decide If Doctors Can Aid in Suicide." *New York Times,* 9 October, A1.

Rosenberg, Charles E. 1987. *The Care of Strangers.* New York: Basic Books.

Sankar, Andrea. 1991. *Dying at Home: A Family Guide for Caregiving.* Baltimore: Johns Hopkins University Press.

Schneiderman, Lawrence J., Nancy S. Jecker, and Albert R. Jonsen. 1990. "Medical Futility: Its Meaning and Ethical Implications." *Annals of Internal Medicine* 112:949–54.

"She Uses Eyes to Ask to Die." 1990. *Philadelphia Daily News,* 26 April, A1.

Smedira, Nicholas G., Bradley H. Evans, Linda S. Grais, et al. 1992. "Withholding and Withdrawal of Life Support from the Critically Ill." *New England Journal of Medicine* 322:309–15.

Solomon, Mildred Z., et al. 1993. "Decisions Near the End of Life: Professional Views on Life-Sustaining Treatments." *American Journal of Public Health* 83:14–22.

Starr, Paul. 1982. *The Social Transformation of American Medicine.* New York: Basic Books.

Steel, Knight. 1991. "Home Care for the Elderly: The New Institution." *Archives of Internal Medicine* 151:439–42.

Steinfels, Peter. 1993. "Help for the Helping Hands in Death." *New York Times,* sec. 4, 14 February, 1.

"They Tortured My Mother: Patronizing Doctors, Agonizing Care." 1991. *New York Times,* 24 January, A22.

Thompson, Ian. 1984. "Ethical Issues in Palliative Care." In *Palliative Care: The Management of Far-Advanced Illness,* ed. Derek Doyle. Philadelphia: Charles Press.

"Trial Begins over Son's Role in Suicide by Ailing Mother." 1992. *New York Times,* 13 February, B14.

Unschuld, Paul. 1979. *Medical Ethics in Imperial China.* Berkeley and Los Angeles: University of California Press.

Wilson, William C., Nicholas G. Smedira, Carol Fink, James A. McDowell, and John M. Luce. 1992. "Ordering and Administration of Sedatives and Analgesics during the Withholding and Withdrawal of Life Support from Critically Ill Patients." *Journal of the American Medical Association* 267:949–53.

CHAPTER 2

Philosophical Debate and Public Policy on Physician-Assisted Death

Carol A. Tauer

Current religious teachings and societal beliefs about the morality of suicide and euthanasia have grown out of centuries of philosophical debate and reflection. Discussions of the morality of suicide and euthanasia go back as far as Western philosophy itself. Socrates, Plato, Aristotle, Hippocrates, and the Stoics all expressed views on whether and when a person ought to choose to leave this life. Two criteria were primarily used: What would a virtuous person do in such circumstances, and what does a person in such circumstances owe the community? Both the individual's responsibility to live a good life and the individual's responsibility for the good of the community were thus considered. The notion of a person's right to freedom of choice did not enter into these discussions, which assumed shared understandings about what was expected of a person and a citizen.

Classical Greek and Roman philosophers often held that there were circumstances in which a virtuous person would request to have life ended, perhaps for the sake of family or community. Within the Jewish and Christian traditions, however, a clear opposition to self-imposed death gradually emerged. It is true that some historical examples of religious self-sacrifice and martyrdom might be interpreted as self-chosen death or suicide, perhaps affirming the moral acceptability of suicide for noble motives (Droge and Tabor 1992). Yet current authoritative documents from a wide range of Jewish and Christian traditions resist this interpretation and express a clear condemnation of both suicide and euthanasia (Hamel and DuBose 1991). These documents argue or claim that both suicide and euthanasia are prohibited by the commandment "Thou shalt not kill." The taking of a human life, even one's own, is interpreted as the most serious violation of God's law and a usurpation of a divine prerogative. Most Christian churches, basing their moral teachings either on a reading of Scripture or on a systematic analysis of the natural law imprinted in us by God, express a condemnation of suicide and euthanasia that they regard as absolute and unchangeable.

In recent years, two American denominations have adopted statements that support an individual's moral right to request assistance in dying: the Unitarian Universalist Church (1988) and the United Church of Christ (1991) (Hamel and DuBose 1991:85–90; Allen 1991). Both statements also encourage legislation that would protect this right. In the Netherlands, where euthanasia is officially illegal but de facto permitted, the Dutch Reformed Church supports the practice. Virtually all other Jewish, Christian, and Eastern religious traditions currently oppose euthanasia and assisted suicide (Hamel and DuBose 1991).

Yet we see that public opinion in the United States appears to favor the legalization of assisted suicide or euthanasia. A 1990 Roper poll, for example, asked the following question: "When a person has a painful and distressing terminal disease, do you think doctors should or should not be allowed by law to end the patient's life if there is no hope of recovery and the patient requests it?" Sixty-four percent replied yes, 24 percent no, and 13 percent were uncertain or did not respond (Marty and Hamel 1991:34). Interestingly, when the respondents' specific religious denominations were identified, the results were approximately the same: 65 percent of Protestants, 62 percent of Catholics, and 70 percent of Jews said yes.[1] I have used this poll question with a number of audiences, mainly church, college, and civic groups, and consistently find a similar percentage of yes answers. I have also found, however, that some people interpret the question as referring to removal of life support rather than assisted suicide or euthanasia, so it is not clear that approval of assisted suicide or euthanasia is actually this high.

Two states have recently considered propositions to legalize physician-assisted death, Washington in 1991 and California in 1992. Although earlier polls had shown the public favoring legalization, the proposition failed in both states by about the same margin, 54 percent to 46 percent. Opposition forces focused their campaigns on the lack of safeguards. These concerns apparently turned the tide in the days immediately preceding each election. Experience gleaned from these elections suggested two things: that the public would approve granting legal status to euthanasia provided it were done "right"; and that groups that believe euthanasia is morally wrong must appeal to secondary factors, such as the possibility of abuse, in order to garner public support.

In November 1994 the state of Oregon, also working through the referendum process, became the first state to pass a law permitting physician-assisted death. The Oregon "Death with Dignity Act" permits physicians to prescribe lethal drugs under certain specified conditions, but does not allow them to administer lethal injections or other forms of euthanasia. The emphasis is on the patient's choice, the patient's request, and the patient's self-administration of the prescribed drugs. The bill somewhat oddly stipulates that a death brought about in accordance with its measures "shall not constitute suicide, assisted suicide, mercy killing or homicide" (*Measure No. 16*, 1994; Capron 1995).

Oregon voters passed the "Death with Dignity Act" by a close margin of 51 to 49 percent. Groups vigorously opposing the law raised an immediate challenge to its constitutionality, resulting in an appeals court decision that struck it down on August 3, 1995 (Associated Press 1995). Further appeals will undoubtedly follow.

Though still highly controverted, the 1994 passage of the Oregon legislation through a statewide citizens' vote indicates widespread acceptance of physician-assisted suicide for terminally ill and suffering persons. This concrete event seems to portend a trend toward greater general acceptance of physician-assisted death.

What social and cultural factors have led so many Americans to alter their attitudes toward assisted suicide and euthanasia? What influences have superseded the moral teachings of the religious traditions to which most of these Americans belong? In general, American culture has influenced the ethos of religious believers much more than the religious traditions have influenced the ethos of American culture.[1] Note, for example, the many ways in which American Christians celebrate the Christmas season and compare the attention devoted to spiritual and charitable concerns with the focus placed on sheer consumerism and other types of excess. Similarly, American social and cultural values appear to be transforming citizens' attitudes toward death and dying that were formerly based in religious traditions.

Several factors can be identified as contributing to increasing public acceptance of assisted suicide or euthanasia. The fact that these practices are more openly discussed and debated may make them seem more acceptable. There has been widespread discussion in the media of such things as the practice of euthanasia in the Netherlands, the Hemlock Society's work and its publication of the book *Final Exit*, the assisted suicides arranged by Dr. Jack Kevorkian, and the referenda on the legalization of physician-assisted dying in Washington, California, and Oregon. Such publicity probably helps make formerly prohibited practices seem more acceptable. But growing acceptance reflects more than just greater familiarity. More significant factors emerge from the philosophical debate within bioethics concerning the importance of patient autonomy, the corresponding change in personal beliefs about patients' rights and control of treatment decisions, and a less-easily-documented change in public attitudes concerning the meaning of suffering and death.

Autonomy, a Central Ethical Principle

During the past twenty years, professional medical ethics has shifted gradually from a paternalistic practice to a patients' rights focus. Patient consent has always been required for surgery, but it used to involve largely the choice of yes or no, often with limited information provided and the signature a formality. For other medical procedures, it was generally assumed that the doctor knew best and that by putting oneself under a doctor's care one had agreed to accept the recommended therapy. With the advent of life-sustaining procedures such as respirators and dialysis machines, doctors generally felt bound to use the technology which was now at their disposal.

Several events converged in the 1970s to initiate radical changes in the physician-patient relationship. In 1972 the case *Canterbury v. Spence* gave rise to a broadened concept of informed consent. This case determined that the patient must be told all risks that would be material to his decision to consent to a proposed procedure; a physician may not withhold such information for fear that it might cause the patient to refuse. While this case applied only to the Washington, D.C., jurisdiction, it spurred national reconsideration of the concept of informed consent. Contemporaneously, both professional organizations and state legislatures began to draft statements of the rights of patients. Most significantly, these statements specified that full information must be given to patients and that patients have the right to refuse any or all medical treatments.

In 1974 a commission established by Congress to deal with abuses in research involving human subjects began a project that had an influence far beyond its assigned sphere. The National Commission for the Protection of Human Subjects of Biomedical and Behavioral Research wisely sought a foundation of ethical principles on which to base its specific recommendations (1978). Recognizing that freedom of choice is an ethical imperative for the participation of a research subject, the commission made autonomy or self-determination its central principle. While the application of other ethical principles might involve nuanced judgment and interpretation, the free and informed consent of the autonomous subject is an absolute and clear-cut requirement for participation in research, according to the commission.

Because ethicists who participated in developing the commission's documents had influential roles in shaping the new field of bioethics, the principle of autonomy or self-determination came to have a central role in that field. The principles enunciated in the commission's *Belmont Report* were expanded in numerous texts and anthologies in bioethics.[2] Autonomy, which had overriding ethical importance in recruiting subjects for participation in research, was often given the same overriding importance in other contexts, thus appearing to be the primary ethical principle. Some authors maintained that patient autonomy trumped all other concerns, paraphrasing the social philosophy of Ronald Dworkin that "individual rights are political trumps held by individuals" (Dworkin 1977:xi).

Meanwhile a series of court decisions at the appellate or state supreme court level also supported autonomy rights, not only for persons able to make their own choices but for persons no longer able to express their wishes. The case of Karen Ann Quinlan in 1976 upheld the right of Karen's parents to choose to have her respirator disconnected, even though physicians testified that they felt it was obligatory to continue life support. A series of changes in legal practice were achieved through a dialectical interchange between the legal system and the community of professional ethicists. As a result, a genuinely shared ethical-legal consensus emerged: A person able to make decisions may refuse any medical treatment, including medically provided nutrition and hydration. If someone is no longer able to make decisions, a proxy or surrogate must choose or refuse medical treatment according to what the patient would have wanted. Lacking an explicit statement, the proxy must try to reconstruct a patient preference from what is known about the patient. Only if there is no way to know what the patient would have preferred (as with an infant, child, or seriously retarded person) should the proxy use his or her own concept of what would be best for the patient.

The ethical-legal consensus as it stands in 1996 clearly continues to emphasize autonomy, even in the case of a person who is no longer capable of self-determination. The privacy right enunciated in 1973 by the U.S. Supreme Court with regard to reproductive decisions, including abortion decisions, similarly gives the heaviest weight to personal autonomy.

To many people who adopt this view of autonomy it may seem natural and inevitable that freedom of choice should be extended to allow the choice of euthanasia or assisted suicide. These persons may argue that if one has a right to refuse life-sustaining medical treatment, knowing that the refusal will result in death, why should one not have a similar right to request that death be caused directly? If individual autonomy is the principle by which refusal of treatment is justified, then why is autonomy limited where suicide or euthanasia is in question? If autonomy to refuse treatment overrides other ethical principles, then why does a patient's wish for assistance in dying not override ethical concerns that other people may have?

A circuit court judge in Michigan used such arguments to support his decision not to prosecute Dr. Jack Kevorkian for assisting suicide: "If a person can refuse life sustaining treatment, then that person should have the right to insist on treatment which will cause death. . . . The prevailing interest should be the constitutionally protected interests of the individual" (*State v. Kevorkian* 1992:13). This ruling relied heavily on assumptions set out in an unsigned law review article: "Current right-to-die case law establishes a legal right of self-determination that can be interpreted to protect patients' interests in receiving suicide assistance from their physicians. The same policies and practices that underlie the current right to die justify the recognition of a right to die with assistance" ("Physician-Assisted Suicide" 1992:2024).

Logically, there are at least three things wrong with these arguments. First, the right guaranteed to patients is not the right to die. None of the earlier cases cited in the article are about the right to die or the right to cause death. Unfortunately, writers of judicial opinions sometimes do characterize their cases as being about "what is in common parlance referred to as a 'right to die'" (Rehnquist, as cited in Annas 1993:89). But even if that term is the common parlance, jurists ought to be more precise. Second, the right to refuse medical treatment is what moralists call a negative right, a right not to be intruded on or imposed upon. In contrast, the "right to insist on treatment which will cause death" would be a positive right, a right to demand that something be done to one or given to one. Between negative and positive rights there is, in general, a clear ethical and legal distinction. Third, the fact that the ethical and legal right of self-determination might be interpreted to grant a right to assistance in suicide by no means implies that it should or must be interpreted that way.

In fact the Michigan Supreme Court, reviewing several judgments of lower courts involving Dr. Kevorkian, concluded in December 1994 that neither Michigan nor the U.S. Constitution prohibited the state from imposing criminal penalties on a person (including a physician) who assisted another in committing suicide (Gostin 1995). Hence the patient cannot have a constitutional liberty or privacy right to obtain such assistance.

A similar succession of legal opinions has appeared recently on the West Coast. In May 1994 a federal judge in Washington state struck down Washington's ban on assisted suicide, on grounds that there is no relevant distinction between refusal of treatment and request for assisted suicide. Since the U.S. Supreme Court in its only decision on life-sustaining treatment (*Cruzan* 1990) had stated that the Constitution guaranteed a competent patient's right to forgo life-sustaining treatment, the judge concluded that the Constitution also protected the patient's right to physician-assisted suicide (*Compassion in Dying v. Washington* 1994).

As in Michigan, this decision was also reversed at a higher level. Judge John Noonan in March 1995 wrote an opinion for the Ninth Circuit Court of Appeals defending the distinction between the right to refuse treatment and the right to assistance in suicide or euthanasia (*Compassion in Dying v. Washington* 1995). However, a request for rehearing before the entire Ninth Circuit was granted, and eleven judges heard arguments on October 26, 1995. A decision is expected in early 1996.[3]

Despite the current emphasis on the ethical principle of autonomy and the legal rights of liberty and privacy, high-level appeals courts continue to distinguish refusal of life-sustaining treatment from assisted suicide and euthanasia. Having a right to the former does not necessarily entail that one has a right to the latter.

Jurists who have conflated the two categories of rights appear to recognize no claims other than those of autonomous choice. Their arguments, however, suggest that a more complex philosophical issue lurks in the background: whether it is possible to make a clear conceptual distinction between acting and omitting to act. This conceptual distinction is related to the moral boundary we have customarily maintained between killing (impermissible) and allowing to die (permissible). In the following section I examine this distinction. If the distinction cannot be sustained, then it would seem absurd to try to maintain the moral and legal prohibition of assisted suicide and euthanasia.

The Possibility of Distinctions: Acting and Omitting

Religious denominations that oppose assisted suicide or active euthanasia often accompany this condemnation with statements that accept withholding or withdrawing medical treatment in some situations. Most denominations consider it unnecessary to use medical means to prolong life—or the dying process—if there is little hope of recovery. Some limit their argument to "extraordinary means," asserting that these sorts of life-preserving measures are not morally required.

The Catholic church for centuries has distinguished suicide and euthanasia from withdrawing treatment in order to allow natural death to occur. When the recommended means of treatment offer greater burdens (pain, suffering, mutilation, and so on) than benefits to the patient, they need not be used. In withholding or withdrawing such measures, one is allowing natural processes to take their course. Death is both a natural and a spiritual event, and at some point it is appropriate for patient and caregivers to accept it. Death need not be held off at all costs.

This position depends on the distinction between killing (through suicide or euthanasia) and allowing to die (through withholding treatment or withdrawing life support). The possibility of clearly making such a distinction has been questioned by a number of philosophers, who claim that there is no "bright line" between the two concepts.

James Rachels argues that many practices are considered permissible because they are interpreted as withdrawing treatment, but they cause death as surely as direct killing does (1975, 1981). Some instances of withdrawing treatment are easily interpreted as actions: disconnecting a respirator, for example. In some scenarios this decision is compassionate, in others malicious. In disconnecting a respirator, one is actively doing something that may be praiseworthy or criminal. On the other hand, there are situations where one may be guilty for *not* doing something. Rachels uses the example of Smith, who sees his young cousin drowning in the bathtub but walks away because he hopes to profit from his cousin's death. In this case Smith is responsible for allowing the young boy to die, and he is just as guilty as if he had actively killed him.

Proponents of such arguments hope to convince us of two things: that it is difficult to determine whether certain practices—such as disconnecting a respirator—are truly acts or merely omissions, and that moral responsibility does not depend solely on whether one has acted or has merely failed to act.

Arguments like Rachels's, however, appear to be based on a misunderstanding of the current ethical consensus, which prohibits assisting suicide and euthanasia but permits refusal of medical treatment.[4] In order to hold to that consensus, it is not necessary to believe that there is always a "bright line" conceptually between killing and allowing to die. There are surely clear acts of medicalized killing (for example, giving a lethal injection of a substance that has no palliative or therapeutic value, no purpose other than to cause death). Likewise, there are clear instances of allowing someone to die (for example, refraining from a new course of chemotherapy that at most could add a few weeks of suffering to the dying process of a cancer patient). The fact that there may be a gray area between clear instances, where the distinction involves some interpretation and subtlety, does not mean that no distinction can be made. Analogies abound: Each twenty-four-hour period clearly includes periods of daylight and nighttime even though the line distinguishing them is not sharply defined. The same is true for the life stages of childhood and adulthood, which clearly exist as distinct stages even though the demarcation between them may be a fluid one.

An even more significant misunderstanding is shown in Rachels's suggestion that the current ethical consensus bases its conclusions on the mere difference between acting and omitting to act. He implies that someone who opposes active euthanasia but accepts withholding or withdrawing treatment would consider any such omission morally acceptable, no matter what the circumstances. But that is clearly not the case. In fact, the "Vatican Declaration on Euthanasia" distinguishes passive euthanasia from allowing to die: passive euthanasia, which is morally no more permissible than active, is defined as an "omission which of itself or by intention causes death in order that all suffering may . . . be eliminated" (1980:155). Allowing to die, in contrast, is morally permissible because the treatment withheld is hopeless or unduly burdensome. In this explication, as in the current secular consensus, the crucial point ethically is the refusal of treatment by a patient or appropriate proxy who assesses the medical measures to be disproportionate to their predictable outcomes.

The Significance of Intention

A second line of argument that calls into question the coherence of the current ethical consensus involves the role and significance of "intention." Note that the Vatican Declaration, as cited above, prohibits omissions that "by intention" cause death. This prohibition distinguishes intended consequences from foreseen but unintended consequences. It assumes acceptance of the principle of double effect, a criterion developed within Catholic theology and now widely accepted as a guide in medical ethics, sometimes in a modified form.

According to the double-effect principle, if an act has two effects, one good and one bad, then the moral acceptability of that act depends on four conditions being satisfied: the act itself is not intrinsically evil; the bad effect is not the means of producing the good effect; the bad effect is not directly intended but is only an indirect or side effect; and there is a proportionate reason for allowing the bad effect to occur. This principle is now invoked nearly universally, both in religious and secular medical ethics, to justify giving morphine or other substances in quantities sufficient to control pain and suffering. Administering large dosages of a drug may have the indirect effect of depressing respiration and thus hastening death (the bad effect). But if the direct intention is to provide the drugs that are needed to relieve pain (the good effect), then the hastening of death is foreseen but unintended. The criteria of the double-effect principle would thus be satisfied, and adequate amounts of pain-relieving medication could be administered.

Acceptance of this moral conclusion is important in forestalling the movement toward assisted suicide and euthanasia. The ability to provide adequate pain control is essential in humane care of the dying, and it has been strongly promoted by the hospice philosophy. In order to respond to arguments proposing assisted death as a solution for patient pain and suffering, the most effective and adequate measures to relieve pain and suffering must be developed and used, coupled with better education of physicians. But the ethical justification for using such measures often depends on the central concept of the double-effect principle: that intention matters, that in this situation it distinguishes what is ethical from what is unethical practice.

Just as questions have been raised regarding the distinction between killing and allowing to die, so questions arise regarding the moral significance of intention. These questions focus on both theory and practice.

Theoretically, the issues are these: Can you foresee that your action will have a particular consequence and at the same time deny that you intended that consequence? Are you culpable if you intended to bring about death, yet not culpable if you did something that brought about death without your intending that outcome? Does the moral quality of your act depend on the interpretation you hold in your mind?

Two national panels that developed ethical recommendations to guide end-of-life decisions took different positions on these theoretical questions. The President's Commission for the Study of Ethical Problems in Medicine did not find it helpful to distinguish between effects that are intended and effects that are merely foreseen. Instead, this commission developed other arguments to justify providing adequate pain medication, even when there is a risk of harm (1983:77–82). In contrast, the Hastings Center's report of 1987 relied on the standard distinction but used the concept of "purpose" in place of "intention": "Providing large quantities of narcotic analgesics does not constitute wrongful killing when the purpose is not to shorten the lives of these patients, but to alleviate their pain and suffering" (Hastings Center 1987:73).

Policy statements of professional organizations and hospitals regarding pain control generally use phrasing based on the double-effect principle, often in a formulation similar to the Hastings Center's statement.[5] At the same time, a vigorous debate on "intention" continues in the philosophic literature (Buchanan 1996:27–31; Frey 1996). The current controversy over physician-assisted death has led some writers to ask: Does the concept of "intention" provide a way for doctors to assist suffering patients to die more quickly, while keeping up a pretense of not directly causing their deaths? If this use of intention is, at least in some cases, a pretense, then would it not be better to be open and admit that euthanasia is actually occurring?

Even if the philosophic problems were resolved, how would we know what is happening in practice? What intention does the physician or nurse actually have when prescribing or administering large doses of analgesics or sedatives? In an attempt to answer this question, empirical studies are being conducted. In a study of forty-four patients who died in intensive care units in two San Francisco hospitals, researchers surveyed physicians and nurses who provided drugs to these patients at the time that life support was withheld or withdrawn (Wilson et al. 1992). (All these patients were expected to die as a result of the decision to remove life support.) On being asked to list their reasons for administering the drugs, 12 percent of the physicians listed "to hasten death," but in each case this was one of at least three reasons listed. Of the nurses, 13 percent listed "to hasten death," and one of these nurses gave only one additional reason.

What health care providers are actually thinking as they administer large doses of drugs is interesting matter for study. But even if every professional's thought processes do not correspond to the reasoning of theoretical ethical arguments, his or her acts may still be justifiable according to those arguments. If a hospital's policy on drug administration carefully distinguishes pain control from euthanasia and specifies procedures and documentation, then a health care provider who follows these requirements will be acting ethically despite specific individuals' having mixed motives. Hospital policy cannot require all practitioners to be skilled in theoretical ethical argumentation.

The previous three sections showed how certain strands within philosophical ethics might be used to support arguments for assisted suicide or euthanasia. Through the central role given to the principle of autonomy, and through questioning the ethical relevance of the distinctions between acting and omitting and between intending versus merely foreseeing, ethical theory has given some support to a gradual shift in public acceptance of assisted suicide and euthanasia. At the level of personal and family life, however, experiential factors are probably more important influences on belief and opinion than are philosophic debates. In the next two sections I examine two areas of experience that have led many people to desire the option of physician-assisted death.

The Medicalization of Death

Today one hears many people saying that they do not fear death but rather the process of dying. These people may have experienced the lengthy dying processes of family members, or they may have read accounts of families who underwent years of suffering.

Among the common concerns about illness and its treatment that are often of concern to the public are the following:

- medical practice often seems to have as its goal the mere preservation of biological life;
- because medical technology enables us to prolong life, sometimes indefinitely, doctors frequently feel they must use every available technology;
- despite the emphasis on patient and family self-determination, the individual loses control within the medical system;
- institutions are sometimes more concerned about liability and other legal threats than about the best interests of patients;

- control of pain and suffering is often inadequate because caregivers lack interest or expertise and because options to control pain and suffering are too limited.

At a conference on euthanasia and the termination of medical treatment held in December 1992, families involved in court cases concerning the removal of life-sustaining treatment shared their experiences.[6] Speakers included members of the Quinlan, Brophy, Cruzan, Lawrance, Delio, and Busalacchi families. All spoke of the heartache of trying to do what their family member would have wanted regarding withdrawal of treatment, despite meeting obstacles at every turn. Often the family's motives were regarded as suspect, by physicians and other caregivers, by prosecutors and judges, by the media, by interest groups, and by members of the public. These families presented themselves as representatives of numerous other families who wanted to make the same choice they did, but who did not have the stamina or resources to carry through the legal struggle.

Many in the audience were touched by the disillusionment expressed by these people who had had faith in the medical system but who felt opposed, misunderstood, and ignored in their time of distress. Fear of a similar fate leads many to welcome the prospect of legalized euthanasia as a way out. It was clear that some of the family members who spoke at this conference had come to that conclusion. Having had the worst kind of experience with medical and legal institutions, some were now open to the alternative of euthanasia.

Undoubtedly assisted suicide and euthanasia are not the only alternatives to what might be viewed as excesses or abuses in the current practice of medicine. Each problem listed has remedies other than killing the patient. In fact, one might ask whether a medical system that is the subject of so many complaints and so much wariness is a system that ought to be entrusted with additional power, the power to kill.

The Meaning of Suffering

Imagine an ideal world of personalized and caring physician-patient relationships, attentive and responsive health care institutions, procedures to support patient and family decision making, treatment options and alternative modes of patient care, adequate pain management, and affordable health care for all. Even in such a world, acute illness, chronic disease, and the dying process would involve pain and suffering. The breakdown of one's body and possibly one's mental faculties indicates that one's life on earth will not go on forever. Over a short or a long period, one must let go of things of importance in this life: strength, vitality, independence, control, talents, achievements, relationships, family, the future. Even if pain is managed well, one's physical suffering may result simply from being immobile or from constantly undergoing medical procedures. Psychological suffering results when one is unable to work, to participate in ordinary family and social life, to give to others as well as receiving from them.

Proponents of the practice of euthanasia in the Netherlands acknowledge that it is suffering rather than pain that is the main problem for those who are ill or dying. Dr. Peter Admiraal states that "pain should rarely or never be the occasion for euthanasia, as pain . . . is comparatively easily treated" (Battin 1991:301). Nessa Coyle of the Department of Neurology Pain Service at Sloan-Kettering reports that in studies ranking patient symptoms in order of the seriousness of distress caused, pain itself averaged only fifth in seriousness (1992; see also Goetz 1989).[7] The four most distressing symptoms were all aspects of psychological suffering.

Suffering presents two challenges: How do others respond to it? How does the suffering person cope with it? In the past, each of these questions would have received an answer grounded in religious faith. The first question still does; faith communities continue to recognize the importance of putting their beliefs into practice through ministering to those who are suffering and needy. But the second question often fails to elicit a spiritual response that is inspiring and understandable to the American mind, even the mind of a religious believer.

Fifty years ago it was common for children to be taught that suffering had a meaning and value. For Christians, suffering enabled them to unite with the suffering of the crucified Christ, to make up for sins committed by themselves and others, to earn blessings for loved ones, and to merit a reward in the afterlife. Other religious traditions had their own understandings of suffering. Suffering has been seen as an opportunity to learn more about life and oneself, to grow in virtue, to test one's strength of character. Since suffering was permitted by God, it required acknowledgment that God knew what was best for us humans. It required acceptance of what one did not understand.

Today many Americans seem to think that they should not have to suffer, that something has gone wrong if there is suffering in their lives, that there must be some means to take away whatever suffering they experience. Some people may turn to therapy and therapy groups, while others choose alcohol or illegal drugs or seek a succession of romantic and sexual encounters.

Today pain and suffering are rarely viewed as having a meaning and value. It is no wonder that a majority of Americans say that assisted suicide or euthanasia should be available when pain and suffering become unavoidable, during the final weeks and days of life. Have the faith communities, in an effort to be positive, warm, and welcoming places, neglected their responsibility to help their members face the darker side of life? And if they do not help people find meaning in the face of suffering, what other institution would have the spiritual resources to do so? Literature and other forms of art are significant sources of reflection, but they cannot take the place of religious affiliation in most people's lives.

The legalization of euthanasia or physician-assisted suicide is an important issue for all religious denominations. But their responses should not be restricted to campaigns against legalization, as they often appear to be. The moral position that each religious community takes regarding suicide and euthanasia is only a part of the complex role it is called upon to play in response to the suffering and tragedies of human life. Besides providing opportunities to explore the spiritual significance of suffering, faith communities have a crucial role in helping the suffering and dying person remain connected with the human community. The presence and compassionate caring of representatives of a religious congregation may be the only links the patient has with the world beyond the sickroom. Religious institutions will be perceived as credible opponents of the legalization of physician-assisted death only if they take an effective positive role in supporting the suffering and dying.

NOTES

1. This point was called to my attention by Charles Ceronsky.
2. See, for example, Beauchamp and Childress's *Principles of Biomedical Ethics*, four editions of which were published within fifteen years (1979–1995).
3. By a vote of 8–3, the Court of Appeals on March 6, 1996, decided that state laws prohibiting assisted suicide were unconstitutional (1996 WL 94848 [9th Cir.]).
4. For a complete discussion of this topic, see President's Commission for the Study of Ethical Problems in Medicine (1983:62–73).
5. See, for example, the position paper on pain management developed by the Hennepin County Medical Society (1990) in response to the county medical examiner's determination that two deaths involving morphine were acts of euthanasia. This document specifically references the Hastings Center *Guidelines* and the principle of double effect.
6. The conference, "Managing Mortality: Ethics, Euthanasia, and the Termination of Medical Treatment," was held in Minneapolis, 3–5 December 1992.
7. Coyle spoke at the Minneapolis conference on euthanasia and termination of treatment (see note 5 above). Videotapes and audiotapes of sessions are available from the Center for Biomedical Ethics at the University of Minnesota.

REFERENCES

Allen, Martha Sawyer. 1991. "United Church of Christ Endorses Right to Euthanasia." *Minneapolis Star Tribune*, 6 July, 8C.

Annas, George J. 1993. *Standard of Care: The Law of American Bioethics*. New York: Oxford University Press.

Associated Press. 1995. "Judge Strikes Down Oregon Suicide Law." *New York Times*, 4 August.

Battin, Margaret P. 1991. "Euthanasia: The Way We Do It, the Way They Do It." *Journal of Pain and Symptom Management* 6 (July): 298–305.

Beauchamp, Tom L., and James F. Childress. 1979, 1983, 1989, 1995. *Principles of Biomedical Ethics*, 1st, 2nd, 3d, and 4th eds. New York: Oxford University Press.

Buchanan, Allen. 1996. "Intending Death: The Structure of the Problem and Proposed Solutions." In *Intending Death: The Ethics of Assisted Suicide and Euthanasia*, ed. Tom L. Beauchamp, 23–41. Upper Saddle River, N.J.: Prentice Hall.

Canterbury v. Spence. 1972. 464 F.2d 772 (D.C. Cir., 19 May).

Capron, Alex M. 1995. "Sledding in Oregon." *Hastings Center Report* 25, no. 1 (January–February): 34–35.

Compassion in Dying v. Washington. 1994. 850 F. Supp. 1454 (W.D. Wash, 3 May).

Compassion in Dying v. Washington. 1995. 49 F.3d 586 (9th Cir., 9 March).

Coyle, Nessa. 1992. "Aggressive Treatment of Suffering: A Clinical Perspective." Paper presented at the conference "Managing Mortality," Center for Biomedical Ethics, University of Minnesota, Minneapolis, 3–5 December.

Cruzan v. Director, Missouri Dept. of Health. 1990. 497 U.S. 261, at 278.

Droge, Arthur J., and James D. Tabor. 1992. *A Noble Death*. San Francisco: HarperSanFrancisco.

Dworkin, Ronald. 1977. *Taking Rights Seriously*. Cambridge, Mass.: Harvard University Press.

Frey, Raymond G. 1996. "Intention, Foresight, and Killing." In *Intending Death: The Ethics of Assisted Suicide and Euthanasia*, ed. Tom L. Beauchamp, 66–79. Upper Saddle River, N.J.: Prentice Hall.

Goetz, Harriet. 1989. "Euthanasia: A Bedside View." *Christian Century*, 21–28 June, 619–22.

Gostin, Lawrence O. 1995. "Law and Medicine." *Journal of the American Medical Association* 273, no. 21 (7 June): 1688–89.

Hamel, Ron P., and Edwin R. DuBose. 1991. "Views of the Major Faith Traditions." In *Choosing Death: Active Euthanasia, Religion, and the Public Debate*, ed. Ron P. Hamel, 51–101. Philadelphia: Trinity Press International.

Hastings Center. 1987. *Guidelines on the Termination of Life-Sustaining Treatment and the Care of the Dying.* Bloomington: Indiana University Press.

Hennepin County Medical Society. 1990. "Position Paper on Management of Pain and Suffering in the Dying Patient." *Minnesota Medicine* 73, no. 6 (June): 36–37.

Marty, Martin E., and Ron P. Hamel. 1991. "Some Questions and Answers." In *Choosing Death: Active Euthanasia, Religion, and the Public Debate,* ed. Ron P. Hamel, 27–50. Philadelphia: Trinity Press International.

Measure No. 16. 1994. Official 1994 General Election Voters' Pamphlet— Statewide Measures. State of Oregon.

National Commission for the Protection of Human Subjects of Biomedical and Behavioral Research. 1978. *The Belmont Report: Ethical Principles and Guidelines for the Protection of Human Subjects of Research.* Washington, D.C.: U.S. Government Printing Office.

"Physician-Assisted Suicide and the Right to Die with Assistance." 1992. *Harvard Law Review* 105 (June): 2021–40.

President's Commission for the Study of Ethical Problems in Medicine. 1983. *Deciding to Forgo Life-Sustaining Treatment.* Washington, D.C.: U.S. Government Printing Office.

Rachels, James. 1975. "Active and Passive Euthanasia." *New England Journal of Medicine* 292 (9 January): 78–80.

———. 1981. "More Impertinent Distinctions." In *Biomedical Ethics,* ed. Thomas A. Mappes and Jane S. Zembaty, 355–59. New York: McGraw-Hill.

State v. Kevorkian. 1992. No. CR-92-115190-FC. Michigan, Oakland County Circuit, 21 July, at 13.

"Vatican Declaration on Euthanasia." 1980. *Origins* 10 (14 August): 154–57.

Wilson, William C., Nicholas G. Smedira, Carol Fink, James A. McDowell, and John M. Luce. 1992. "Ordering and Administration of Sedatives and Analgesics during the Withholding and Withdrawal of Life Support from Critically Ill Patients." *Journal of the American Medical Association* 267 (19 February): 949–53.

CHAPTER 3

Knocking on Heaven's Door:
Medical Jurisprudence and Aid in Dying

Ann Dudley Goldblatt

"Give me leave. Here lies the water—good. Here stands the man—
good. If the man go to this water and drown himself, it is, will he
nill he, he goes; mark you that. But if the water come to him and
drown him, he drowns not himself. Argal, he that is not guilty of
his own death shortens not his own life."
  "But is this law?"
  "Aye, marry, is't—coroner's quest law."
  —Shakespeare, *Hamlet* 5.1.15–23

The men who dug Ophelia's grave found some of the legal and ethical
distinctions surrounding death difficult to accept; so do we. The decision that permitted Ophelia to lie in consecrated ground seems artificial, a form of intellectual legerdemain designed to reach a result we
believe to be just because we know the suffering of this young woman
and the circumstances of her death. The sleight of hand is easily discovered. Suicide is morally wrong; therefore we will recast the definition of suicide.

During the past twenty years, many Americans' attitudes toward
assisted suicide and euthanasia have seemingly undergone a similar
shift.[1] Now some members of our society want to change definitions,

66

definitions of morality rather than action, to conclude that assisted suicide and euthanasia are ethical and legal, at least within limited boundaries. Recent medical jurisprudence has been much concerned with the acceptability, both ethical and legal, of assisted suicide and euthanasia. The first part of this chapter addresses the question of why this change is occurring at this time. The second part considers why assisted suicide and euthanasia are typically expected to be physician controlled when and if they are permitted by law.

Why Now?

At present, assisting a suicide is a crime in almost all states, and consensual homicide is a crime throughout the country. There is no federal limitation on state legislation prohibiting or permitting assisted suicide and euthanasia. Legislation to legalize assisted suicide and euthanasia, such as the "Death with Dignity" model statute defeated by Washington and California voters in 1991 and 1992, would be constitutional; the Constitution, as currently interpreted, would not invalidate such laws.[2] The Constitution also does not offer any implicit right to seek or obtain assisted suicide and euthanasia. The federal constitutional rights to privacy and to individual liberty, as presently interpreted by the United States Supreme Court, do not include a right to request or receive aid in dying. New legislation specifically aimed at prohibiting physician-assisted suicide or euthanasia would also be permitted under the U.S. Constitution, although it is possible that such prohibitions could be held to violate an express or implied right to privacy under a particular state constitution.[3] Thus, the legal issues do not involve constitutionally protected rights or prohibitions.

Why is the idea of a patient's requesting assisted suicide or euthanasia and a physician's acceding to that request now offered as an appropriate addition to the doctor-patient relationship? Physicians have always had the knowledge and means to end life, yet for most of history, medical professionals have had little ability to restore, to cure, to ameliorate suffering, or to control pain. It is strange that now, when medicine has a much greater ability to cure and control disease, dysfunction, and pain, there is also increased demand for physician-aided death.

There are many partial answers to the question of "Why now?" These include growing consumer awareness and higher expectations, the increase in the amount of medical care provided by strangers, the AIDS epidemic, fear of advanced technology, and the problems of health resource allocation and health care costs. Analysis of recent common-law and constitutional jurisprudence casts additional light on this question. Extensive common-law, statutory, and constitutional litigation involving termination of life-sustaining treatment has resulted in more than fifty court decisions, culminating in the Supreme Court's decision in *Cruzan v. Director, Department of Health* (1990).

The legal journey to *Cruzan* begins with the traditional doctor-patient dyad. The doctor-patient relationship is validated and limited by the fundamental common-law concept that every touching without consent is a battery. A battery, a nonconsensual touching, is both a crime against the state, which can be punished by imprisonment or fine, and a private wrong or tort against the person who did not consent to the touching, for which financial damages may be assessed against the batterer. This rule applies to physicians as it applies to all others. Generally, physicians cannot provide medical treatment without consent; beneficent motive is irrelevant. There are a few limited medical exceptions to the fundamental concept of requiring personal consent to legitimate a touching, but almost all apply only to an incapacitated or incompetent patient requiring immediate and temporary lifesaving medical care.

Is there ever a situation in which a competent patient must accept life-preserving medical care? A 1964 District of Columbia federal appellate court decision held there were four exceptions to the basic rule requiring voluntary consent to medical treatment. A patient's refusal to consent to necessary medical treatment can be overruled if the refusal contravenes one of the following fundamental governmental duties: the preservation of life, the protection of third parties, the prevention of suicide, or the promotion of the ethical integrity of the profession of medicine (*Application of the President* 1964:1005). These exceptions have been construed narrowly; their application almost always has presumed that the refused lifesaving medical care would restore the patient almost immediately to good health.

The fundamental concept of Anglo-American common law that a physician cannot treat a patient without obtaining the patient's consent underlies the termination-of-treatment cases. Courts have declined to establish a legal difference between refusing to consent to the initiation of medical care and refusing to consent to the continuation of medical care. The patient's continuing consent is essential, and it may be withdrawn at any time. This is a basic requirement of legal and ethical medical treatment and of all physical contact by a physician.

Why then were these termination-of-treatment cases initially so troublesome for the law? One reason was that the plaintiff patients in most cases were unconscious; their refusals to consent to further treatment were established or imputed by proxy and were therefore indirect and uncertain. A second reason was that in the 1960s, for the first time, permanently unconscious patients could be maintained indefinitely on life support. Prior to the 1960s, life-sustaining treatments were viewed as temporary. Life-sustaining treatments either enabled the patient to return to physiological self-sufficiency, or the patient died. Because these treatments were thought to be temporary, it was much less common for a patient or a proxy to refuse life-support technology.

In 1976, Karen Ann Quinlan's father challenged the traditional understanding that consent to life-sustaining medical treatment should be presumed, a traditional understanding based on the assumption that such treatment would be short term (*In re Quinlan* 1976). Mr. Quinlan argued that there should be a presumed refusal of long-term life-sustaining medical treatment when the sustained life was unconscious and unaware. The physicians caring for Karen Ann disagreed. They did not contend that Karen Ann would consent to continued treatment if she were able to do so, but they argued that terminating treatment would result in death and that this was therefore life*saving* treatment for which legal and ethical tradition and normal medical practice presumed consent. These physicians also argued that terminating treatment would be an illegal abandonment of the patient and a violation of their professional duties.

Karen Ann's father turned to the common law requiring consent to all medical treatment and to the recently enunciated constitutional concept of personal privacy. His attorneys argued that the common-law right to refuse unwanted medical care is a fundamental, historically authenticated, and traditionally accepted right, one that is implicit in a concept of ordered liberty and one that can be asserted by proxy. The New Jersey Supreme Court accepted these two arguments. Almost all the other jurisdictions that have faced this controversy from 1976 until 1990 agreed with the New Jersey Supreme Court, although most termination-of-treatment decisions have been based solely on the common-law right to refuse medical treatment. In 1990, a controlling determination of the common-law ability to refuse life-sustaining medical care by proxy was made by the United States Supreme Court in *Cruzan*.

The *Cruzan* decision held that there is a common-law right to refuse even life-sustaining medical care, that a refusal can be based on evidence of personal desires, and that the required degree of certainty as to personal desire is controlled by state law. *Cruzan* determined that the common-law right to refuse medical care extends to the termination of life-sustaining measures, including the provision of artificially administered food and fluids, and that the exercise of this right in the case of incompetent patients is appropriately limited by state legislation when such legislation is reasonably related to protecting the interests of the incompetent patient by ensuring that the proxy refusal reflects what the patient would decide on his or her own behalf, if he or she could. The court stated that a common-law right to refuse medical treatment was "a protected liberty interest" but was not a fundamental constitutional right.

There is an important difference between protected liberty interests and fundamental constitutional rights. A fundamental constitutional right may not be invaded or limited unless the government has a compelling reason to limit the right and the proposed statutory limitation is as minor as is possible in order to achieve the state's compelling reason to constrain the fundamental right. A protected liberty interest may be limited or even eliminated so long as the statute that affects the protected liberty interest is reasonably related to any legitimate state interest. Liberty interests are only weakly protected against governmental incursions; fundamental rights are extremely well protected against statutory constraints. Freedom of speech is a fundamental right; the right to refuse life-sustaining medical treatment is a liberty interest protected only against unreasonable statutory limitations. While almost all the judicial decisions in the termination-of-treatment (also called right-to-die) cases found that patients had a liberty interest in refusing medical treatment, none considered the possibility that a patient might have a coexisting liberty interest in demanding or receiving specific medical care or medically mediated procedures. This is important because the conventional legal distinction between a termination of treatment that results in death and assisted suicide or euthanasia has historically been based on the distinction between the right to refuse treatment and the nonexistence of a right to demand treatment.

How then is the right to refuse life-preserving medical treatment linked to legitimating a request for assisted suicide or euthanasia? How has our society formulated a bridge from refusing treatment to requesting death as a medical management option? One possibility is that assisted suicide and euthanasia might be described as just another modern innovation in medical care. Contemporary medical "services" include many patient-requested elective procedures such as cosmetic surgery and the prescription of mood-enhancing drugs. But no one has a right to demand an elective medical procedure. Moreover, those in favor of assisted suicide and euthanasia do not view these death-providing procedures simply as additional medical options. Most advocates of assisted suicide and euthanasia consider the right to control the time of one's death a fundamental aspect of individual autonomy, a matter of human dignity.

Viewing assisted suicide and euthanasia as an extension of a traditional, fundamental right to refuse medical treatment rather than as an extension of elective medical procedures is also unsuccessful in providing a link between the recognized right to refuse treatment that forestalls death and a right to demand treatment that will cause death. Refusals are enforceable; demands are not. No one has a common-law, much less a constitutionally protected, right to demand treatment. But some bridge attaching the potential legitimacy of assisted suicide and euthanasia to an acknowledged common-law or constitutional "right" to request medical services is required. Surprisingly, the United States Supreme Court's decision in *Roe v. Wade* (1973) provides that bridge.

Roe v. Wade held that there is a fundamental, constitutionally protected right to seek a legal abortion. Justice Blackmun, who wrote the Court's decision in *Wade*, wanted to resolve public concerns about the moral appropriateness of abortion by characterizing the abortion procedure as a normal part of a traditional doctor-patient relationship, that is, a typical and therefore morally acceptable medical treatment. The words *elective* and *nontherapeutic* never appear in *Wade*; agreeing to perform the procedure is seen as a purely clinical decision. As the Court viewed abortion, a pregnant patient sought medical advice from her attending physician, and, if the physician determined that an abortion was medically indicated, the procedure was performed. In the words of *Wade*, the abortion decision "in all its aspects is inherently and primarily a medical decision" (1973:166). Many, perhaps even most, abortions were medically atypical: an elective abortion is a patient-determined need arising from a condition other than physical disease or dysfunction, a patient-desired outcome, and a patient-determined medical treatment. These aspects of the actual practice of abortion were virtually ignored in the Supreme Court decision, which portrayed abortion as a mainstream medical treatment. The abortions legalized in *Wade* did not involve a medical treatment suggested by the physician to which a patient could refuse or consent; they were medically mediated options that patients requested and that physicians could consent to or refuse to perform. *Wade* created not a right to abortion but a right to request a legal abortion from a willing physician.

Although Chief Justice Burger's concurrence specifically denied that *Wade* legitimated abortion on demand (1973:208), abortion on demand was the practical result of the decision, because there were physicians willing to perform every abortion a "patient" requested. *Wade* therefore seemed to allow patients to demand this single medical treatment, although the "demand" was importantly conditioned on the physician's agreement. The Court ignored or suppressed any awareness that the physician's agreement was assumed. As the existence of for-profit abortion clinics demonstrated, there were sufficient numbers of physicians willing to meet the demand as a demand, with no exercise of clinical judgment or standard of medical need other than (usually) a medical examination or diagnostic test to confirm that the patient was, in fact, pregnant. Our society was introduced to constitutionally protected, patient-driven medical treatment indirectly, under the guise that it was a typical aspect of a traditional physician-dominated doctor-patient relationship. The Court's attempt to dissipate the controversy over the morality of medical abortion in this manner was unsuccessful, but that is another matter.

Although an elective abortion is an atypical medical procedure, elective abortion is a typical patient "demand" for treatment. It requires medical aid, but its choice depends on nonmedical, nonphysical determinations of needs and wants, and access to it is represented primarily as an issue of self-determination, not of health. In public opinion, the abortion decision legitimated patient-initiated medical procedures, even though many people disputed the legitimacy of abortion itself. There is a direct and important connection between a perceived right to have a legal abortion and the right to obtain legal medical aid in dying. Except for the right to request and obtain a legal abortion acknowledged in *Wade*, there is no common-law or constitutional precedent for the right to request and obtain legal aid in dying. There is, of course, another important connection between requesting aid in dying and requesting abortion: both involve death. Regardless of one's opinion on the moral acceptability of either abortion or aid in dying, the connection provided by the intentional destruction of life and of potential life cannot be ignored.[4]

Physician Control

Theologians and philosophers discuss the distinction between omission and commission, much as the gravediggers in *Hamlet* did, considering whether terminating life-sustaining treatment is morally distinguishable from providing direct aid in dying. The law does distinguish the two, and so do most patients. Refusing medical treatment, even life-preserving treatment and even treatment previously accepted, is supported by a strong common-law tradition. The permissibility of assisted suicide and consensual homicide, a request for aid in dying, has no common-law, statutory, or constitutional history. Public acceptance of assisted suicide and euthanasia requires the bridge from refusing medical treatment to requesting medically mediated procedures that cause death that the Supreme Court abortion decisions provide. Overruling *Wade* would not eliminate this bridge. The public understanding of the potential legitimacy of patient requests for medical procedures including medically mediated death is a concept independent of its original application.

The Supreme Court's decision on abortion required the participation of a physician. This requirement helped depict the procedure as a normal medical practice and invested the procedure with the moral capital of the profession of medicine. Yet there is no inherent reason to require the participation of a licensed physician in the performance of abortion. Abortions were historically provided as frequently or more frequently by laypersons and midwives than by licensed physicians. The procedure itself is not technically difficult; the training of paramedical abortion providers is practicable. Similarly, requiring physician participation in assisted suicide and euthanasia also seems nonessential; nonetheless, the need for a medical expert to provide aid in dying as well as to determine the appropriateness of the request has been unquestioned. Assisted suicide and euthanasia require physicians, some proponents argue, because doctors have expertise in the means of providing medical death, in quantifying and alleviating pain, and in judging when a patient's request is appropriate. These arguments are unconvincing. Expertise in the means of bringing about death is easily learned, but such training is not a traditional element of medical education or practice. Current professional pain control practices are often challenged as inadequate, and poor pain management is often cited to support a demand for aid in dying. Professional expertise in prognosis and diagnosis often generates results that are far from certain.

Physician certification of the appropriateness of a request for assisted suicide and euthanasia may provide safeguards, but I doubt that this alone explains why the concept of physician control makes assisted suicide and euthanasia more acceptable to the public. Having a physician determine the appropriateness of death as a medical option validates the decision of suicide and medicalizes death. It makes the requested death a form of medical treatment, even a cure. It creates a semblance of control over death and launders the less acceptable aspects of imposed death. Physician approval and mediation of assisted suicide and euthanasia make this kind of death, when deemed appropriate, a matter of clinical judgment in much the same way that the Supreme Court depicted elective abortion as a typical medical treatment. Physician-mediated aid in dying helps to portray death as a form of healing, even though it results in the elimination of the patient rather than the disease, an elimination of the sufferer rather than an amelioration of his or her suffering.

Such a depiction of medically mediated death as a curative procedure is not unprecedented. There is a quietly expanding practice in this country of inflicting capital punishment by means of lethal injection. At such executions, a person in a lab coat, in some states by law a licensed physician, carefully swabs the location of the injection with an antiseptic and introduces an intravenous drip; death ensues in a matter of minutes. The irony of sterilizing the injection site, of ensuring that the wound will not become infected, is overwhelming. Execution by lethal injection is reasonably quick and relatively painless in purely physical terms; its quasi-medical technique provides society with the opportunity to view capital punishment as a "cure" for the criminal. This metaphorical depiction of imposed death as an ultimate medical treatment rather than a legal homicide, exchanging the black hood of the executioner for the white coat of the physician, has strong appeal. But it also has detrimental aspects. Medicalizing death, making it a patient management option, a form of medical treatment, would radically change our conception of the doctor-patient relationship, weaken our presently perceived ability to rely on the judgment and good will of the physician, and call into doubt the image of the physician as the patient's personal advocate.

The decision in the *Barber* case (1983), in which a California appellate court dismissed a murder indictment against two physicians for withdrawing intravenous food and fluids from an unconscious patient who was not brain-dead, was the first to declare as a matter of law that artificially administered food and fluids are "typical" medical treatments, treatments that can be refused and also, importantly, treatments that can be withheld or withdrawn by medical personnel from irreversibly ill incompetent patients without proxy consent if they are determined to be medically futile (*Barber v. Superior Court* 1983; *Rasmussen v. Fleming* 1987).[5] The Nevada Supreme Court, in a 1990 case authorizing a quadriplegic's refusal to continue the medical treatment provided by a respirator, agreed with a 1989 Georgia Supreme Court decision that medication necessary to make a disconnection from a ventilator pain-free was "inseparable from a right to refuse medical treatment" (*McKay v. Bergstedt* 1990; *State v. McAfee* 1989). Mr. McAfee could not discontinue mechanical ventilation because oxygen deprivation caused him severe pain. The court ordered his doctors to provide a sedative to make the termination of treatment pain-free. "His right to have a sedative . . . administered before the ventilator is disconnected is part of his right to control his medical treatment" (*State v. McAfee* 1989:652). These recent expansions of the patient's right to adequate pain control and the physician's right not to be required to offer or to continue medically futile treatment are the current extremes of the judicial interpretation of the right to refuse medical treatment.[6]

A Michigan county court judge dismissed a murder indictment in a suicide assisted by Dr. Jack Kevorkian (*Michigan v. Kevorkian* 1992). The dismissal concluded that even though assisted suicide is a "common law crime," physician-assisted suicide is different and is not a crime. This is a bizarre conclusion. Exceptions to common-law crimes, as well as to statutory crimes, are in derogation of the law; they must be narrowly drawn and authoritatively supported. The *Kevorkian* opinion rested the distinction solely on the absence of past criminal convictions of physicians assisting in suicide. But the absence of precedents creates no evidence of legality; a negative does not prove the opposite positive. The *Kevorkian* dismissal further stated that "if a person can refuse life sustaining treatment, then that person should have the right to insist on treatment which will cause death. . . . The distinction between assisted suicide and the withdrawal of life support is a distinction without merit"

(1992:12). This statement, also, has no precedent. It contradicts common-law and constitutional jurisprudence, and it is entirely unsupported. If physician-assisted suicide and active voluntary euthanasia are to be legalized, they must be legislated; they cannot be judicially construed.[7]

These suggestions of the reasons for the current surge in public opinion favoring assisted suicide and euthanasia, and for assuming a physician to be an essential part of this proposed practice, are based on contemporary legal concepts and practices. The legal and constitutional aspects of the abortion controversy have helped to create an association between the traditional right to refuse medical treatment and the unprecedented proposal of the appropriateness of requesting and receiving medically mediated death. This association makes a request for aid in dying appear less innovative than it is. The proposal that medical professionals assess the appropriateness of requests for aid in dying comes in part from a desire to medicalize and sanitize the procedure in much the same way that execution by lethal injection attempts to medicalize and sanitize capital punishment. Legalizing a practice does not make that practice morally appropriate, but Americans tend to associate legality and morality. America has historically (and unsuccessfully) attempted to legislate morality, as in Prohibition, and Americans often tend to accept as moral what the professions of law and medicine authorize. Our legal and social history demonstrates that effective public debate must occur *before* a morally controversial practice is authorized by law. We have lived with the anger and violence that followed the constitutional protection of elective abortion. Assisted suicide and active voluntary euthanasia raise equally controversial issues of morality and propriety. These issues should be discussed now, before any supreme court permits assisted suicide and euthanasia, so that the bitter, divisive consequences of the abortion decision may be eliminated or at least controlled.

NOTES

1. For the purposes of this chapter, euthanasia is defined as the intentional killing of a mentally competent individual in response to that individual's voluntary request for death.

2. *Lee v. Oregon*, civil no. 94-6467-HO, decided on August 3, 1995, by the United States District Court for the District of Oregon, held that the Oregon Death with Dignity Act, a ballot initiative approved in 1994, was unconstitutional. The Oregon Death with Dignity Act permitted competent, terminally ill adults to obtain physician aid in dying. The district court found that the act violated the equal protection clause of the Fourteenth Amendment because it does not contain adequate safeguards to ensure the competency and autonomy of the terminally ill who seek aid in dying. Oregon residents who are not terminally ill are protected by statutes that make assisting in suicide a crime. The district court held that there was no reasonable state purpose in eliminating the protection of the law against assisted suicide for all terminally ill persons. "[The act] . . . provides a means to commit suicide to a severely overinclusive class who may be competent, incompetent, unduly influenced, or abused by others. The state interest and the disparate treatment are not rationally related and . . . [the act], therefore, violates the Constitution of the United States." *Lee v. Oregon* has been appealed to the Ninth Circuit Court of Appeals. The circuit court may or may not agree with the district court that the safeguards of the Oregon act are insufficient. In either case, the decision in *Lee v. Oregon* does not state that permitting aid in dying is unconstitutional but only requires that a statute permitting aid in dying be carefully worded to eliminate the potential for abuse.

3. *Compassion in Dying v. Washington* (1995) declared that a Washington statute prohibiting assisted suicide did not violate the United States Constitution even as applied to competent, terminally ill adults who seek aid in dying from licensed physicians. The court held that the statute was consistent with a rational distinction between a refusal of medical treatment that results in a natural death and a request for aid in dying that results in an intentionally premature death.

4. It is important to note that the United States Supreme Court specifically stated in *Wade* that fetal life is not constitutionally protected; abortion does not involve a death of a constitutionally protected person (*Roe v. Wade* 1973:113).

5. The definition of medical futility is beyond the scope of this chapter. One definition is that the treatment does not provide a physiological benefit to the patient. Given this definition, it is difficult to conclude that a decision to terminate or withhold artificial nutrition and hydration from a competent patient against his or her wishes is justified. But in *Rasmussen v. Fleming* (1987), the Arizona Supreme Court held that DNR (do-not-resuscitate) and DNH (do-not-hospitalize) directions made on behalf of a severely compromised but not unconscious elderly patient whose personal desires were entirely unknown

were in her best interests. The petitioners in this case originally requested authorization for removing artificially administered food and fluids from this same patient; however, the decision did not address this problem because the food and fluids were withdrawn without specific permission while the case was pending. The court held that hospitalization and treatment provided no benefit to this person, that she would if she could (or should because she ought?) refuse all further treatment.

6. Even if the physician has a legally enforceable right not to offer medical care if it will provide a patient with no physiological benefit, this decision does not answer the question of whether a patient may demand treatment that will provide that patient with a physiological benefit. The judiciary so far has refused to conclude that a physician can withdraw life-sustaining treatment in the face of the patient's or a proxy's belief in the possibility of a miraculous recovery. A trial jury has, however, decided after the fact that a unilateral termination of life-sustaining treatment despite the clearly stated desires of the patient was not inappropriate. In an unreported case, physicians at Massachusetts General Hospital made a unilateral decision to extubate and not reintubate a terminally ill incompetent patient because further treatment was, in the opinion of the physicians, medically although not physiologically, futile. See "Court Ruling Limits Rights of Patients" 1995.

7. This case was reversed by the Michigan Supreme Court in *People v. Kevorkian* (1994). The Michigan Supreme Court held that there is no bar to criminalizing assisted suicide and that licensed medical practitioners are not exempted from such criminalization. See also *Compassion in Dying v. Washington* (1995).

REFERENCES

Application of the President and Directors of Georgetown College. 1964. 331 F.2d 1000 (D.C. Cir.; *rehearing denied*, 331 F.2d 1005).

Barber v. Superior Court. 1983. 147 Cal. App. 3d 1006.

Compassion in Dying v. Washington. 1995. 49 F.3d 586 (9th Cir.)

"Court Ruling Limits Rights of Patients." 1995. *New York Times*, 22 April.

Cruzan v. Director, Department of Health. 1990. 58 U.S.L.W. 4916 (26 June).

In re Quinlan. 1976. 335 A.2d 647, *cert. denied*, 429 U.S. 992.

Lee v. Oregon. 1995. 1995 U.S. Dist. LEXIS 12011.

McKay v. Bergstedt. 1990. 801 P.2d 617 (S. Ct. Nev.).

Michigan v. Kevorkian. 1992. CR 92-115190-FC, Circuit Court, Oakland Cty., Michigan (21 July).

People v. Kevorkian. 1994. 527 N.W.2d 714 (Mich.).

Rasmussen v. Fleming. 1987. 741 P.2d 674 (S. Ct. Ariz.).

Roe v. Wade. 1973. 410 U.S. 113.

State v. McAfee. 1989. 385 S.E.2d 651 (S. Ct. Ga.)

CHAPTER 4

The Language of Principle and the Language of Experience in the Euthanasia Debate

Arthur W. Frank

"My answers don't all agree, do they?" Thus an intensive care nurse commented on the interview responses she gave during a study of attitudes toward euthanasia (Kelner and Bourgeault 1992). A woman with terminal cancer told an interviewer: "I am still totally determined to take my life. . . . I know from experience that I often formulate elaborate plans and then when the time comes I do something entirely different" (Shavelson 1995:178). Ambivalence has characterized virtually every discussion I have ever had about euthanasia, the only difference being the individual's awareness of his or her own ambivalence. Mark Siegler and Carlos Gomez (1992:1164) have noted that "there is no sign yet of a consensus [on euthanasia] in the medical, legal, and ethics communities of the United States." A review of forty years' survey studies of public attitudes toward euthanasia (Blendon et al. 1992) observes marked changes over the years surveyed, but the meaning of these changes is not clear. Commentary trying to sort out the 1991 Washington euthanasia referendum (Carson 1992) suggests the difficulty of knowing what voters thought they were voting on. These same difficulties pervade survey responses.

When the answers don't all agree, it is time to examine the rhetoric in which the issues are presented. My goal here is not to argue a position but rather to suggest one dimension of the rhetorical impasse that debate seems to have reached. Social theory both anticipates such an impasse and provides guidance in dealing with this impasse.

While the course of discussion will show my own preferences concerning euthanasia, let me be clear at the outset that I share the ambivalence of the nurse quoted above: my own answers don't agree either. But the more I study the issue, the less I am concerned with the possibility, or even the desirability, of consistency. Ambivalence may be the best response.

The Discourse of the Euthanasia Debate

Social scientists increasingly study an issue by examining the rhetoric— the spoken and written discourse—in which that issue is framed and debated.[1] The presuppositions of this discursive turn can be briefly summarized as follows:

1. The term *discourse* implies that written and oral language reflect and perpetuate specific "forms of life," in Wittgenstein's phrase. Discourse presupposes an interpretation of reality, and discourse then perpetuates this interpretation *as* reality. This interpretation is all the more powerful because it is invisibly embedded in language that purports only to describe reality.

2. Discourse perpetuates assumptions about *power*, which is shaped and sustained through symbolic acts, including speech and written texts. Discourse is never politically neutral but rather historically situated, culturally biased, gendered, and open to contest.

3. Thus discursive practices are exercises in power, and to effect a change in discourse is to *redistribute access* to social resources, including the meanings people attach to actions and objects.

4. There is no privileged position outside of discourse: what is called *truth* is always a discursive production. Thus critical analysis turns to the claims and effects of discourse.

5. Finally, and significantly for the present inquiry, discourse is particularly powerful in shaping the experience we have of our *bodies*. Through various discourses, society controls the body (see Frank 1991).

With this summary as background, I suggest that the rhetoric of euthanasia has three discursive modes. In this section I discuss the first mode, the empirical, and introduce the other two, the language of principle and the language of experience.

The rhetoric of the empirical mode is statistical; "how many?" is the dominant question. Blendon, Szalay, and Knox's (1992) review of opinion surveys on euthanasia exemplifies this discourse. The authors are sensitive to difficulties of sampling, to variance in the respondents' understanding of the questions, and to differences of experience among respondents. Most important, they seem to recognize that however provocative and informative empirical studies can be, quantified responses necessarily raise more questions than they resolve.

Blendon et al. suggest that "Americans think about right-to-die questions in two very distinct ways—as a public policy issue and as an issue of personal choice for themselves" (1992:2659). This distinction returns us to ambivalence: there are contradictions between what respondents advocate as policy and what they believe or say they would do as personal practice. With regard to policy, Blendon et al. summarize survey findings of a "major change" toward a desire for "legislation that would permit more personal control over the quality of life" (1992:2659). Much of this change refers to withdrawal of life-support systems (that is, allowing to die), not to the legality of choosing to have one's own life ended (euthanasia). The survey clearly illustrates the distinction respondents make between public policy and personal choice. On *policy* questions concerning withdrawal of life-support systems and legalizing euthanasia, those who had personal experience of irreversible coma or terminal illness and those who had no firsthand experience responded similarly. Their *personal* choices, however, showed significant differences. Those with firsthand experience were more likely to have discussed their own wishes for treatment with family and friends, and they were more likely to believe families would honor these wishes, including stopping life-support systems (Blendon et al. 1992:2661–62).

These differences between what people perceive as policy decisions and personal decisions affect other survey responses. When interpreting surveys, we must ask whether respondents were answering a question with reference to social policy or with reference to what they want for themselves. My point here, however, is that this policy/personal distinction mirrors what I found, independently, in my own analysis of arguments for and against active euthanasia. These arguments fell into two distinct discourses: those argued on the basis of principle and those argued on the basis of experience. Ultimately the "facts" of the empirical discourse resolve nothing: statistics by themselves are amoral, and only our interpretations bring them into the context of moral argument. The other two discourses of the euthanasia debate, what I call the language of principle and the language of experience, are explicitly moral rhetorics.

The language of principle rests on (a) belief in the competence and accountability of professional knowledge; (b) belief in the progress of technical achievement and the matching progress of ethical implementation; (c) the primacy of logic and reason, applied universalistically; (d) a complementary suspicion of embodiment as a source of unreason, requiring "control"; and (e) consequently a willingness to make decisions for others. The core assumption of the language of principle is the benevolence of expertise, whether scientific or ethical.

The language of experience is (a) local in its reference and particular rather than universal in its intended scope of applicability; (b) "thick" in its description of personal values and context; (c) embodied in its primacy of both physical descriptions and its willingness to accept visceral responses; and (d) dependent on *Verstehen* for its intelligibility: the reader/hearer of this language must be willing to suspend his or her usual way of seeing the world and entertain the worldview of the other as plausible. The core assumption of the language of experience is the necessary singularity of personal situations, yet it remains possible for each of us, based on our own experience, to enter the circumstances of the other, to share that other's world, and to be changed by it.

That the euthanasia debate should split into these two rhetorical positions is not surprising. Let me describe only two social theories that predict a split between the languages of principle and experience. In the early 1960s the sociolinguist Basil Bernstein theorized that persons speak in two codes, which he called *elaborated* and *restricted* (1970). The elaborated code is universal and cosmopolitan. Its references are transportable in their intelligibility; thus academics can have closer communication with colleagues in another country than with their neighbors. The restricted code is particularistic, embedded in local reference to persons and places, and dependent on the shared significance of those references. Speech in the restricted code does not make much sense, or at least the same sense, to outsiders. For my purposes, the language of principle is a form of elaborated code, and the language of experience has affinities to a restricted code.

More recently, the social theorist Jürgen Habermas (1987a, 1987b) has argued that society is split between levels of *lifeworld* and *system*. The lifeworld is based on understandings that evolve through sharing traditions, living in communities, and raising children to take their places in these communities. The lifeworld is formed and reformed through what Habermas calls communicative agreement: social life proceeds by discussion and consensus formation in that discussion.

What Habermas calls the level of system is based on noncommunicative media, principally money and votes. These can only be tallied; elections and markets can produce winners and buyers, but they cannot achieve mutual understandings. Thus, understandings that remain necessary at the level of system depend on the lifeworld, since only in the lifeworld is communicative consensus possible. The legitimacy of the system level of markets and politics depends on the lifeworld, because legitimacy requires consensus, and communicative consensus can be grounded only in the commonalities of shared experience and talk that are part of the lifeworld.

Habermas's argument is embedded in other social theories (see Frank 1989, 1992b), but the issue comes down to his observation that we live in a period of the colonization of the lifeworld by the system. The system level increasingly crowds out the lifeworld, forcing its exchanges to proceed through noncommunicative media such as money. Decisions once based on common understandings become responses to "functional" imperatives reflecting the needs of an administrative system that is elsewhere. Habermas does not oppose administrative systems—this is not a Luddite theory—but he does observe the paradox that administrative legitimacy simultaneously depends on lifeworld consensus and undermines the resources necessary for this consensus. When administrative systems destroy the basis of communicative consensus, they destroy their own legitimacy and themselves.[2]

The lesson Habermas suggests for the euthanasia debate, and for medical ethics generally, can be simply stated: When ethical principles lose touch with local narratives of experience, then their attempted universalism has no popular moral consensus behind it. When principles lack consensus, they lose legitimacy. "Ethics" becomes an activity for specialists: abstract, administrative, and perceived as just another imposition on people's lives.[3]

Theories like those of Bernstein and Habermas lead us to expect the kind of rhetorical impasse that can be observed in the euthanasia debate. We learn from these theories that the two codes, whether elaborated and restricted or system and lifeworld, depend on each other *and* are always in tension with each other. The issue is not to choose one or the other, but rather to understand how each can find its proper complementarity to the other. For there to be the "overlapping consensus" on euthanasia that writers like Siegler and Gomez (1992) call for, the languages of principle and experience must be reconciled—but *they never can be*. Learning to create at least a productive tension between these two codes can begin with an analysis of their respective rhetorical claims.

In the examination of rhetoric that follows, my bias is that Habermas is right: our present crisis is the colonization of the lifeworld by system. One implication of this imbalance in the sphere of medical ethics is that the language of principle about euthanasia must bend in the direction of the language of experience.

The Language of Principle

"*Within* these outer limits," writes Leon Kass about decisions in the care of the terminally ill, "no fixed rules of conduct apply; instead, prudence—the wise judgment of the man-on-the-spot—finds and adopts the best course of action in light of the circumstances. But the outer limits themselves are fixed, firm, and non-negotiable" (1991). The statement exemplifies the central features of the language of principle. Kass appears to concede to the local and particular, but he holds back more than he allows.

First, Kass's concern, in this article as elsewhere, is with physicians' interventions in active euthanasia. The question for him is one of *professional* practice; "ethics" is thus an issue for the medical profession. The "man-[*sic*]-on-the-spot" is a physician, no other. Thus the statement presupposes—but renders invisible—a hierarchy. At the lowest level, but unmentioned in the discourse, is the dying person, whose spot the physician is on. Then comes the physician, who is wise but whose judgment extends only to certain limits, which are "fixed, firm, and non-negotiable." These "limits" do not derive out of nothing, although that is often the implication of the language of principle. If the dying person is invisible at one end of the hierarchy, equally invisible are those at the top of the hierarchy who set the "non-negotiable" limits for the physician's care of the dying person.

The rhetoric of Kass's statement thus presupposes professional dominance and hierarchy. The one who sets the outer limits is effectively insulated from the invisible patient at the bottom of the hierarchy, so the question becomes, how flexible are the principles that regulate the practicing physician? For all Kass apparently concedes to the practitioner, the limits on practice remain "non-negotiable." Consensus, to use Habermas's terms, is not to be reached within a situation of communicative exchange, but rather it is imposed from above; ethics are administered. The individual on the spot is praised but not entirely trusted.

Kass could certainly claim that his emphasis on medical centrality in active euthanasia reflects popular attitudes as reported in survey results, but these attitudes are ambivalent. Blendon et al. (1992:2661) report that twice as many respondents would ask a physician for help in ending their lives as would ask a family member (24 percent to 11 percent), a finding that seems to support the centrality of the physician. But physical intervention is not the same as decision making. "Thirty percent would want the family to decide alone, and a mere 3 percent would want a physician or the courts to make the decision on their behalf" (Blendon et al. 1992:2661). As always, the answers do not entirely agree: respondents want families to have the power to decide but not the responsibility to carry out the decision. The point is that the physician is understood as implementing the family's wishes, not as the one making the judgments, much less as one implementing judgments handed down from elsewhere.

If the language of principle seeks to reserve decision making on the termination of life for professionals, it does so on the assumption that only professionals exemplify the standards of rationality that must inform these decisions. Edmund Pellegrino calls arguments favoring euthanasia "logically inadequate" (1992:95). Pellegrino focuses on the burden of proof—who bears it and what sustains it. A problem of suffering for Pellegrino is that it "makes rational thought difficult" (1992:97), which may be true but implies that those who are in pain are not to be trusted in their wishes.

These phrases delimit what arguments are admissible in euthanasia decisions. The key terms are *logic*, *proof*, and *rationality*. Pellegrino argues, correctly in my view, that "the medical profession is a moral community" (1992:99), but the morality he seems to propose for this community is a cool, procedural one. Nor do Pellegrino's own answers add up either, at least on my reading. He claims that one of the most negative effects of euthanasia would be to "reinforce this objectification of death and dying, and further desensitize [physicians] to killing" (1992:99). But what is objectification other than reducing the individual physician's response to her patient's suffering to matters of proof, logic, and rationality?

As we will see below, when caregivers write of being with the dying, they do not present their responses as an "argument" subject to these formal considerations. Pellegrino, whatever informs his personal practice and experience, does not write his prescriptive ethics from a position at the bedside, and that is the whole issue.

Pellegrino hardly devalues the communication between physician and patient. He writes that "physicians must work out with each patient that patient's definition of a good death, and determine—before a crisis comes on—what life-support measures will and will not be acceptable to the patient" (1992:101).[4] But for Pellegrino the resolution of these discussions depends on his belief in the power of technology. "There are many reasons for the request to be killed," Pellegrino states, "and *many remedies* once we know the reason" (1992:101; emphasis added). Here is a perfect example of systems media—technological remedies in this case—pushing out lifeworld, communicative consensus. Pellegrino begins with communication between persons, doctor and patient, but what will ultimately be done to the patient hinges not on what the patient or even the primary-care physician wants, but on what remedies can be provided. The communication between the dying person and her physician is not the basis of a *mutual* understanding; instead the physician reduces the patient's speech to a set of demands to be remedied.

Pellegrino's statement about remedies introduces his discussion of pain control, its current inconsistency, and the need for higher medical standards.[5] But pain, even when "controlled," is not suffering. Blendon et al. (1992:2660) report that only 20 percent of respondents anticipate pain as a possible reason for requesting euthanasia, compared to 47 percent who fear burdening their families. "Remedies" only go so far. The ideal of a multiprofessional team "mobiliz[ing] the forces necessary to remove or ameliorate these causes" (Pellegrino 1992:101) is noble rhetoric, but it *is* rhetoric. The world presupposed is one where expertise can mobilize forces to effect any remedy. This ideal should hardly be dismissed, but neither should any ideal be confused with reality. Too much suffering cannot be remedied, and too many remedies are unavailable to too many people. But the language of principle is concerned with sustaining ideals, not coping with people and their situations.

Probably the most disturbing aspect of the language of principle is its willingness to make decisions for others, particularly decisions about their suffering. Pellegrino certainly realizes that remedies will not remove all suffering, and so his rock-bottom argument has to be the nobility of this suffering. The passage is worth quoting in full.

> We can justify euthanasia for our pets precisely because they cannot possibly understand suffering or dying. They cannot die in a "human" way. But humans can grow morally even with negative experiences. A good death contributes something valuable to the whole human *community*. It enables us to assess our human relationships and to come to grips with the important and ultimate questions of human destiny, which believers and nonbelievers alike must confront. A good death is the last act of a drama, which euthanasia artificially terminates before the drama is really completed. (1992:97)

Pellegrino does not bear the weight of this argument alone; Daniel Callahan (1992:55) writes much the same thing: "It is not medicine's place to lift from us the burden of that suffering which turns on the meaning we assign to the decay of the body and its eventual death."[6]

The irony of this language is that Pellegrino's "good death" is precisely what pro-euthanasia advocates also seek. Their argument is that artificial termination is necessary to provide that good death.[7] Pro-euthanasia advocates would describe actual deathbed scenes—the delirium, incontinence, and agony—and ask how these could possibly be understood as what anyone would want for the "last act" of the drama of his life.[8] The language of principle eschews such description, or any description of actual deaths.

Callahan and Pellegrino both suggest that medicine has no right to intervene in the course of dying, but both omit noting that dying and its attendant sufferings have been constructed by medicine and medicalized circumstances long before an actual request for euthanasia is considered. Medicine has *already constructed the meaning we assign to our bodies and their decay,*[9] medicine not just as practiced in hospitals and doctors' offices but as adjunct to corporations and governments, as fronting the pharmacology industry, as depicted in popular culture and "health promotion," and as sponsor to a constant self-surveillance of our bodies and lives.[10]

As important as recognition of this political economy of medical knowledge is, the moral argument about suffering may be more significant. I agree with Callahan and Pellegrino that suffering gives meaning to life; my contention with them is how people discover this meaning. Pellegrino (1992:97) quotes Miguel de Unamuno: "Suffering is the substance of life and the root of our personality. Only suffering makes us persons." Before applying this statement to euthanasia decisions, we must remember that Unamuno wrote as a philosopher reflecting on the human condition in general. His ideas are a theoretical resource, the specific meaning of which readers are left to discover in moments of their own lives. When we are suffering, Unamuno's words may come back to us, and as we realize their relevance to our own present moment, we may experience that suffering differently and respond differently to it. But his words do not *prescribe* that meaning or response; they only *provide for* their discovery.

This same issue of discovering moral meaning for oneself applies to Pellegrino's observation that "the lives of many of the handicapped, the retarded, and the aged teach us much about courage and personal growth" (1992:97). I certainly agree, but these lives are not lived for our edification; again, living in suffering cannot be prescribed. If people choose to live and die in ways that teach us about suffering, then we should be grateful. But this gratitude hardly implies we can dictate their choices for our benefit or, more presumptuous still, for their own good.

This chapter will certainly not resolve the issue of what a "good death" can be. Pellegrino describes the ideal as well as possible, and our species will always have the challenge of putting that description into practice. The language of principle would prescribe at least the "outer limits" of that practice. I now turn to the language of experience, which trusts individuals to choose the practice of their own deaths.

The Language of Experience

The language of experience speaks not in logical arguments but in narratives of dying (see, for example, DuBose and Wolters 1991; Seguin 1994; Shavelson 1995). These narratives no longer refer to "the dying" or "the terminally ill" but to Steve, Michael, Martha, and Ron. Writers express a relationship to the dying person—my mother, my grand-father—and the sense of this relationship pervades the story. "Patients" are no longer some ideal type; instead, physicians write of their care for persons with names, families, and particular fears and wishes (see Quill 1991, 1993).

The emphasis is not on physicians as members of a profession but on caregivers who can include physicians but are more usually family caregivers. The relation of caregiver to ill person is a fully embodied one, as described by the physician Marcia Angell: "Most of us know someone who took on the back-breaking and soul-destroying job of caring at home for a spouse or patient with Alzheimer's disease. This means round-the-clock attendance, including diapering, feeding and bathing. When the patient is put in an institution (where the care is often indifferent at best), the family must 'spend down' to qualify for Medicaid."[11] Here is Callahan's "decay of the body" in its embodied reality. Callahan is technically correct: the meaning we assign to this bodily decay is a meaning we assign, but this statement is mere tautology when confronted with the "back-breaking and soul-destroying job" of care. Can anyone tell those doing this care that the meaning of their work is what they assign to it? Can we tell an elderly person in the early stages of Alzheimer's that he will "grow morally" by having his adult child change his diapers?

The language of experience is thus about people living with suffering that they, unlike the professional, cannot go home from; home is the scene of the suffering. Realities like incontinence might be details beneath notice to the language of principle, but to the language of experience these details are what life consists of. The details of the body are what dying is about, and the toll that care for one body takes on another is the reality for families.

The language of experience recognizes that this situation was set in place by medicine. Angell expresses this clearly: "Our [physicians'] ability to extend life through new technologies will certainly grow, and with it will grow the dilemmas created by the extension of intractable suffering" (1988:1350). To return to Pellegrino's metaphor, medicine has already extended the drama; does it not have some responsibility for the ending?[12]

Finally, the language of experience recognizes the limits of medical care. Harriet Goetz, a nurse, writes, "But there are some terminal patients whose suffering goes beyond anything the medical profession can alleviate" (1989:619). Allow one case to illustrate this statement. The inquiry of the British Medical Association in describing the condition of Lilian Boyes (who was given a lethal injection by her physician, Nigel Cox) called her pain "constant and unmanageable" (Dyer and Mihill 1992:25).[13] Can we who are now healthy imagine the lived reality expressed in those words? But this reality of pain is what principles are supposed to address.

What do we *not* find in the language of experience? No promises of future technologies, no abstractions about the possible meaning of categories of experience—in short, no deferral of response to suffering. The situations described go on for long periods before voluntary death is contemplated, but there is no deferral of responsibility to an authority that is insulated from the embodied experience of the people involved. Instead of questioning the ability of those involved to make rational choices, we find trust in the capacity of people to make decisions for themselves and to respond to the needs and wishes of others. Of course these decisions will involve mistakes, self-recrimination, and constant "what if" questions, but so will action based on principle. Error is endemic to care in moments of crisis, but if the context of care is defined by relationships of respect and, wherever possible, love, and if care is not constrained by bureaucratic intervention, these errors will not be perceived and remembered as sources of recrimination.

What marks the language of experience is precisely the communicative consensus that Habermas associates with the lifeworld. Barbara Brack's narrative of her mother's voluntary death gives an eloquent illustration of Habermas's theory: "After watching her [own] mind deteriorate slowly over five years, and after ten months of prayerful discernment and planning, my mother quietly and with great dignity and grace ended her life. She had my support and the help of a compassionate physician who prescribed sleeping pills for her. For over 40 years my mother was my closest confidante, guide and friend. To help her die was the only thing she ever asked of me. I sought guidance in prayer and from Christian friends before agreeing to help her" (1991:1055).[14] Here, surely, is the wise judgment of the person on the spot.

My obvious bias in favor of the language of experience is not as total as it might appear. It is, rather, a situational bias. Brack's description displays a strong orientation to principles, but to principles the outer limits of which *are* negotiable. The theoretical rationale for a bias toward such local negotiation of principle is Habermas's argument that the lifeworld is, at present, the colonized discourse. We do not make decisions about euthanasia in a historical vacuum but in particular circumstances where the balance of lifeworld and system is always, to some extent, in need of correction.

Euthanasia as a Response to the Colonization of Dying

The rhetoric of the euthanasia debate recapitulates the situation the dying find themselves in, that is, the colonization of experience by administrative principle. What people fear in hospitals is being treated as they are written about in the language of principle: as "cases" whose personal sufferings are subordinated to other needs to sustain a certain rationality of professional practice.

As I suggested above, the issue of appropriate medical pain control is only part—albeit an important part—of a much larger problem of the medical response to suffering. Medicine, as an industry, is increasingly perceived as incapable of responding to individual particularities of suffering. Medicine has become, in Habermas's terms, a system, colonizing the lifeworld of the ill and dying.

Technological advances have centralized medical treatment in tertiary-care facilities, and increased costs have proliferated medical bureaucracies. "Medicine" is no longer the physician making house calls but an industry driven by functional, administrative imperatives. Richard McCormick is one of the few anti-euthanasia writers to perceive that the problem of responding to demands for euthanasia goes far beyond pain control. Like Pellegrino, McCormick believes medicine should be a moral community, but he is less optimistic about attaining this ideal.

By "secularization" I mean the divorce of the profession of medicine from a moral tradition. Negatively, this refers to the fact that medicine is increasingly independent of the values that make health care a human service. Positively, it refers to the profession's growing preoccupation with factors that are peripheral to and distract from care (insurance premiums, business atmosphere, competition, accountability structures, government controls, questions of liability and so on).

Quite practically, the secularization of the medical profession means that it is reduced to a business and physicians begin acting like businesspeople . . . in the marketplace. (1991:1133)

If Habermas's lifeworld is evoked by Brack's "months of prayerful discernment and planning" leading to her mother's death, McCormick's "marketplace" of medicine describes what Habermas calls the system. At present, this system is colonizing the lifeworld: Brack, her mother, and their physician must act surreptitiously, as Timothy Quill had to do when he treated Diane. The wise judgment of the person on the spot is suspect, restricted, ensnared.

In the euthanasia debate the languages of principle and experience seem to speak past each other, neither able to attend to the other's discourse. Habermas's theory would lead us to expect this impasse and understand it as one symptom of a larger social crisis. Social theory does not hold out any immediate solutions for "overlapping consensus." Habermas's point is that the conditions of consensus formation have been deformed by colonization. So long as system colonizes lifeworld, then neither in euthanasia debates specifically, nor in medical ethics more generally, will consensus be recovered. In medicine as elsewhere, a crisis of legitimacy will weaken the link between experience and authority.

If we take Habermas seriously, the colonization of the lifeworld by systems will not be reversed in this generation. But in this period of colonization, some responses to suffering can effect provisional reversals of system dominance. Where possible, the language of experience, emanating from the lifeworld, can be honored and nurtured. Consensus about these responses can only be local, which in this instance means at the bedside, because only in this lifeworld context do the communicative conditions for consensus formation remain.

Of course the person on the spot cannot act without principles. The issue between the languages of principle and experience will never be either/or, but rather which language is now foreground and which is background. Euthanasia decisions cannot be made without principles, and ethicists like Kass, Pellegrino, and Callahan make valuable contributions. But the principles they advance must constantly be held accountable to the experiential narratives of people with real names, in real relationships, suffering both in their bodies and in the dramas of their lives.

Postscript: A Final Narrative

Essays like this one are not written in a vacuum, either. My call for ethics to follow a language of experience would be disingenuous if I did not add something of the context in which I write. Right now, here in Canada, headlines feature a forty-two-year-old woman, Sue Rodriguez, who is petitioning the courts to allow her a physician-assisted death. Ms. Rodriguez has advanced amyotrophic lateral sclerosis, and she wants to be able to decide when to die before she loses the power to speak, then to swallow, and finally to breathe.

By the time this is published, Sue Rodriguez will almost certainly be dead, assisted or not.[15] Perhaps another case will capture the headlines. But as I write, Sue Rodriguez is not a case; she is a woman whose testimony I have read, whom I have seen on television, with whom I share a mutual friend, and whose picture sits on my desk, making me ask if I am writing anything that I could not say directly to her, at any stage of her decline. Sue is a living person, acting out the drama of her life in public statements that lend meaning to many other lives.

My own answers on the extent to which euthanasia, or assisted suicide, should be legalized don't add up; legalization as a response implies
a recourse to system over lifeworld. But the following news report carries a demand that cuts through the theoretical ambivalences: "After listening for two days to legal arguments concerning how she should die,
Sue Rodriguez said she felt weary, frustrated and resentful that others
could interfere in her death" (Matas 1992). No one should have to
spend her last days listening to others debate how she ought to die.

NOTES

I would like to express my appreciation to my colleague Marja Verhoef and to John
Hofsess, editor of *Last Rights*, for providing many of the articles and books quoted
in this paper.

1. The sources of this discursive turn include the later philosophy of
   Wittgenstein, the French philosopher Michel Foucault, the German philosopher Jürgen Habermas, North American and British "conversation analysis,"
   the feminist conceptualization of "voice" as a political category, and the growing interdisciplinary importance of "cultural studies." Probably the greatest
   single effect of poststructuralism and postmodernism in social science has
   been the turn toward investigating both social life and science as discursive
   constructions.

2. Habermas's (1987b) primary empirical example of system colonization of the
   lifeworld is "juridification," or how a sense of justice, grounded in lifeworld
   moral consensus, is replaced by administrative fiats of procedural law. The
   legitimacy of this law rests on lifeworld justice, but law substitutes its own
   abstract criteria in place of community morality, thus undermining its own
   legitimacy. The example can be readily transposed to the common observation
   that more complex medical edifices do little to improve our health. *Health* is
   increasingly defined in administrative terms—for purposes of insurance, com-
   pensation, and employment—and the lifeworld sense of bodily fitness for
   meaningful tasks is reduced to these terms and thus colonized.

3. As one example of such a lay attack on medical ethics, see Derek Humphry's
   Dying with Dignity (1992:63–65). Humphry's popular appeal should warn medical ethics scholars that something is going wrong.

4. The practical problem with this excellent statement is whether the conditions
   of the contemporary hospital allow the physician who participated in the original discussion to retain effective control of the dying person's treatment.
   Dubler and Nimmons (1992) describe the hospital ethicist's frequent difficulty
   as a staff member trying to determine who a patient's primary physician is.
   Miles (1990) describes a dying patient being moved from her nursing home,

where her nonaggressive treatment preferences were known, to a hospital where she was subjected to aggressive intervention. An anonymous author describes her mother's move from a hospice where her pain was under control to a hospital where the doctors "admitted they knew little or nothing of the drugs given to her by the hospice team" ("Pain That Passes" 1992). Frank (1992a) describes a case where physicians had left their dying patient in the care of a junior nurse, with advance directives that proved inadequate to cover the contingencies that followed. Of course, Pellegrino might reply that these are problems of institutional organization and should not prejudice *reasons* for and against euthanasia, but this kind of separation of issues is exactly what the language of experience refuses. For the persons affected, the analytical separation hardly counts.

5. One contribution of the euthanasia debate has been increasing recognition of the need for better pain control. In her plenary presentation at the Ninth International Conference on the Care of the Terminally Ill (Montreal, 1992), Dr. Margaret Somerville argued that inadequate pain control should be grounds for malpractice suits, and this in the Canadian medical system that values a far more restrictive approach to malpractice than in the United States. Her proposal received warm applause from the 1,200 international delegates. Examples of inadequate pain control are the Achilles' heel of anti-euthanasia arguments, and most ethicists include proposals for higher standards in pain control.

6. Pellegrino's and Callahan's arguments bear haunting similarity to nineteenth-century opposition to the use of anesthetic in childbirth, on the grounds that God intended Eve's daughters to suffer; see Lebacqz 1991.

7. This argument is best stated by Ronald Dworkin (1993), whose work goes further than any in bridging the languages of principle and experience. For an extended discussion of Dworkin, see Frank 1994.

8. For one very powerful description, see "Pain That Passes All Understanding" (1992), in which a woman describes her mother's death, "contorting in agony, at times so bad she nearly jerked out of bed."

9. For an overview of how medicine constructs our knowledge and perception of the body, see Freund and McGuire 1991. A more theoretical discussion is found in Turner 1987.

10. Such self-surveillance includes diet and body weight, cholesterol levels, blood pressure, and the recent growth industry related to "stress." Computer-chip technology makes home-monitoring devices cheaper and more pervasive, and self-help expands beyond groups and books into audio and video cassettes. Thus "medicine" defines health and its commodification as self-surveillance far beyond those activities in which physicians are directly involved.

11. This quote was taken from a newspaper editorial titled "Don't Criticize Doctor Death." The editorial was distributed with a packet of reading materials at a 1992 conference on euthanasia, and I have not been able to track down a complete citation.

12. Barbara Brack (1991:1055) expresses this medical responsibility in her narrative of her mother's voluntary death: "Suicide is also frowned upon because it seems to be playing God or flouting the sovereign will of God. But so does all of medical science. Every vaccination of a baby interrupts the natural course of events."

13. Despite what the press described as "huge doses of heroin," Boyes was in such pain that she could not be touched. The British Medical Association did not revoke Dr. Cox's license, although its finding reiterated its stance against legalizing euthanasia: physicians acting as Dr. Cox did must "be prepared to justify their actions in court and before their peers" (quoted in Dyer and Mihill 1992). In his testimony Dr. Cox made a point of presenting his actions not as a test case for euthanasia but rather as his only possible response in an extreme case. But as Goetz (1989), Angell (1988), and others write, the situation is extreme but not unusual.

14. Brack goes on to point out that if euthanasia had been legal, her mother could have delayed her death longer and would not have had to die alone, so as to avoid legal liabilities for others.

15. Early in 1994 Rodriguez died, assisted by an anonymous physician and attended by a member of parliament, Svend Robinson. Robinson was investigated by police but not charged. Little attempt was made to find out the identity of the physician. Those who might explain Rodriguez's desire to die as her engagement in a political cause should consider the story of Kelly Niles, a person with very different disabilities and commitments, as told by Shavelson (1995:105–57).

REFERENCES

Angell, Marcia. 1988. "Euthanasia." *New England Journal of Medicine* 319 (17 November): 1348–50.

Bernstein, Basil. 1970. "Social Class, Language and Socialization." In *Language in Social Context*, ed. P. G. Giglioni, 157–78. Middlesex, England: Penguin.

Blendon, Robert J., Ulrike S. Szalay, and Richard A. Knox. 1992. "Should Physicians Aid Their Patients in Dying?" *Journal of the American Medical Association* 267, no. 19 (20 May): 2658–62.

Brack, Barbara. 1991. "Rational Suicide: My Mother's Story." *Christian Century*, 13 November, 1054–55.

Callahan, Daniel. 1992. "When Self-Determination Runs Amok." *Hastings Center Report* 22 (March–April): 52–55.

Carson, Rob. 1992. "Washington's I-119." *Hastings Center Report* 22 (March–April): 7–9.

Dubler, Nancy, and David Nimmons. 1992. *Ethics on Call.* New York: Harmony Books.

DuBose, Edwin R., and Margaret Wolters. 1991. "Personal Narratives." In *Choosing Death: Active Euthanasia, Religion, and the Public Debate*, ed. Ron P. Hamel, 1–13. Philadelphia: Trinity Press International.

Dworkin, Ronald. 1993. *Life's Dominion: An Argument about Abortion, Euthanasia, and Individual Freedom.* New York: Knopf.

Dyer, Claire, and Chris Mihill. 1992. "Mercy for Doctor Who Killed." *Guardian Weekly,* 29 November, 25.

Frank, Arthur W. 1989. "Habermas's Interactionism: The Micro-Macro Link to Politics." *Symbolic Interaction* 12, no. 2: 353–60.

———. 1991. "For a Sociology of the Body: An Analytical Review." In *The Body: Social Process and Cultural Theory,* ed. M. Featherstone, M. Hepworth, and B. S. Turner, 36–102. London: Sage.

———. 1992a. "Not in Pain, but Still Suffering." *Christian Century,* 7 October, 860–62.

———. 1992b. "Only by Daylight: Habermas's Postmodern Modernism." *Theory, Culture and Society* 9, no. 3: 149–65.

———. 1994. "Is Compromise Possible? Medical and Philosophical Views on Euthanasia." *Journal of Palliative Care* 10, no. 4: 35–39.

Freund, Peter E. S., and Meredith B. McGuire. 1991. *Health, Illness, and the Social Body.* Englewood Cliffs, N.J.: Prentice Hall.

Goetz, Harriet. 1989. "Euthanasia: A Bedside View." *Christian Century,* 21–28 June, 619–22.

Habermas, Jürgen. 1987a. *The Philosophical Discourse of Modernity.* Cambridge, Mass.: MIT Press.

———. 1987b. *The Theory of Communicative Action.* Vol. 2, *Lifeworld and System: A Critique of Functionalist Reason.* Boston: Beacon Press.

Humphry, Derek. 1992. *Dying with Dignity.* New York: Birch Lane Press.

Kass, Leon R. 1991. "Why Doctors Must Not Kill." *Commonweal,* 9 August, 472–76.

Kelner, M. J., and I. L. Bourgeault. 1992. "Competing Images of Dying: Patients and Health Care Professionals." Paper presented at the Images of Aging Conference, Trent University, May 1992.

Lebacqz, Karen. 1991. "Reflection." In *Choosing Death: Active Euthanasia, Religion, and the Public Debate,* ed. Ron P. Hamel, 114–17. Philadelphia: Trinity Press International.

McCormick, Richard A. 1991. "Physician-Assisted Suicide: Flight from Compassion." *Christian Century,* 4 December, 1132–34.

Matas, Robert. 1992. "Rodriguez Tires of Arguments about How She Should Die." *Toronto Globe and Mail,* 19 December, A9.

Miles, Steven H. 1990. "The Case: A Story Found and Lost." *Second Opinion* 15 (November): 55–59.

"Pain That Passes All Understanding." 1992. *Guardian Weekly,* 29 November, 25.

Pellegrino, Edmund D. 1992. "Doctors Must Not Kill." *Journal of Clinical Ethics* 3, no. 2: 95–102.

Quill, Timothy. 1991. "Death and Dignity—A Case of Individualized Decision Making." *New England Journal of Medicine* 324 (7 March): 691–94.

———. 1993. *Death and Dignity: Making Choices and Taking Charge.* New York: Norton.

Seguin, Marilynne. 1994. *A Gentle Death*. Toronto: Key Porter.

Shavelson, Lonny. 1995. *A Chosen Death: The Dying Confront Assisted Suicide*. New York: Simon and Schuster.

Siegler, Mark, and Carlos F. Gomez. 1992. "U.S. Consensus on Euthanasia?" *Lancet* 339 (9 May): 1164–65.

Turner, Bryan S. 1987. *Medical Power and Social Knowledge*. London: Sage.

CHAPTER 5

Moral and Religious Reservations about Euthanasia

William F. May

Two groups in Western medical ethics dominate the current debate on the question of euthanasia. In their extreme forms, "pro-lifers" tend to see death as the absolute evil; "quality-of-lifers" define suffering as the absolute evil.

I cannot wholly side with either extreme party in the debate. My values have been shaped by the biblical tradition, and my reluctance derives from theological grounds. The Judeo-Christian tradition recognizes that neither life nor wealth of life is an absolute good; they are creaturely goods, fundamental goods, derived from God, not God himself. Further, neither death nor suffering is an absolute evil, that is, powerful enough to deprive human beings of that which is absolutely good. Therefore, the goods and ills we know in life are finally creaturely and relative—we are free to enjoy goods but not irrevocably desolate at their loss; we are commissioned to resist evil, but not as though this resistance alone provides our final meaning and resource.

This position would not inevitably establish in ethics a unique set of guidelines. It would not always call for its own distinctive path of action, but it would open up a somewhat brighter sky under which to act—a sky cleared of the despair of those who believe that except for life, there is only death, or except for quality of life, there is nothing but the final humiliation of poverty. We should not view the moral life as a grim struggle of life against death or quality of life against poverty. Neither should our political life disintegrate into a fierce conflict between pro-lifers and quality-of-lifers, each heaping epithets on the other, each charging the other with moral blindness. Both absolutistic positions are ultimately too shrill to control their advocates' own excesses: one group clamors for life at all cost; the other proclaims, give me quality of life or give me (or them) death.

A less rigid theological perspective suggests that decisions should vary in different cases, sometimes to relieve suffering, at other times to resist death. But in any event, decisions should not spring from the fear and despair that often create the absolutist in ethics.

(I do not want to argue that only a theist can hold to this perspective on ethics. Supporters of a variety of other religious and secular positions might also criticize the absolutist commitments of the pro-lifers and the quality-of-lifers. I have simply attempted to acknowledge the theological source of my own reservations about the two movements.)

In the debates over public policy, a theist ought not, in my judgment, side with either party in its extreme form. The first group would define the medical profession wholly by a fight against death. Yet physicians should be free to respond to patients' requests to cease and desist in the struggle to prolong life when treatment can no longer serve the health of the host. Maximal treatment is not always optimal care. Sometimes it makes sense not only to withhold but to withdraw treatment. A physician does not always have the duty to fight pneumonia if such death has become acceptable to the patient in preference to imminent death by irreversible cancer. To be sure, the commandment states, "Thou shalt not kill," but there is, after all, a time to live and a time to die, and a fitting time for allowing someone to die.

Nonetheless, I cannot side with the opposite extreme. Neither physicians nor our society at large ought to prize so highly the quality of life that we try to end suffering by eliminating the sufferer. Advocates of euthanasia seek to relieve the evil of suffering by shortening the interval between life and death, by hastening death.

The impulse behind the movement for euthanasia is understandable in an age when dying has become such a protracted, inhumanly endless business at the hands of people committed to the first extreme. But euthanasia goes beyond the middle course of the right to die and insists upon the right to be killed. It solves the problem of a runaway technological medicine with a final resort to technique. It opposes the horrors of a purely technical death by using technique to eliminate the victim. It insufficiently honors the human capacity to cope with life once terminal pain and suffering have appeared. It tends to doubt that dying itself can be suffused with the human.

I am in favor of policies that accommodate the terminally ill patient who requests to be allowed to die, but I have serious reservations about policies that establish routines and protocols for mercy killing.

Some would argue that the distinction between allowing to die and mercy killing is hypocritical quibbling over technique; they would collapse the distinction. Since the patient dies—whether by acts of omission or commission—what matters the route the patient took there? By either procedure he ends up dead. Medical advances have made dying at the hands of the experts and their machines a prolonged and painful business; why not move beyond the patient's right to die to the right to be killed?

Ethicist John Fletcher has called the distinction between allowing to die and euthanasia a "worn-out" distinction. He argues that it is arbitrary and misleading. Have we not held to the distinction partly because fatal *actions* seem worse than fatal *omissions?* But each of us can think of exceptions to that rule. Some actions that lead to death can be acceptable. For example, large doses of morphine to relieve severe pain may be quite appropriate even though they may also hasten death. In contrast, some omissions that lead to death would be very serious wrongs—for example, deliberately failing to treat an ordinary bacterial pneumonia in a patient who, with treatment, could recover and live productively.

The existence of exceptional cases that cross the boundary we use to distinguish one category from another does not of itself argue against respecting a line between the two. A particular fifteen-year-old may be more mature than the average seventeen-year-old, but that does not of itself invalidate setting some threshold, usually age sixteen, for a driver's license. On a given piece of land, one may not see where one passes from the United States into Canada; nevertheless, substantial reasons may exist for drawing territorial boundary lines, even in the absence of such obvious markers as a lake, a river, or a mountain range. Upon such fine lines civilized life often depends.

But where, in grave medical issues, should we draw the line? Is the boundary between allowing to die and euthanasia the right place?

Two of the five major arguments for euthanasia surface in the terms *voluntary euthanasia* and *mercy killing*. Supporters of euthanasia believe that, first, respect for the patient's autonomy and, second, compassion for the sufferer should figure foremost in the care of the dying. By not providing the option of euthanasia, we fail to respect the liberty of those who want the doctor's assistance in bringing their lives to an end. In a country that values freedom, individual liberty ought to extend to the choice of one's final exit. Since the patient who consents to being killed or asks assistance in suicide presumably harms no other person, a legal prohibition against assisted suicide or euthanasia seems unjustified and arbitrary. Further, in prohibiting euthanasia we do not act as compassionately as we might; we impose gratuitous suffering on the terminally ill.

Patients in severe pain, chronic or terminal, or individuals contemplating the prospect of such a condition offer a third argument: they do not want "to be a burden to others." This argument, in effect, once again appeals to the value of liberty and to the moral importance of compassion. But the roles of the players reverse. In this case, the patient wants to exit life out of compassion for the caregivers— to relieve them of the terrible burdens of giving care and the daily limitations upon their liberty. Since, moreover, awareness that she is a burden compounds the patient's own suffering, euthanasia or assisted suicide appeals doubly as an act of mercy: the act mercifully provides caregivers relief from their burdens and the care receiver relief from being a burden.

The fourth and the fifth arguments for euthanasia surface not in the terms themselves but in the rhetoric and literature. The fourth rests on the conviction that dying is a private, personal, intimate event, at most, a matter for the patient in relation to his or her family, friends, and physician. The public has no business or interest that justifies regulating or interfering in this private event.

The fifth argument, which overlaps with the insistence upon the patient's autonomy, reflects the general fear of losing control over one's life, control which a "how to" book on killing oneself or arranging assistance in suicide seems to reinstate. This last argument reflects a very American aspiration, which the numerous self-help books lining the shelves of drugstores, bookstores, and libraries seek to exploit. As a people we prize independence and abhor dependency and loss of control. Why not then a book that reasserts total control over life, even over the last gasp of suffering, letting us design our own death? Furthermore, opening up the option of euthanasia might also help to restore a sense of control to physicians who have seen their powers reach an intractable limit in the patient beyond the reach of their remedies.

Opponents of policies that would establish the option of euthanasia have grounds for skepticism about each of these five arguments.

Patient Autonomy

First, behind the emphasis on the voluntariness of the act lies what ethicist Richard McCormick has called the "absolutization of autonomy" (McCormick 1991:1132). A libertarian insistence on the unconditional right of self-determination (except for those actions that would limit the freedom of others or harm them without their consent) would, carried to its logical extreme, lift prohibitions not only against consensual acts of killing, such as voluntary euthanasia and assisted suicide, but also against dueling. It would also provide no grounds for prohibiting slavery, should the enslaved person consent to his or her own degradation.

Not all libertarians would push to that extreme, but they do tend to honor men and women simply as individuals and neglect the doubleness of human existence. We are individuals, to be sure, but we are also parts of a whole. The whole, the society, has an interest in us, not simply when we harm others but when we harm ourselves, an interest which grows in proportion to the magnitude of the harm. As Daniel Callahan wryly has observed, "Consenting adult killing, like consenting adult slavery or degradation, is a strange route to human dignity" (Callahan 1992:52).

Further, the notion of voluntary euthanasia—viewed as an expansion of the patient's right to determine his or her own destiny—may harbor an extremely naive view of the uncoerced nature of the decision. The plea to be killed is hardly a free decision if the terms and conditions under which we deliver care for the dying are already woefully mistargeted, inadequate, or downright neglectful. When elderly patients have stumbled around in apartments, alone and frightened for decades, when they have spent years warehoused in geriatrics barracks, when they have not been visited by relatives for months or when relatives dump them off in emergency rooms to be rid of them for a holiday, then the decision to be killed for mercy hardly reflects an uncoerced decision. Their alternative may be so wretched, repellent, and disgusting as to push some patients toward this resolution of their plight.

Compassion for the Sufferer

It is a huge irony and, in some cases, hypocrisy, to talk suddenly about a compassionate killing, when the aged and dying may have been starved for compassion for many of their declining years. To put it bluntly, a country has not earned in good conscience the moral option to kill for mercy if it has not already sustained and supported life with compassion and mercy. Euthanasia could be a "final solution" for handling the problem of the abandoned. (We have some 37 million Americans without health care insurance, the only industrialized country other than South Africa that so neglects a major portion of its citizens in the provision of acute care. We have another 37 million people underinsured. The possibility of euthanasia provides too many people with an offer they might feel, given the alternative, that they cannot refuse.)

The test of compassion lies not in the investment of yet more money in acute-care facilities (we already spend too much of the health care dollar on acute-care facilities), but rather in the shift of substantial amounts to preventive medicine, rehabilitative medicine, chronic care, terminal care, and strategic home services, which provide patients with a humane alternative to a quick death. Otherwise we kill for compassion only to reduce the demands on our compassion. My point here is not to question the motives of any doctor or family members who may feel that they have reached the limit of their resources. Lacking adequate provision for chronic care and home assistance, we nudge toward the exit not only the solitary, neglected patient but also the patient who watches his overburdened family struggle to give him care without respite. The test of compassion is not simply the individual case but the cumulative impact of a social policy.

Admittedly, this argument is partly culture-specific. One can imagine societies that provide adequately for the stricken and the elderly and also provide legal permission for euthanasia in those instances when a person may opt out of that care. But one hesitates to make legal provision for a form of care that provides simply a convenient final solution for a society's general carelessness. While at the level of policy this argument is culture-specific, it is not relativist at the level of moral principle. It argues that we owe care always. Most of the time care takes the form of treatment. At some point, treatment becomes futile, but, while we cease to treat, we do not cease to care. That is the moral principle behind allowing to die.

Allowing to die, as I conceded at the outset, is also subject to abuse. No line-drawing solves any and all problems. But, at least, abuses of passive euthanasia clearly indicate the underlying principle that justifies allowing to die, that is, the principle of care.

Continued prohibitions against euthanasia should be accompanied by full and proper use of allowing to die. The tests of the patient's welfare and her rights of self-determination should apply not only to withholding treatment but also to withdrawing it, not only to starting the machines but also to stopping them, not only to the use of extraordinary means but also to the employment of ordinary means. A too-narrow definition of allowing to die can lead to inappropriate treatment and patient abuse.

Furthermore, a prohibition against euthanasia carries with it an even more intense responsibility to make sure that no patient, especially those who are being allowed to die, should be abandoned. As efforts to treat cease, efforts to care for, make comfortable, and console must intensify. Joanne Lynn, the distinguished geriatrician and hospice physician who served on the President's Commission for the Study of Ethical Problems in Medicine and Biomedical and Behavioral Research, wrote a fine appendix for the commission's report, *Deciding to Forego Life-Sustaining Treatment*. Her essay fully details that care which our obsession with spectacular medicine has tempted us to neglect: the effective use of drugs to control pain, even though the drugs may hasten death; the adroit management of various symptoms—gastrointestinal, respiratory, and agonal; treatments for skin problems, fever, and weakness; and aids to mental function. These prosaic tasks, which high-tech medicine has tended to dismiss as hand-holding, are, in fact, an integral part of high-quality care.

Medical research and education have not fully focused on the pressing needs of the dying. As Dr. Lynn has complained, "it is easier to get a heart transplant or cataract surgery than supper or a back rub" (*New York Times*, 14 February 1993). Dr. Kevorkian may engage in overtreating his drop-in patients with assisted suicide because he has attracted those who have been undertreated for depression. Apparently the zealous missionary never bothered to have the first nine of his patients psychiatrically evaluated before he helped them die. A 1991 editorial in the *New England Journal of Medicine* noted that 90 percent of suicides among the thirty thousand suicides a year suffer from depression. "One study of 45 terminally ill patients showed that only three patients considered suicide, and when they were examined psychiatrically, it was discovered that they suffered from major clinical depression" (*New York Times*, 14 February 1993). We generally underevaluate and thus mistreat the dying. In a survey reported in a *New York Times* editorial (25 January 1993), some 81 percent of doctors conceded that "the most common form of narcotic abuse in the care of the dying is the undertreatment of pain." Only one in ten physicians, according to a 1989 study conducted by Dr. Jamie H. Von Roenn of Northwestern University, "said they received good training in managing pain" (McCormick 1991:1133). Only one-fifth of 1 percent of the billion-dollar budget of the National Cancer Institute goes to research on the reduction of pain. Instead of caring appropriately for the dying, the euthanasia movement tempts us to swing smoothly from aggressive treatment to keep alive to equally aggressive treatment to kill.

Compassion for the Caregiver

Patients, especially aging patients, offer a third argument for euthanasia (less an argument than an expressed wish): they do not want to end up a burden to others. At first glance, this argument seems far removed from the underlying individualism of those who argue for euthanasia on the basis of the patient's autonomy. It reflects the moral sense that we are not merely individuals but parts of a larger whole. We do not want to impose on others. Far from making an imperial claim to autonomy, the person so disposed insists only on her freedom to make a decision that she deems to be for the benefit of others.

Without denying the self-sacrificial character of such a patient's sentiment or action, one might question whether the total moral setting that gives rise to it actually reflects the sense that we are parts of a whole. I am truly and fully a part of a community not only when I am willing to make sacrifices for others but also when I am willing to accept their sacrifices for me. Community is a two-way street of giving and receiving, not giving alone. In some circumstances and stages of life, we are primarily givers; at other times we should not be too proud to be receivers. At its healthiest, community depends upon interdependence, upon a reciprocity of giving and receiving.

The desperate plight of the chronically dependent patient who seeks death in order to relieve her caregivers reflects the failure of our society to support caregivers or provide them with adequate respite from their labors. Our lack of social supports for home care and long-term care reveals a harshly atomistic health care system. It demands from the unlucky a level of sacrifice that only the most saintly could sustain. While we may admire the unselfish responses of the disabled or the dying who would spare members of their immediate circle from heroic sacrifices, we must doubt the moral commitment of a nation that would allow individuals and families to be pushed to these extremes.

The Privacy of Death

The fourth argument defines dying as an intimate, private, at most familial act, one that is therefore not properly subject to public regulation and scrutiny. This argument overlooks the public element in all of human life from birth to death. Birth is our first caterwauling public appearance; and death, our final exit from the public scene.

A society cannot plausibly wash its hands of the practice of euthanasia and say that the doctor's cooperation in killing is a purely private matter. A huge public investment supports the training of doctors and places medical resources at their disposal. Further, the very nature of the decision to euthanize perforce implicates the society in the deed. Daniel Callahan has analyzed the public dimension of the decision as follows: "If doctors, once sanctioned to carry out euthanasia, are to be themselves responsible moral agents—not simply hired hands with lethal injections at the ready—then they must have their own *independent* moral grounds to kill those who request such services" (Callahan 1992:52). Simple appeal to the patient's declaration that he suffers unbearably does not supply independent grounds. Doctors experienced with the complexities of euthanasia in Holland concede that "there is no objective way of measuring or judging the claims of patients that their suffering is unbearable. . . . Three people can have the same condition but only one will find the suffering unbearable" (Callahan 1992:53). The judgment reflects not simply the medical condition but the values of the patient. In effect, then, the doctor will be treating the values of the patient, not simply the disease. A doctor could not responsibly accede to the request unless she shared the values. Inevitably, this transaction pushes the decision out into the public arena. "Euthanasia is not a private matter of self-determination. It is an act that requires two people to make it possible, and a complicit society to make it permissible and acceptable" (Callahan 1992:53).

Further, the denial of the public significance of dying intensifies the problem of the slippery slope, the thin edge of the wedge, or the camel's nose under the tent (pick your own metaphor). Advocates of euthanasia argue that they have protected against the slippery slope. In the Netherlands, for example, the law requires that the patient's condition be irreversible and terminal, with death imminent. The patient should also authorize his or her being killed by explicitly granting consent. The act should be performed only by doctors, and it requires the authorizing signature of at least two doctors. These various regulations protect against bizarre whims, malice, or the neglect of third parties. Similar protections have been incorporated into proposed legislation here and elsewhere.

Yet, despite Holland's many regulations governing euthanasia, including the prohibition of *involuntary* euthanasia, the Dutch Governmental Committee on Euthanasia reported in September 1991 that, out of 130,000 deaths in the Netherlands over a year, nearly 6,000, or 4.6 percent of all deaths, were cases of involuntary euthanasia. (This figure includes not simply the 1,000 explicitly identified and reported cases of involuntary euthanasia but also the 4,941 cases in which doctors report giving morphine not simply to relieve pain but for the express purpose of terminating life.) Further, "in 45 percent of the cases in which the lives of hospital patients were terminated without their consent, this was done without the knowledge of the families" (Fenigsen 1991:343). Of the 4,941 cases of morphine overdoses given with the intent to kill, 27 percent were done without the knowledge and consent of a fully competent patient. Sixty percent of practitioners failed to consult another physician before killing without patient consent, and these doctors, "with a single exception, never stated the truth in the death certificates" (Fenigsen 1991:343). Physicians also flouted the rules governing *voluntary* euthanasia: 19 percent of physicians disregarded the rule to consult another physician; 54 percent failed to record the proceedings in writing; and 72 percent concealed the fact that patients died by voluntary euthanasia (Fenigsen 1991:343).

The tendency of practice to slip from the moorings originally supplied by Dutch regulations may follow from the appeal to the intimacy and privacy of the act of dying. To insist that dying is a private act places it, in principle, beyond public regulation and control. In his foreword to Carlos Gomez's *Regulating Death: Euthanasia and the Case of the Netherlands*, Leon Kass explores the difficulty of setting public standards for personal decisions:

> how can one insist that euthanasia is and ought to be a private choice, best handled privately between patient and doctor, and yet expect there to be appropriate oversight, public accountability, and control? Must we, can we, should we, rely solely on the virtue of the medical profession—and each of its unregulated medical practitioners—to protect the exposed and vulnerable lives of the infirm, the elderly, and the powerless, who, incapable of real autonomy, will be deemed by others to have lives no longer worth living or, more likely, no longer worth sustaining at great medical expense? (Gomez 1991:x)

Gomez rejects the idea of euthanasia as a strictly personal decision, basing his argument on the public nature of medicine itself: "To suggest that what transpires between a physician and a patient, even at the hour of the patient's death, is an entirely private matter is, however, to overlook the public institutional quality of the profession of medicine. . . . For all its necessarily private and intimate aspects, . . . [medicine is] necessarily a *public* enterprise. . . . The claim to a right to death at the hands of a physician is essentially a private claim to a public good" (Gomez 1991:134).

The slippery slope that concerns me is not the one conventionally feared: a lethal slide like that from the early Nazi practice of euthanasia to Hitler's genocide. The chief danger we face is not the demonic, totalitarian, political ideology but rather marketplace seduction. We need fear less the dictator who makes us do what we do not want to do

(George Orwell's *1984*) than the seducer who stirs our desires to do what we ought not do (Aldous Huxley's *Brave New World*). We are probably less vulnerable to the bark of the dictator's command than to the sweet talk of money, which tells us we have better uses for our money than to make Grandpa's life bearable. "If the Netherlands—with its generous [health care] coverage—has problems controlling euthanasia," Gomez says, "it takes little effort to imagine what would happen in the United States" with a population dedicated to its own quality of life (1991:138).

Now why should we be so concerned about the slippery slope? One of the original justifications for euthanasia is control of one's own dying. But the crossing of the boundary from voluntary to involuntary euthanasia means the loss of control over one's dying. It means putting to death someone against her will or without her will. The bottom of the slope contradicts the justifying ideal at the top of the slope.

Controlling Our Lives

The fifth argument for euthanasia reflects the American obsession with solving problems through technical mastery and a corresponding fear and sense of resourcelessness before the uncontrollable. So obsessed, we seek to solve the problem of diminishing control over our lives by controlling the exit.

No response to this argument can dismiss technical problem solving as an important moral task in life. But many of the problems confronting patients and their families do not admit of a technical solution. They must be faced rather than solved. The lack of a solution to a problem, however, does not automatically condemn us to resourcelessness before it. We sometimes assume, to our impoverishment, that we have only two options: controlling our lives or submitting passively to them.

Unfortunately, narrowing our moral lives to the options of control and passivity overlooks an important range of human responses—particularly to events like death that are tinged with the sacred. Sacred occasions or holy days are set apart from other days. They are the days in which the ordinary canons of mastery and control do not work. Theologian Karl Barth once distinguished work days from holidays in the sense that on work days we make things happen, while on holidays we let things happen. Letting things happen is not a state of mere passivity. By "taking in" the sacred occasion—the puberty rite, the marriage, the public gathering, the day of atonement, the Good Friday service—we let the occasion, in a sense, do the work, as it defines us.

Serious illness and death often resemble the holiday and other defining moments in life that call for decorous response rather than control. The wife of a college president once said to me, "I could do nothing about the death of my husband. The chief question I faced was whether I could rise to the occasion." With one stroke, his death altered the very terms of her daily life and intimacy and transformed her from a person with a clear-cut public role in the college to a supernumerary. How could she rise to an occasion that redefined every moment of her daily life?

It is not only the bereaved who may need to rise to the occasion but we ourselves in the course of our own dying. The community needs its aged and dependent, its ill and its dying, and the virtues they sometimes evince—humility, courage, and patience—just as much as it needs the virtues of justice, courage, and compassion in the agents of its care.

We might plausibly read the movement on behalf of euthanasia as a religious recoil against all the medical busyness and officiousness with which we have surrounded death—all the tests and protocols and contingency plans and codes and charts and tubes. While seeking in our busyness to save a life or delay the dying, we sense that we have profaned the person dying. We have refused to open ourselves to what is happening by frantically making things happen. But, ironically, the euthanasia movement seeks to halt all these furious efforts at control by one more assertion of control. The last word is control, not a breakthrough to another level of human existence and meaning beyond the urgencies of control. This last consideration does not of itself justify the prohibition of the practice of euthanasia, but it suggests the existence of some responses to death that may make the prohibition justified on other grounds a little more tolerable.

Taking the arguments cumulatively and on the whole, I am in favor of a social policy that would permit the practice of allowing to die, rather than killing for mercy, that is, a policy that would recognize the moment in illness when it is no longer meaningful to take every action to cure or to prolong life, when it is fitting to allow patients to do their own dying, with gentle assistance in the management of pain. This policy seems most consonant with the obligations of the community to care and the patient to rise to the occasion.

I can, to be sure, imagine rare circumstances in which I hope I would have the courage to kill for mercy—when the patient is terminally ill, utterly beyond human care, and in excruciating pain. I cannot forget the picture a neurosurgeon once showed me of a Vietnam casualty who had lost all four limbs in a land-mine explosion. The catastrophe had reduced this person to a trunk; his face was transfixed in horror. On the battlefield, I hope I would have the courage to cross the boundary and kill the sufferer with mercy. But hard cases do not always make good laws or wise social policies. Regularized mercy killings would too quickly relieve the community of its obligation to provide good care.

Further, we should not always expect the law to provide us with full protection and coverage for what, in rare circumstances, we may need morally to do. Sometimes, the moral life calls us out into a no-man's-land where we cannot expect total security and protection under the law. But who ever said that the moral life was easy?

REFERENCES

Callahan, Daniel. 1992. "When Self-Determination Runs Amok." *Hastings Center Report* 22, no. 2 (March–April): 52–55.

Fenigsen, Richard. 1991. "The Report of the Dutch Governmental Committee on Euthanasia." *Issues in Law and Medicine* 7, no. 3: 339–44.

Gomez, Carlos. 1991. *Regulating Death: Euthanasia and the Case of the Netherlands.* Foreword by Leon Kass. New York: Free Press.

Lynn, Joanne. 1983. Appendix B to *Deciding to Forego Life-Sustaining Treatment.* Report of the President's Commission for the Study of Ethical Problems in Medicine and Biomedical and Behavioral Research. Washington, D.C.: U.S. Government Printing Office.

McCormick, Richard A. 1991. "Physician-Assisted Suicide: Flight from Compassion." *Christian Century* 108 (4 December): 1132–34.

CHAPTER 6

Physician Assistance at the End of Life: Rethinking the Bright Line

Christine K. Cassel

Many central controversies in bioethics are characterized by clearly articulated views argued systematically by the different sides, with little or no expectation that these arguments will change anyone's mind. The arguments seem rather to be contributions to those on each side of the debate, whatever it is, to enlarge and strengthen their own already-held views. Academic delight is taken not so much in the rightness or wrongness of one's position as in the complexity, originality, or craft of the arguments. This process is grounded in the artfulness of deductive arguments, where the essence of debate centers on which of competing principles takes precedence. Although this is an exaggerated portrayal of principle-based ethics, it nevertheless is true that oversimplification in arguments from rules has limited the exploration of many issues.

Physician-assisted dying is one of them. Physician-assisted suicide differs from most bioethics issues in important and instructive ways. A few prominent spokespersons who strongly oppose or favor the practice have outlined the extreme positions. Those most firmly opposed agree that assisting a patient to die goes against the very core of the principled profession of medicine; those strongly in favor argue the patient's right to relief of suffering, especially when no cure is possible. But most health professionals and bioethicists do not adhere to either of these strong and principled positions. In informal discussions, they admit to a deep ambivalence or uncertainty. They will acknowledge the value of one or both principled positions but quickly point to exceptions, often drawn from personal experience with actual cases. This degree of uncertainty is unusual, and it suggests either a shift in fundamental values or limits to the conventional philosophical approaches to end-of-life concerns. The issue of assisted suicide, therefore, is very much in evolution; policies, arguments, and even values are in the process of formation. In the face of so much uncertainty, most thinkers welcome a chance for extensive thoughtful exploration.

I will invoke a medical custom and tell a case of a patient—so that we place this discussion in the human context where so much ambivalence arises, and so that we have specifics in mind as we think about these important but abstract rules and value conflicts. This issue and the debate that surrounds it are indeed characterized by a gap between the rules orientation and the experiential narrative. It thus can be seen in terms of the structural debate that has emerged in ethics theory over the past decade between an ethics based on principles and rules applied to individual situations as opposed to an ethics that arises from detailed descriptions of individual situations (or "cases"), where values are understood as profoundly relative to the cultural and interpersonal context of the case. Putting a human face on the patient asking for help in dying allows a more accurate consideration of these theoretical frameworks in understanding physician-assisted suicide.

This is a true story of a man who died of AIDS; in discussing his case with medical groups I usually describe him as a physician. Imagine this middle-aged man who has been infected with the HIV virus for ten years and who is now nearing the end of his long, heroic struggle. Though he was able to maintain a full, active life for the first eight years of his illness, the last two years have been dominated by a series of losses—many infections, hospitalizations, unemployment, and progressive loss of strength and vitality. Once athletic, independent, and highly creative, he is now physically wasted and incapable of caring even for his own bodily functions. A viral infection has taken his sight, and his memory is beginning to fail. His most overwhelming fear has always been of the dementia associated with the end stage of AIDS. He has helped to care for several friends who died of this disease. He has seen bad deaths in spite of excellent hospice care. He feels physically and spiritually exhausted by this fight and sees no purpose in living out its final chapter. He is not religious in a traditional sense, but he has a clear sense of spirituality related to human dignity and compassion. His fight so far has embraced enough human interaction to compensate for the profound losses, but for him the future promises only further degradation and loss. The only relief he can see is death. He has thought deeply about his options and has reached an acceptance of his own dying. His view of the future is realistic and not distorted by depression. He is not in pain. His physical symptoms include profound weakness, chronic nausea, incontinence, and confusion. Every medical approach to these problems exacerbates his confusion. He pleads with his doctor to give him a lethal dose of medication to help him die with what little dignity remains, before he loses the competence to have his request taken seriously and to carry it out himself.

This case is not bizarre or unusual. To the contrary, it has elements that are common and basic to the moral debate about physician-assisted dying. These elements include the undeniable prognosis of terminal illness, the competence of the patient, the clarity of his own context of personal meaning, and the unambiguous nature of the request to the physician. Cases like this engender the greatest ambivalence among those opposed to physician-assisted dying, and the clearest certainty among those who support a moral role for physicians, however rare it may be, in assisted dying. For this reason it is a starkly instructive narrative.

Care of the Dying Patient

We have made a good deal of progress in respecting the values of patients in treatment toward the end of their lives. This progress should not be minimized. It is now clear to almost everyone that competent patients have a right to refuse life-sustaining interventions and even to exert control over the future through advance directives like living wills and durable powers of attorney, although appropriate interpretation and documentation remain barriers to their effectiveness. We have also made progress in the clinical standards of comfort care. Comfort care, also called palliative care, is the aggressive care of people who are dying, aimed toward making them comfortable rather than extending their lives. Clinicians now are less troubled by senseless worry about using addictive drugs to treat people who are dying and suffering from pain. Major efforts in education and setting of clinical guidelines have reinforced the principles of patient-controlled analgesia, regular rather than "as needed" dosing, and use of easier-to-take oral formulations of long-acting narcotics. We also worry less about the so-called double effect—that what we do to bring patients comfort may in some way hasten their deaths—although it is possible that recent controversies about a physician's role in assisted dying may have revived fears of legal reprisals if pain treatment or other symptom control seems to hasten death.

We still have a lot of work to do, however, and that's part of what this physician suffering from advanced AIDS fears. He has witnessed inadequate palliative care and suffering that might have been prevented. Especially in tertiary-care hospitals, for some reason, dying with dignity becomes harder to achieve. This has to do with deep-seated attitudes of health care professionals as well as institutional structures and behaviors. Many physicians are not very knowledgeable about palliative care, and medical education clearly needs to do better in that area. One argument against allowing physicians actively to help patients die is that caring for the dying patient this way is too easy. It could be an easier way of dealing with a difficult situation, particularly for inexperienced or technically focused doctors who are uncomfortable in engaging with dying patients. They would avoid learning what they need to learn in order to confront their own mortality and the profound aspects of the experience of being with a dying person, to really engage the meaning of that experience, to be with their patients during the dying process—not just write lethal prescriptions. Some ethicists fear that if we are too quick to allow assisted suicide we won't force doctors to try every effort to relieve suffering first.

Thus the argument goes that maintaining a "bright line" over which physicians should not step in causing death will allow—perhaps even encourage—physicians to be more aggressive in providing comfort care to dying patients, because they will not fear being confronted with a request to cause death. It is possible, however, that this logic works in the opposite direction. It is possible that drawing the bright line as we have and particularly highlighting it in the context of the current public debate has made physicians even more fearful about the potential double effect. Many of us have heard a doctor express concern about being "accused of euthanasia" in situations where aggressive (and appropriate) comfort care may also lead to the shortening of life. Indeed, it seems that in many teaching hospitals aggressive comfort care is not being offered. Confusion about where the bright line is located and fear of legal or moral transgression are barriers to good comfort care, and such fear and confusion are widespread among physicians. This may explain why people are so afraid that they will not be treated with compassion and dignity in their dying days but rather will be "hooked up to machines" or allowed to suffer pain needlessly. If the profession were to acknowledge that this line is not so bright and that there is indeed a significant gray area, and if the profession were to reinforce the physician's responsibility to ensure the patient's comfort and dignity rather than to avoid rigidly any treatment that might *appear* to be euthanasia, a more positive approach might be taken to the care of dying patients.

Death with Dignity and the Limits of Comfort Care

Still, it is true that in the best of situations, for most people who are dying and who have access to good medical care, thoughtful and competent comfort care *can* make the dying process gentle and free of physical suffering. But dignity is harder to achieve. *Dignity* and *meaning* are unfamiliar terms in medical parlance, terms rarely used in medical discussions about euthanasia. Experts argue that if we just treat the pain correctly the person will not want to die, and therefore more adequate pain treatment will eliminate the demand for physician-assisted dying, and with it the complex ethical and policy problems. There is, however, no evidence that all physical suffering associated with terminal illness can be relieved. Most symptoms of dying are not well understood. They are often protean, and their causes difficult to diagnose. Pain is only one of them, and it alone can have many sources and require complex approaches. But there are also many other symptoms: nausea, shortness of breath, urinary and bowel incontinence, episodic and sometimes terrifying delirium and hallucinations (sometimes coming from the disease itself, sometimes coming from the medications used to treat it), and immobility. As described in our case history, these kinds of symptoms cannot always be effectively treated by medication. In some cases, as with shortness of breath, the appropriate treatment—morphine, the most effective known agent to relieve air hunger—inevitably hastens death because it lessens the drive for breathing. So while there is both an art and a science to symptom control, it is unlikely that we can abolish all these symptoms, short of abolishing consciousness (Doyle et al. 1993). Some have in fact proposed as an alternative to assisted dying that we offer a permanent state of general anesthesia until death occurs from dehydration. This would avoid the direct involvement by physicians in helping people die. But who really is benefiting from such a choice? The profession of medicine, some would argue. No one could successfully argue that this is best for the patient.

But even if we could effectively treat the physical suffering of dying, we must remember that suffering is not merely physical. This is all too often neglected in the medical literature. Many of these symptoms threaten personhood itself or the dignity of the person. They cause fear of the loss of that dignity, of the loss of the self; they cause fear of a loss of meaning, a kind of descent into absurdity and degradation. That is what the patient in our case history worries about. He does not want to die in anesthetic coma or AIDS dementia because he recognizes that death *can be* a profound and meaningful part of life. This meaning is something too often forgotten in modern medical settings. Death has meanings that are personal and universal. It is importantly mysterious, and it is something that, in a way, defines our humanity. If we try to deny or avoid it, we lose a central part of what it means to be human. Unfortunately, modern ways of dying, especially in hospitals, have made it harder to recognize and capture that meaning. The social historian Philippe Ariès describes the way in which modern medicine has fragmented death so that personal meanings are difficult or impossible to recognize or achieve. "The process of dying has been so cut up into different segments, and the process of trying to keep someone alive so often goes on so long that when you look back in retrospect, it's not even clear when the person actually died" (Ariès 1974). In this context it does not seem eccentric or selfish for a dying person to want to have some control over how he or she leaves this world. It seems rather to be an understandable reaction of someone seeking meaning, some existential relationship to that most profound event, in a social context that threatens to degrade the event to the purely corporeal and anonymous.

Some religious commentators have claimed that the desire to have control over one's own dying is a peculiarly American phenomenon because suffering and debility are not socially acceptable. They caution us to remember that suffering—especially in the Judeo-Christian tradition—is thought to be ennobling and that one should seek transcendent meanings in the reflective reality of giving up control and allowing God to determine the time and mode of one's own demise. This certainly is one coherent way of thinking about the meaning of dying. For those whose religious beliefs are consistent with these ideas, we can only exhort the medical world to refrain from unnecessarily prolonging the dying process but not to support active intervention. According to the historical context painted by Ariès, however, the foreseen and planned farewell was considered a noble exit during many eras even of Christian history, although active suicide was not necessary because medical treatment was so ineffective. Nevertheless, in a society dedicated to respect for self-determination and tolerance of pluralistic values and religions, it seems that we ought to allow those who do not believe in the Christian ideals of ennobling suffering to choose their own approach to the dignity and meaning of this profound experience. While many of us may believe that suffering and physical humiliation are meaningful life experiences, we cannot prescribe them for those who do not agree with our views.

Public Opinion and Medical Mores

Although it is difficult to assess the accuracy of polls, they repeatedly have shown significant public support for something like physician-assisted dying. The National Opinion Research Center's general social survey has asked this question repeatedly: "When a person has a disease that cannot be cured, do you think doctors should be allowed, by law, to end the patient's life by some painless means if the patient and his family request it?" (NORC 1992). In 1977, 60 percent of those surveyed responded yes, and that number has increased steadily since then. By 1991, 72 percent responded positively. According to a survey conducted by the Harris Association in late 1993, a majority of the public (72 percent) approves even Dr. Jack Kevorkian's notorious and sensational actions in assisting suicides by several people, most of whom did not have terminal illness. One person whom Kevorkian assisted in committing suicide, Janet Adkins, was not terminally ill but was in fact in the early stages of Alzheimer's disease. A *New York Times* survey conducted just after her death asked, "If a person has a disease that ultimately destroys that person's mind or body and the person wants to take his own life, should a doctor be allowed to assist in this?" Fifty-three percent of the respondents said yes. In the 1992 Washington State Initiative 119 the public was asked to vote on a referendum that would make physician-assisted suicide legal in Washington, for at least a three-year period. The Harvard School of Public Health, together with the *Boston Globe*, conducted a national survey prior to the vote and found that 64 percent of those polled approved of physician-assisted dying. Interestingly, the survey also asked whether people thought family members should ever help a person to die; only 42 percent approved of family involvement. Some physicians would argue that helping people die is not the doctor's business; if people want to die they should get someone else, perhaps a family member, to help. Against this is the argument that family members have very complex relationships, one to the other, so that family-assisted suicide raises concern about inappropriate motives. The physician is understood to be professional and therefore more objective.

Somewhat surprisingly in the face of public opinion data, the Washington initiative failed to pass, although narrowly. The California initiative in 1992 also failed in a close vote. In 1994, a public referendum in Oregon was passed that made it legal for physicians to write prescriptions for lethal drugs for patients facing terminal illness. The law stipulates careful scrutiny, accountability, and necessary assessments to ensure optimal treatment of depression and attention to symptom management, which has led hospitals in Oregon to establish palliative care teams to improve the quality of end-of-life care. The new statute is currently under a court injunction after challenges by a "right-to-life" group. Interestingly, many physicians there feel that attention to palliative care has already improved even though the ultimate fate of the law remains in doubt.

The medical profession as such took no public position on the Oregon referendum, although it had opposed both the California and Washington initiatives. Perhaps the most persuasive conclusion to be drawn is that the polls and initiatives indicate a great deal of public interest in, and confusion concerning, the possibilities of physician-assisted suicide. In the medical profession itself, there seems to be an equal amount of confusion and considerable ambivalence but no consensus.[1]

Most medical ethics literature also does not support physician-assisted dying. Writers appeal to the Hippocratic oath: "I will neither give a deadly drug to anyone if asked for it, nor will I make a suggestion to this effect. In purity and in holiness I will guard my life and my art." Yet physicians who say "This is not what we do, this is not healing people" are not addressing the patients' expressed concern. Physicians and ethicists are in some way more concerned with the "purity and holiness" of the profession than with some of the agonizing realities in the care of patients. In a profession whose sole purpose is supposed to be the care of the patient, this distinction seems contradictory. The contradiction can be clarified, however, as a trade-off between principles and cases. Many writers argue that just because there are exceptional cases where many people will agree that assisted suicide would be morally acceptable, *in general* the threat to the integrity of the profession is too great to allow for open acceptance or disclosure of such practices. Many physicians believe they might make a morally permissible exception to the rule in assisting the death of a patient, but they would not want to trust their colleagues, in general, with the same power.

Those who would accept the idea of physician-assisted dying do not deny that the value of life is central to our profession. We value the patient's life explicitly; its quality and preservation are at the heart of this profession. In the face of terminal illness we especially value the quality of life over the prolongation of life for its own sake. There is often a crucial moment when the physician makes that distinction, so this valuing of life is not simply a vitalist devotion to biological life itself but an acknowledgment of the meaning of that life inherent in the person and which we relate to that person. Although less often explicit, we also acknowledge the inevitability of death in some situations, such as the case of our physician with advanced AIDS. Accepting the finitude of human life enhances rather than diminishes respect for life.

Double Effect and the Bright Line

The acceptance of inevitable death undergirds the principle of double effect, which is central to the ethics of end-of-life care and which has become a source of confusion in the current debate. The confusion centers on the question of intention. In the process of providing comfort care for the person who is dying, we accept that an intervention may have two effects. For example, giving morphine to a woman who is dying of lung disease soothes her terrible sense of air hunger, but it also may suppress her breathing, and she may die somewhat sooner because of the treatment. But it would be torture to withhold relief of suffering just so the patient could live a few hours or days longer. As long as the physician does not intend the treatment to cause the patient to die, then "unintentional" hastening of death is acceptable if the treatment is necessary to relieve suffering. Most people accept this—at least theoretically—but fear of "euthanasia" still unduly concerns many physicians.

One clinical scenario in which it becomes harder and harder to distinguish between intending comfort and intending death is exactly this decision to discontinue mechanical ventilation in a conscious patient with end-stage lung disease. When it is clear that the disease is irreversible and the patient or his surrogates have decided that the life-support system is no longer wanted, a morally acceptable decision is made to discontinue the ventilator, knowing that the person cannot live without it. A period of minutes or hours follows during which the patient is in a desperate state of air hunger—a terrible feeling thought to be far worse than most kinds of cancer pain. The physician in this situation should give morphine in combination with other medications to sedate the gasping patient and make him more comfortable. The quieting of the drive to breathe relieves the sense of suffocation but also hastens death. The physician who orders such treatment cannot help knowing that she is causing death in some way (Edwards and Tolle 1992). To say that she intends to make the patient comfortable but does not intend to make the patient die is a rationalization at best. At worst, it is a self-deception that limits the physician's ability to be fully present and caring for the patient and the grieving family.

Consider individuals in a persistent, irreversible state of unconsciousness, such as Nancy Cruzan, for whom surrogates seek to discontinue the artificial nutrition and hydration keeping them alive. The discontinuation of intravenous food and water leads inevitably to death, so it is illogical to say that one's intention is not to make death happen.

Consider an ethics committee hearing the case of a middle-aged woman with metastatic ovarian cancer. The patient was competent but in terrible distress; she had cancer throughout her body, she had open, draining wounds that smelled terrible, and fluid had built up in her abdomen and legs so that she could not move out of bed. When treated with pain medication, she became delirious with frightening hallucinations. She hated her condition, and she requested a lethal overdose from her physician. She was competent. She had said her good-byes and was ready to die. Her attending physician, with the support of the ethics committee, thought it would be best that she be sedated to the state of coma and not be provided artificial nutrition and hydration but be allowed to die. Is this a rationalization (that death is not "intended"), or is it a way of protecting some very important psychological or moral line that we should not cross in medicine? Would it have been so bad simply to have given her a larger dose of morphine to hasten death, especially if this was her last request? Certainly the intention in some fundamental way is the same. Are we really avoiding the *causing* of death? Are we allowing the disease to kill the patient, or are we simply not facing the truth about what we are doing? And is there something cruel in this self-deception? And again, for whose benefit is this decision?

Consider an anthropological report on aging in a primitive society (Albert and Cattell 1994). A 1928 account of a preliterate society in which elderly people were highly regarded and respected relates that when an elder became frail and couldn't keep up with the others, the family would get together and make a decision; the particular case reported concerned an elderly woman whose family decided to "cover her up." They buried her up to the neck in dirt; she couldn't move, and she was left behind to die, but no one "killed" her. She was in a worse state than our patient with ovarian cancer because she was conscious and surely capable of suffering. This may be the same kind of thing we are doing with this double-effect argument. Is this action, "covering her up," morally superior to direct killing? For whose benefit is the distinction? In addition to the moral question, there are also the psychological issues such as the fact that it feels different to cause someone's death rather than to "allow" it. But we should not confuse the avoidance of psychological discomfort with a moral standard.

Many argue that it is necessary to maintain this bright line between allowing to die and causing death in order to alleviate physicians' fear of becoming close to the dying patient, confronting their own mortality, and engaging fully in the comfort care of patients at the end of life. It is possible, however, that this strategy has backfired because the clear distinction between allowing and causing death is seen to be something of a fiction. Every physician in practice knows that there are many situations where the line is gray and extremely hazy. Acknowledging this and accepting a strict proscription against any active involvement in death, the physician is likely to retreat from aggressive care of the dying patient, to hold back on comfort care if it seems to push too close to the edge, and to find a convenient excuse not to confront the painful reality of human mortality. Perhaps if we allow ourselves to acknowledge that discontinuing mechanical ventilation in a patient with end-stage lung disease is in some way recognizing an intention that the patient die *and* that there is nothing morally objectionable in that intention, then physicians will learn to accept that death is not optional and that it is not always a personal failure. Patients too may learn that they do not have to demand miracles from medicine in order to receive caring, compassion, and consideration.

The Slippery Slope

Besides concern for the integrity of the profession and its underlying values, social concerns are also raised as objections to allowing assisted dying. We are cautioned to avoid taking a first step onto a "slippery slope." Opponents argue that if we make assisted suicide legal, abuses will occur, especially in this society where we have so many categories of people who are undervalued. Because we do not have national health insurance, there is risk of undue pressure to reduce the cost of caring for uninsured dying patients by hurrying the process along, not always with their consent. Certainly there would be risks of the abuse of the practice of assisted dying, especially with disadvantaged and undervalued people, but one could argue that this is a reason to enact national health insurance rather than a reason to limit compassionate treatment for people who are dying. It's as if we have to construct moral limits for ourselves because we cannot, in another realm, do something that our country ought to do. We hold dying patients hostage to the moral failing of our society. In fact, many people argue that physicians and the public in Holland accept euthanasia exactly because physicians don't feel pressured by external factors such as lack of insurance. Everyone is insured. This also means that individuals don't feel pressure to ask for euthanasia to protect their families from a huge medical debt. Even if we risk abuses, an open process might be a better way of keeping the profession accountable in preventing abuses compared to what we have now, which is essentially a covert practice. Within the current framework of "allowing to die," the poor and disadvantaged already receive fewer expensive and potentially lifesaving interventions such as coronary artery bypass surgery (Langa and Sussman 1993).

Another argument has it that legalizing assisted dying would lead to a loss of trust in the medical profession because patients would never know whether their doctor might kill them. In the face of critical illness one wants to know that the physician is unequivocally on one's side, beneficently concerned to save one's life. Yet physicians are already losing the trust of those people who do not trust us to care for them at a most important time—when they are dying. If the public felt more confidence in their doctor's ability to care for them and willingness not to abandon them at the end, people might not have bought Derek Humphry's (1992) suicide book at such record rates. If Janet Adkins had had a physician whom she really trusted to let her die when the time came, when her Alzheimer's disease got so bad that she wouldn't want to live, she might not have felt it necessary to take her life prematurely.

Some people argue that legalizing assisted dying might erode the respect for life so fundamental to the medical profession, yet we may find that, within specified and special circumstances, allowing doctors to help a person die may increase our reverence for life, within both our profession and our society. Accepting mortality is something that physicians need to learn. Being with people who are confronting their own deaths is a way of doing that—creating better rituals, talking about death, and exploring the dimensions of its personal meaning might in fact give us a renewed appreciation for the meaning of life and death. The fiction of a bright line between allowing and causing death is probably bolstering our ability to avoid this confrontation with the intrinsic and powerfully meaningful connection between life and death.

Physician Practice and the Law

The reality, of course, is that physician-assisted suicide *is* happening and has probably been happening since the beginning of medicine, even perhaps since the time of Hippocrates. Nobody knows how widespread the practice is because we do not discuss it openly. In response to an article in the *New England Journal of Medicine* (Cassel and Meier 1990), I received one hundred personal letters from doctors who were eager to discuss the matter openly and to tell their own stories. In response to a survey by the American Society of Internal Medicine, 20 percent of respondents acknowledged that they had at least once actively caused a patient's death. Another 20 percent said they would do so under certain circumstances. Some physicians help their patients in this way, thinking it is the right thing to do but feeling that they cannot talk about it with their colleagues (Quill 1993). Even people who think it is not morally correct for doctors to assist in suicide found Quill's account compelling in its description of how deeply he cared for this person who was his patient (Quill 1991). Many physicians also reserve control for themselves in the event of their own confrontation with terminal illness; they expect to use their knowledge to control their own end-of-life decisions, whether or not they provide the same choice to their patients.

Research is needed not just to learn "hypothetical" attitudes but to find out in a scientific way how many physicians are engaged in assisted suicide and what they really think about it. This is difficult research to do, because of the legal issues and because the practice of physician-assisted dying has been very covert. Helping people die is homicide under the law. No gentle language is used in that realm, nor does the law take a relativist approach of respecting differing individual preferences. Many physicians may be sympathetic to requests for assisted suicide, but they are understandably frightened by the serious consequences of the act. It is thus important to consider the legal aspects of this issue rather than to nod glibly to the different worlds of ethics and law, as if they are irrelevant to one another.

It is also important to note that when we review the legal cases in this area, we get a sense that society is saying one thing and doing another. Those who have reviewed all the cases in the United States of physicians or family members who had helped people die in some way or another show that juries and judges will not hold physicians accountable if it is clear they helped the patient die out of compassionate motives (see Gostin 1993).

In cases of consenting terminally ill patients where the doctor knew the patient, there has never been a conviction in the United States. The grand jury has failed to hand down an indictment (which is what happened in the case of Dr. Timothy Quill), the jury has acquitted the physician, or, in a couple of cases where there was not an acquittal, the judge waived the sentence. So here the law says one thing and the human beings, the people who carry out the law, are concluding quite another thing. We have rules on the books, but in practice we don't follow the rules. Some people believe this is good public policy—keep the laws against physician-assisted suicide or euthanasia, and assume that, in those few exceptional cases where it might be justified, the physician will follow his or her conscience and act in the best interests of the patient, even at risk of breaking the law. To most physicians this is not a viable policy; they are likely to avoid the risk of committing a felony even if they believe the action would be best for the patient. It is also difficult to argue that it is sound public policy to maintain a law that is not respected, followed, or enforced. One could argue that this is a kind of social hypocrisy that prevents us from understanding the need for better care of dying patients and that undermines public respect for the law.

I believe there are situations when it is morally acceptable for a physician to help someone die by taking action to hasten death or providing the patient the means to do this. Such situations are few and far between, and if we took better care of dying people, there would be even fewer. Justifiable cases should be rare, but they will never disappear altogether. Whether we as a society should remove the legal proscription against assisted suicide is a much more difficult question. If we were to legalize the practice, I would argue that it should be allowed only in very limited and circumscribed situations (Quill et al. 1992). There should first be maximum symptom control, and there should be a very clear and documented process with diverse professionals involved to make sure that all medical treatment that could relieve the person's suffering has been tried. Most important, the patient must be competent, because the greatest potential for abuse arises when we start making these decisions for other people.

The question about legalization really is, Is it better to maintain a covert practice, relying on the courage of physicians willing to commit an illegal act so that we can maintain the social fiction that we don't assist patients in dying? My guess is that surveys would show that the practice actually has become *less* rather than more common in recent years because of the legal attention and notoriety. Physicians who might have been willing to help one of their patients die ten years ago would be much more nervous about it now because there has been so much attention. In any case, we cannot know as long as the practice is covert. We have no way of better understanding or regulating this practice as long as it is secret. We could instead make it an open but strictly regulated and limited practice; to do so would allow professional and public scrutiny. What we lose is some degree of intimacy and privacy—an important loss—but we gain perhaps in reducing the risk of abuses and in allowing the public and the profession the opportunity for proper assessment and honest discourse about this most important subject.

NOTE

1. Thanks to W. D. White for this insight.

REFERENCES

Albert, S. M., and M. G. Cattell. 1994. *Old Age in Global Perspective: Cross-cultural and Cross-national Views.* Toronto: Maxwell Macmillan Canada.

Ariès, Philippe. 1974. *Western Attitudes toward Death.* Baltimore: Johns Hopkins University Press.

Cassel, C. K., and D. Meier. 1990. "Morals and Moralism in the Debate over Euthanasia and Assisted Suicide." *New England Journal of Medicine* 323, no. 11 (13 September): 750–52.

Doyle D., G. W. C. Hanks, and N. MacDonald. 1993. *Oxford Textbook of Palliative Medicine.* New York: Oxford University Press.

Edwards, M. J., and S. W. Tolle. 1992. "Disconnecting a Ventilator at the Request of a Patient Who Knows He Will Then Die: The Doctor's Anguish." *Annals of Internal Medicine* 117, no. 3 (1 August): 254–56.

Gostin, Lawrence O. 1993. "Drawing a Line between Killing and Letting Die: The Law, and Law Reform, on Medically Assisted Dying." *Journal of Law, Medicine and Ethics* 21, no. 1 (spring): 94–101.

Humphry, Derek. 1992. *Final Exit.* New York: Dell.

Langa, K., and E. Sussman. 1993. "The Effect of Cost-Containment Policies on Rates of Coronary Revascularization in California." *New England Journal of Medicine* 329, no. 24 (9 December): 1784–89.

National Opinion Research Center. 1992. General Social Survey. Chicago: University of Chicago.

Quill, Timothy E. 1991. "Death and Dignity: A Case of Individualized Decision Making." *New England Journal of Medicine* 324, no. 10 (7 March): 691–94.

———. 1993. *Death and Dignity: Making Choices and Taking Charge.* New York: W. W. Norton.

Quill, Timothy E., Christine K. Cassel, and Diane E. Meier. 1992. "Care of the Hopelessly Ill: Proposed Clinical Criteria for Physician-Assisted Suicide." *New England Journal of Medicine* 327, no. 19 (5 November): 1380–84.

PART TWO

Assisted Death in American Society:
Theological Responses

CHAPTER 7

Assisted Death: A Jewish Perspective

Elliot N. Dorff

Killing oneself or others has always been technically possible. It is thus not surprising that the Jewish tradition, like many others, has much to say about those possibilities. Among other things, it delineates a prohibition against murder, a positive obligation of self-defense, and varying penalties for acts of homicide, depending upon the circumstances. In our time, however, the matter has been complicated by our new ability to sustain almost indefinitely people who would otherwise die. Moreover, we can now predict the course of a disease with greater accuracy, and so people have less room for unrealistic hope. That knowledge and the increasing secularization of America have together prompted some people to take their own lives, sometimes asking others to assist them, when they are faced with an incurable disease. That knowledge has also led some individuals to kill a dying spouse or relative to keep their loved one from suffering further. Thus, even though the issues raised by suffering and sickness are age-old ones, the contexts are sufficiently new to warrant a thorough reexamination of the traditional rules and the theological grounding for them. We need either to be reassured that the old directives are still right and proper or to identify reasons and directions for changing them.

This chapter examines aspects of the Jewish tradition relevant to euthanasia. Like other authors in this section, I focus on four theological themes that set the context for the contemporary discussion of euthanasia. Our collective hope is to identify the perspectives and values that give us guidance and yet cause us conflicts as we all grope to find moorings in very murky moral waters.

Freedom and Responsibility

> We hold these truths to be self-evident, that all men are created equal, that they are endowed by their Creator with certain unalienable Rights, that among these are Life, Liberty, and the pursuit of Happiness.—That to secure these rights, Governments are instituted among Men, deriving their just powers from the consent of the governed.
> —United States Declaration of Independence

> See, this day I set before you blessing and curse: blessing, if you obey the commandments of the Lord your God that I enjoin upon you this day; and curse, if you do not obey the commandments of the Lord your God.
> —Deuteronomy 11:26–28

American Jews are the product of two cultures. Nowhere is the contrast between the American and the Jewish cultures stronger than in the issue of authority. Am I, as the Declaration of Independence proclaims, a creature born with inalienable rights, or am I, as Deuteronomy would have it, a person born into a host of obligations? The two are not contradictory, but they certainly present two very different ways of thinking of oneself, ways which have a direct effect on how one thinks of euthanasia.

The clashes between Judaism and American democratic theory appear in several forms.[1] The first concerns the assumptions that I as a human being and a citizen make about myself and others. If rights are the primary reality of my being, the burden of proof rests upon anyone who wants to deprive me of those rights or restrict them. Since other people are born with the same rights, there are times when my rights are legitimately restricted, and there are even times when I have a positive duty to others. In each case, however, the duty arises out of a consideration of the other person's rights. If, on the other hand, the prime fact of my being is that I have obligations, as it is in Judaism, then the burden of proof rests upon me to demonstrate that I have a right against another person as a result of his or her duties to me. My rights exist only to the extent that others have obligations to me, not as an innate characteristic of my being.

The source and purpose of my obligations also divide Judaism from American democracy. It is "We, the people" who create the Constitution of the United States; the government must be "of the people" and "by the people" in Lincoln's words, not just for them. The people institute rules "to secure these rights," as the Declaration of Independence says; American individualism can be set aside by American pragmatism, in this case the practical need to insure that all can enjoy what is theirs by right.

For Judaism, the author of the commandments is God, not the governed. The Bible delineates several reasons to obey God's laws: to avoid divine punishment and to receive divine reward; to fulfill the promises of our ancestors to abide by the Covenant, promises to which we too are subject; to have a special relationship with God, thereby becoming a holy people; and to express our love for God (Dorff 1989). None of these aims, however, is to secure rights. Judaism and American democracy differ completely, then, in the initial assumptions of the legal system (rights or obligations), the source of the law, and its goals.

Moreover, the ways in which a person views the world differ in the two systems of thought. In the one, I owe God; in the other, the world, or, at least, the government, owes me. In Judaism I begin with the assumption that things can be expected of me; in the American system, I begin with the assumption that I have "an unalienable right" to "life, liberty, and the pursuit of happiness," a right which the government is established to secure.

These differences between Jewish and American ideology derive at least in part from disparate basic assumptions about the nature of the individual. American democratic principles were shaped by the Enlightenment, which saw the individual as the fundamental reality. All individuals are independent agents who may or may not choose to associate themselves with others for specific purposes. Religious congregations, for example, are voluntary associations to which individuals belong and from which they may dissociate themselves at any time. That is one manifestation of the enduring individuality of existence in this system of thought, for even when people join groups, they do not lose their primary identity and privileges as individuals. That is why Locke's and Jefferson's rights are "unalienable" by any government. Another corollary of this view is that even if other people happen to belong to a group to which I too belong, what they do is none of my business unless it has a direct effect on me.

This metaphysic stands in stark contrast to the traditional Jewish view that the individual is defined by his or her membership in the group. Membership in the group is not voluntary and cannot be terminated at will; it is a metaphysical fact over which those who are born Jews have no control. This indissoluble linkage between the individual and the group means that each individual is responsible for every other (Maimonides' *Mishneh Torah* [hereafter M.T.], *Laws of Repentance* 3:4; see also Babylonian Talmud [hereafter B.] *Rosh Hashanah* 17a) and that virtually everything that one does is everyone's business. As the Talmud puts it: "Whoever is able to protest against the wrongdoings of his family and fails to do so is punished for the family's wrongdoings. Whoever is able to protest against the wrongdoings of his fellow citizens and does not do so is punished for the wrongdoings of the people of his city.

Whoever is able to protest against the wrongdoings of the world and does not do so is punished for the wrongdoings of the world" (B. *Shabbat* 54b).[2] At the same time, the communal view of traditional Judaism does not swallow up the individual's identity but in fact gives it greater scope by linking it to the larger reality of the group. Milton Konvitz has expressed the resulting viewpoint well:

> The traditional Jew is no detached, rugged individual. Nor is his reality, his essence, completely absorbed in some monstrous collectivity which alone can claim rights and significance. He *is* an individual but one whose essence is determined by the fact that he is a brother, a *fellow Jew*. His prayers are, therefore, communal and not private, integrative and not isolative, holistic and not separative. . . .
> . . . This consciousness does not reduce but rather enhances and accentuates the dignity and power of the individual. Although an integral part of an organic whole, from which he cannot be separated, except at the cost of his moral and spiritual life, let each man say, with Hillel, "If I am here, then everyone is here." (Konvitz 1980:143, 150)[3]

There are also, of course, some important points of convergence between Judaism and American democratic theory. Both systems protect individuals, minorities, and aliens. Both see the individual as a human being first and a member of the society second, thereby limiting the opportunities for political abuse. Both strongly emphasize the rule of law, even over kings and presidents. Both invoke God and human beings, albeit in varying degrees, in shaping the law and in motivating obedience to it (see Dorff 1987).

The case of euthanasia, though, brings into sharp contrast the factors dividing the Jewish from the American traditions. If freedom is emphasized, a person, it seems, should be allowed to request or effect a "mercy killing," at least under the proper circumstances. On the other hand, if responsibility is the core reality in the world—especially one's responsibility to God—then the duty to preserve the body as God's creation seems paramount, even if that entails pain.

Neither the American nor the Jewish system of thought values freedom or responsibility exclusively, but it is precisely the different emphasis that each puts on those values that shifts the burden of proof to opposite parties. In the contemporary American setting of individualism and rights language, those who would deny the freedom to engage in euthanasia must show why, while in the Jewish context the one who wants to justify this form of homicide must demonstrate that it does not violate God's commandments.

Healing and Caring

Judaism's positions on issues in health care generally and on euthanasia in particular stem from two underlying principles—that the body belongs to God and that human beings have both the permission and the obligation to heal.

For Judaism, God owns everything, including our bodies.[4] God loans them to us for the duration of our lives, and they are returned to God when we die. The immediate implication of this principle is that neither men nor women have the right to govern their bodies as they will; since God created our bodies and owns them, God can and does assert the right to restrict the use of our bodies according to the rules articulated in Jewish law. These rules require us to take care of our bodies through proper diet, exercise, sleep, and hygiene[5] and to avoid danger and injury (B. *Shabbat* 32a; B. *Bava Kamma* 15b, 80a, 91b; M.T. *Laws of Murder* 11:4–5; Joseph Karo's *Shulhan Arukh* [hereafter S.A.], *Yoreh De'ah* 116:5 gloss; S.A. *Hoshen Mishpat* 427:8–10). Indeed, Jewish law views endangering one's health as worse than violating any ritual prohibition (B. *Hullin* 10a; S.A. *Orah Hayyim* 173:2; S.A. *Yoreh De'ah* 116:5 gloss); this tenet underlies, for example, contemporary rabbinic rulings that forbid smoking.[6]

Ultimately, human beings do not, according to Judaism, have the right to dispose of their bodies at will, for that would obliterate that which belongs not to them but rather to God.[7] In the laws of most American states, suicide is not prohibited, but abetting a suicide is. It is frankly difficult, though surely not impossible, to construct a persuasive argument that it is in the state's interest to prohibit suicide, especially if the person is not leaving dependents behind. In Judaism the theoretical basis for this prohibition is clear; we do not have the right to destroy what is not ours.

God's ownership of our bodies is also behind our obligation to help other people escape sickness, injury, and death (*Sifra* on Leviticus 19:16; B. *Sanhedrin* 73a; M.T. *Laws of Murder* 1:14; S.A. *Hoshen Mishpat* 426). The obligation does not derive from general humanitarian grounds or from anticipated reciprocity. Similarly, the special duty of physicians to heal the sick is not a function of their oath, an obligation of reciprocity to the society that trained them, or a contractual promise in exchange for payment. It stems from God's commandments, as interpreted by the rabbis, to try to preserve, heal, and protect what belongs to God. Moreover, the fourteenth-century rabbi Nahmanides understands the obligation to care for others through medicine as one of many applications of the Torah's principle, "And you shall love your neighbor as yourself" (Leviticus 19:18).[8]

It is this obligation to help God in restoring health that must be limited in some way if allowing to die is to be permitted, and it must be waived entirely if euthanasia is to be permitted. As we shall see in the sections that follow, classical and contemporary Jewish sources do the former but not the latter.

Healing and caring are not restricted to physical ministrations; they include psychological, emotional, and spiritual support as well. One can be cured and not emotionally healed, as, for example, when a young child suffers a bruise that heals quickly but leaves the child worried about the vulnerability of his or her body. Conversely, physical cure may be impossible, but emotional healing may be available nonetheless as the patient learns to live with the illness for as long as life lasts.

Emotional healing and caring is always an important component in healing the sick, but it takes on special meaning in cases where euthanasia might be contemplated, that is, those where no physical cure is possible. As the *Zohar*, a thirteenth-century work of Jewish mysticism, says, "If a physician cannot give his patient medicine for his body, he should bring it about that medicine [at least] be given him for his soul" (*Zohar* 1:229b).

Embedded in the codes of Jewish law and in the ethos of the Jewish people is God's commandment, as interpreted by the rabbinic tradition, to visit the sick (*biqqur holim*). This, in fact, is one of the ways in which we imitate God: "The Bible teaches that the Holy One visited the sick, as it says [after Abraham circumcised himself and the other males of his household], 'The Lord appeared to him by the terebinths of Mamre' (Genesis 18:1), [and therefore] you too should visit the sick" (B. *Sotah* 14a). Moreover, in a passage included at the very beginning of the morning service each day, the rabbis considered visiting the sick important enough to be numbered among the things for which a person enjoys the fruits of the action in this world (through the boons it creates for both the visitor and the patient) while the principal remains for him in the World to Come (as one of the good deeds that will redound to his benefit in the ultimate judgment of God).[9] One is therefore to visit the sick of all peoples without regard to race, color, or creed (S.A. *Yoreh De'ah* 335:9). These rules apply to every Jew (not just the rabbi, doctor, or nurse); and so at least as early as the fourteenth century and continuing today in many contemporary congregations of all denominations, synagogues have established Biqqur Holim societies, comprising members who have taken it upon themselves to make sure that sick people are visited.[10]

The rabbis, however, were sensitive to the fact that visits could become a burden to the sick as easily as they could be a benefit. They therefore laid down rules for visitors. Unless one is a member of the patient's immediate family or the illness is serious, one should not visit the sick as soon as they fall ill but rather wait until the third day lest they become frightened that the illness is worse than they thought. As a general rule, according to the codes, one should not visit in the early morning hours, when medical staff is likely to be treating the patient, or in the evening hours, when the patient is probably tired, but rather in the late morning or afternoon. One should not make the patient sad by bearing bad news and should not stay too long, making the patient uncomfortable.[11]

Finally, in the spirit of Nel Noddings's book *Caring* (1984), I would like to pose some questions.[12] Do male and female patients need different kinds of emotional caring? Do male and female visitors, as a rule, offer different forms of caring to patients, whether male or female? Put more broadly, are gender issues relevant to emotional caring?

Apart from the contemporary work of Noddings, Carol Gilligan (1982), Deborah Tannen (1990), and many others, there is one hint in the Jewish tradition that gender does affect one's mode of caring and one's need for specific types of care. Traditionally, one's Hebrew name consists of one's first name and then "son of" or "daughter of" one's *father*, for it is the man who represents the family in the community; however, when a prayer is said in the synagogue to ask God to heal an ill person, that person is usually referred to as son or daughter of his or her *mother*. The usual explanation for this custom in the folklore is that when one is ill, one needs the kind of caring that mothers are known to give.[13] While fathers can and should be involved in caring for their sick children just as mothers are, it may be the case that in illness, as in other areas of life, fathers care for their children somewhat differently than mothers do. The traditional practice at least hints in that direction, and it is a direction worth exploring.

The duties to heal and care for others, both physically and spiritually, are clear and important ones within Judaism, devolving upon both individuals and the community as a whole. If we were more successful in fulfilling them, the very temptation to hasten one's own death or that of another would, at least in many cases, no doubt diminish.

Suffering and Dying

Just as healing and curing are not accomplished in physical terms alone, so too the suffering involved in the dying process is not just physical, although that can be considerable in and of itself. It includes feelings of alienation, abandonment, perplexity, vulnerability, and loss of self. Although the words *pain* and *suffering* are colloquially used for both physical and emotional distress, for clarity in what follows I shall use *pain* to designate physical discomfort and *suffering* to mean emotional agony.

Judaism does not value pain. Quite the contrary, it is only on Yom Kippur (the Day of Atonement) and, by extension, the other fast days of the Jewish year that God commands, "afflict yourselves" (Leviticus 23:26–32; Numbers 29:7), traditionally understood to mean through fasting and sexual abstinence. Those, however, are only temporary measures to call attention to the seriousness of the occasion. On all other days, it is actually considered a sin to deny oneself the pleasures that God's law allows. Just as the Nazarite must bring a sin offering after denying himself the permitted delight of wine (Numbers 6:11), so we will be called to account in the World to Come, according to the rabbis, for the ingratitude and haughtiness involved in denying ourselves the pleasures that God has provided.[14] We instead attain holiness by using our body, mind, emotions, and will according to the instruction (*Torah*) that God has graciously and lovingly given us to guide our path in life. Thus bodily pleasures are most appropriately enjoyed when we have the specific intent to enhance thereby our ability to do God's will, as Maimonides explains:

> He who regulates his life in accordance with the laws of medicine
> with the sole motive of maintaining a sound and vigorous physique

and begetting children to do his work and labor for his benefit is not following the right course. A man should aim to maintain physical health and vigor in order that his soul may be upright, in a condition to know God. . . . Whoever throughout his life follows this course will be continually serving God, even while engaged in business and even during cohabitation, because his purpose in all that he does will be to satisfy his needs so as to have a sound body with which to serve God. Even when he sleeps and seeks repose to calm his mind and rest his body so as not to fall sick and be incapacitated from serving God, his sleep is service of the Almighty. (M.T. *Laws of Ethics* 3:3)

The medical implications of this are clear. Jews have the obligation to maintain health not only to care for God's property but also to accomplish their purpose in life, that is, to live a life of holiness. A most important corollary of Judaism's insistence on the divine source of our bodies is its positive attitude toward the body and the prevention of pain.

As people live longer and increasingly die of chronic diseases rather than acute ones, it is becoming ever more evident that the distress involved in dying is more than physical. Patients often are assured that their physical pain will somehow be controlled, but they fear most the abandonment and isolation of death. Franz Rosenzweig, an early-twentieth-century Jewish philosopher who suffered from increasing debilitation for a period of seven years before he died, bases his whole approach to life on the ultimate loneliness with which we face death. For him, all our lives—not just our last days or weeks—are an attempt to overcome this surd fact of human existence, a fact which becomes ever more evident as we near death (Rosenzweig 1970:3–5; Glatzer 1953:179–82).[15] No wonder, then, that the High Holy Day liturgy, in which we confront our sins and God's ultimate decree of "who shall live and who shall die," asks of God, in one of its most poignant moments, "Do not cast us off at the time of our old age; when our powers have failed, do not abandon us."

But it is not only God who, we pray, should not forget us when our health is failing; we need the company of other people as well. Hence the *commandment* to visit the sick, described above, so that the patient should not feel abandoned or forgotten.

The suffering of dying, though, is not only a function of loneliness; it also involves feelings of vulnerability, shame, embarrassment, perplexity (Why is this happening to me? What is going to happen? What should I do now?), anger, worry, frustration, and, ultimately, loss of self as one is alienated from one's community, God, and even one's own disintegrating body. Some of these feelings are unfounded (for example, we should not feel ashamed for what we cannot control), but many are perfectly fitting responses to the distressing elements of the situation, and, in any case, the ultimate fact is that patients often have such feelings, rational or not. When dying, one also tends to see one's whole life in perspective, perhaps for the first time, and that may lead to disturbing questions about its value.

Just as Judaism does not revere pain, it also does not honor suffering. There is a rabbinic doctrine of *yissurim shel ahavah*, "the sufferings of [God's] love," but this is always used to explain ex post facto why the good suffer. It is *not* a statement of the inherent worth of emotional (or physical) distress. Consequently, in cases of assault, Jewish law specifies that, along with payments to repair other aspects of the wound, the assailant must compensate the victim for the embarrassment involved, and the Talmud discusses how the shame of disfigurement stems both from other people's altered perception of the victim and from the victim's own diminished self-perception (B. *Bava Kamma* 86b).

Besides recognizing the suffering of disease, however, Judaism has developed a helpful mechanism to allay at least some of it. The ethical will, an institution that first emerges in full form in the Middle Ages, is a document in which the dying person describes his or her personal history, values, favorite sayings, hopes, and fears. There are no legal requirements surrounding it, and so it can be in any form; contemporary Jews, in fact, often find it easier to talk into a tape recorder rather than write this all out on paper. Ethical wills can be created at any time of life, but when dying people do this, it gives them something important to do each day as they leave a spiritual legacy for their children and other family and friends. In the very process, some of the usual feelings of worthlessness and emptiness that accompany the dying process can be supplanted by a new goal to leave many memories behind.[16]

As we move now to apply these views of pain and suffering to euthanasia and related issues at the end of life, a few definitions will set the stage for the discussion. *Murder* is the malicious taking of another's life without a legal excuse (such as self-defense). *Euthanasia* is a positive act with the intention of taking another's life, but for benign purpose (for example, to relieve the person from agonizing and incurable pain). *Allowing to die* or *forgoing life-sustaining treatment* is a refusal to intervene in the process of a person's natural demise.

Judaism prohibits murder in all circumstances, and it views all forms of euthanasia as the equivalent of murder (M. *Semahot* 1:1–2; M. *Shabbat* 23:5 [151b]; B. *Sanhedrin* 78a; M.T. *Laws of Murder* 2:7; S.A. *Yoreh De'ah* 339:2 and the commentaries of the Shakh and Rama there). That is true even if the patient asks to be killed. Because each person's body belongs to God, the patient does not have the right either to commit suicide or to enlist the aid of others in the act, and anybody who does aid in this plan commits murder. No human being has the right to destroy or even damage God's property.[17]

The patient does have the right, however, to pray to God to permit death to come, for God, unlike human beings, has the right to destroy his own property.[18] Moreover, Judaism does permit allowing to die in specific circumstances, and in our day defining those circumstances is of extreme medical and moral interest in all four branches of American Judaism.[19]

In classical rabbinic literature, death was held to be the consequence of sin, and a sinless person would thus necessarily be immortal.

"There is no death without sin," according to the Talmud. "If a man tells you that had Adam not sinned and eaten of the forbidden tree, he would have lived forever, answer him that that actually happened with Elijah" (B. *Shabbat* 55a; *Leviticus Rabbah* 27:4; see also B. *Shabbat* 55b).

On the other hand, the rabbis sought to minimize people's fear of death by emphasizing that it is a perfectly normal process. On the scriptural words, "There is a time to be born and a time to die" the rabbis say, "From the moment of birth there is always the possibility of death" (*Midrash Kohelet* [Ecclesiastes] on Ecclesiastes 3:2). Moreover, noting that the Bible describes each of the first five days of Creation as "good" and only the sixth day's creations as "very good," the rabbis say that death was one of the things God created on that day to make it very good (Genesis Rabbah 9:5)—a remarkable statement, in light of the rabbis' emphasis on the value of living life to its fullest. Undoubtedly, they had in mind precisely the kinds of cases that lead to serious contemplation of euthanasia, when death is genuinely a blessing.

Death may also be "very good," though, because it makes the purpose of life clear. Striving after material possessions is senseless: "When a person enters the world, his hands are clenched as though to say, 'Everything is mine; I will inherit it all.' When he departs from the world, his hands are open, as though to say, 'I have acquired nothing from the world'" (*Kohelet* [Ecclesiastes] *Rabbah* 5:14; see also M. *Avot* 6:9). Since God's purpose in creating human beings was to afford them an opportunity to glorify the Maker of the universe, life must instead be lived in that light. The biblical phrase "The dead do not praise the Lord" (Psalms 115:17) was used to make that point: "A man should always occupy himself with Torah and the commandments before he dies because at his death he is exempt from Torah and the commandments, and the Holy One, blessed be He, can no longer derive praise from him" (B. *Shabbat* 30a). Therefore the rabbis, with both humor and wisdom, exhorted people, "Repent one day before your death!" (B. *Shabbat* 153a).

Death, then, is not to be welcomed or hurried and is, in fact, the product of sin. At the same time, it is sometimes a blessing, either because it puts life into perspective or because it releases a dying person from great pain. In any case, it should ultimately be a time for rejoicing, as one contemplates the achievements of the life the person lived:

> "Better is the day of death than the day of one's birth" (Ecclesiastes 7:1). When a person is born, all rejoice; when he dies, all weep. But it should not be so. On the contrary, when a person is born, there should not be rejoicing because nobody knows what will be his lot and career, whether righteous or wicked, good or bad. When, on the other hand, he dies, it is an occasion for rejoicing if he departed with a good name and left the world peacefully. Consider the parable of two ships making their way through the ocean, one leaving the harbor and the other entering it. People rejoiced over the ship on its departure, but not over the one which was arriving. A clever man stood there and said to them: "My opinion is the opposite of yours. You should not rejoice over the ship which has set out as nobody knows what lies in store for it, what rough seas and storms it may encounter; but when a ship reaches its harbor, all should rejoice that it arrived in safety." (*Ecclesiastes Rabbah* on Ecclesiastes 7:1)

The Jewish tradition follows the way the rabbis (that is, the Pharisees) interpreted and applied the Bible. One issue that sharply divided the Pharisees from the Sadducees is whether there is a World to Come. The Pharisees insisted not only that there will be resurrection of the dead but that the Torah, which, in truth, knows nothing of that doctrine, proves there is! (M. *Sanhedrin* 10:1).[20] There are varying descriptions among the rabbis concerning what happens in the World to Come. Common elements in every description, though, are the assurance that the righteous will get their just reward and the evil their just punishment at that time (although only the most evil will be punished for more than a year, said Rabbi Akiba, for greater punishment would

be inconsistent with God's mercy), and the righteous will merit study-
ing Torah with God as their teacher.[21]

Although these doctrines are firmly implanted in the Jewish tradition, they are not nearly as central in Judaism as they are in Christianity.
Thus, if devout Christians were asked what is at the core of their faith,
they undoubtedly would answer that Jesus was and is the Christ, and
this response immediately puts one into the context of death and resurrection. If observant Jews are asked the same question, though, they
would probably begin by talking about Torah, God, commandments,
the Jewish people, et cetera, and, if they even thought of Judaism's doctrine of life after death, it would come toward the bottom of the list. As
a result, the attitudes and behavior of the majority of Jews when facing
death are not mollified or influenced in any way by Judaism's faith in a
life after death. A *Los Angeles Times* poll taken in December 1991, for
example, found that 67 percent of Christians and 45 percent of those
with no religious identity believed in life after death, but only 30 percent of Jews said that they did (Maller 1992:5).[22] This, plus Jews' strong
commitment to medical care throughout life, will typically mean that
Jews will have a hard time acquiescing to death, that, indeed, they will
fight it as vigorously as they can, passing from one doctor to the next in
search of a medical cure. In some ways, this is evidence of an admirable
commitment to life, but at some point one needs to prepare for the
inevitable.

Even if a Jew accepts the traditional doctrine of life after death,
that in no way suggests that one should acquiesce to pain or suffering,
let alone prize them; on the contrary, Jewish sources, as we have seen,
strongly affirm the duty to alleviate both pain and suffering. That duty
derives from at least three sources: our obligation to be sympathetic and
compassionate to others; the need to enable people to fulfill the divine
mission of living a life of holiness, a mission they cannot strive to
accomplish if they are racked with pain or suffering; and respect for the
divine image and value implanted in every human being, making each

of us worthy of a life free of such torment. Dying is inevitable, and, in some respects, even good, and we may withhold or remove impediments to it when its time has come. It is not to be hastened, though, for euthanasia or suicide would be destruction of God's property and therefore arrogation of God's prerogatives to ourselves; it would also be an ungrateful denial of the divine gift and value of life.

Justice and Mercy

The first Hebrew patriarch, Abraham, addressed the deity as "the Judge of the whole earth" (Genesis 18:25), and the Talmud depicts God that way too. As the creator of the world and of the human species, God holds his creatures to account for the manner of their living. God's judgments are always just. "With Him there is no unrighteousness, nor forgetfulness, nor respect of persons, nor taking of bribes" (M. *Avot* 4:29).

This does not mean that the rabbis were insensitive to the injustice in the world. One of the main reasons they believed in the World to Come, in fact, was that their faith in God's justice and their frank recognition that "the righteous suffer and the wicked prosper" together forced them to conclude that God must reconcile the accounts, as it were, in a World to Come. They also developed other theodicies to explain how a just God could allow apparent injustice to occur, but ultimately they took refuge in God's mystery: like Job, we simply cannot know the ultimate plan of the universe and the place of what seem to us patent injustices in it. With all this, Abraham, Jeremiah, Job, the classical rabbis—and indeed the overwhelming number of Jewish thinkers to this day, even after the Holocaust—complained to and against God but stopped short of denying divine justice.[23]

In biblical and rabbinic literature an eternal conflict is represented as being waged between God's justice and mercy. So, for example, the divine appellation *Elohim*, translated "God," was understood to denote God's aspect of judgment, and God's proper name, JHWH, translated

"Lord," indicated God's aspect of mercy (for example, *Genesis Rabbah* 33:3). The combination of the two names in the verse, "These are the generations of the heaven and earth when they were created, in the day that the Lord God (*JHWH Elohim*) made earth and heaven" (Genesis 2:4) indicates, according to the rabbis, that the world could never have been created in the first place if God had failed to temper justice with mercy:

> It may be likened to a king who had empty vessels. The king said, "If I put hot water into them, they will crack; if I put icy cold water into them, they will contract." What did the king do? He mixed the hot with the cold and poured the mixture into the vessels, and they endured. Similarly said the Holy One, blessed be He, "If I create the world with only the attribute of mercy, sins will multiply beyond all bounds; if I create it only with the attribute of justice, how can the world last? Behold, I will create it with both attributes; would that it might endure!" (*Genesis Rabbah* 12:15)

If mercy was necessary to create the world, how much more so was it required to create human beings, who know good and evil and who have free will: "When the Holy One, blessed be He, came to create the first man, He foresaw that both righteous and wicked would issue from him. He said, 'If I create him, wicked people will issue from him; if I do not create him, how can righteous people spring from him?' What did God do? He deliberately ignored the way of the wicked, allied the attribute of mercy with Himself, and created Adam" (*Genesis Rabbah* 8:4).[24]

Mercy, in the Jewish tradition, is not only being excused in God's judgment from what one deserves under the law. It is also the quality that God uses in giving us the law in the first place. As the daily morning liturgy states:

> Great is your love for us, Lord our God, boundless Your tender compassion. You taught our ancestors life-giving laws. . . . For their

sake graciously teach us, Father, merciful Father, show us mercy; grant us discernment and understanding to study Your Torah, heed its words, teach its precepts, and follow its instruction, lovingly fulfilling all its teachings. Open our eyes to Your Torah, help our hearts cleave to Your commandments. Unite all our thoughts to love and revere You. Then shall we never be brought to shame. Trusting in Your awesome holiness, we will delight in Your deliverance. Bring us safely from the ends of the earth, and lead us in dignity to our holy land.[25]

Note that the prayer states *why* God's law is experienced as an act of mercy: by following it, "we shall never be brought to shame," for we shall know how to live rightly, as even non-Jews may recognize (following Deuteronomy 4:6–8); and, furthermore, by living according to the law, "we will delight in Your deliverance," both because we shall experience firsthand what kind of life God wants us to live and because we shall merit ultimate redemption in messianic times, with its promise to unite all Jews in the holy land. Thus the law is not simply a decree coming from God's power or justice, but the product of God's love and mercy.

Within Judaism, God's attributes of justice and mercy have immediate ramifications for human action, for God serves as the model for us:

"To walk in all His ways" (Deuteronomy 11:22). These are the ways of the Holy One: "gracious and compassionate, patient, abounding in kindness and faithfulness, assuring love for a thousand generations, forgiving iniquity, transgression, and sin, and granting pardon . . ." (Exodus 34:6). This means that just as God is gracious and compassionate, you too must be gracious and compassionate. "The Lord is righteous in all His ways and loving in all His deeds" (Psalm 145:17). As the Holy One is righteous, you too must be righteous. As the Holy One is loving, you too must be loving.

"Follow the Lord your God" (Deuteronomy 13:5). What does this mean? Is it possible for a mortal to follow God's

Presence? The verse means to teach us that we should follow the attributes of the Holy One, praised be He. As He clothes the naked, you should clothe the naked. The Bible teaches that the Holy One visited the sick; you too should visit the sick. The Holy One comforted those who mourned; you too should comfort those who mourn. The Holy One buried the dead; you too should bury the dead.[26]

In our context, this has implications on two levels: the social level, where justice and mercy must combine to provide medical care for everyone; and the individual level, where mercy *may* temper what the law demands.

Many who have written about euthanasia point out that their evaluation might be different if medical care were affordable and available for all. As it is, many who ask to be killed do so because they do not want the financial legacy they hope to leave to their children "squandered" on their own medical care. Others ask to be killed because they do not have the money or insurance to get necessary pain relief in the first place and therefore prefer a quick death to a long, painful one. The lack of affordable health care for everyone thus makes a request for assisted suicide less than a pure moral choice concerning how one wants to die, and so questions about the cost and availability of medical care have a direct bearing on the morality of euthanasia.

Jewish sources on the cost and availability of medical care, of course, come out of a very different historical and social context, but they still can offer at least some guidelines for our present dilemmas. There is great concern that medical services be available to the poor. The sick, in fact, enjoy priority over other indigent persons in their claim to private or public assistance (S.A. *Yoreh De'ah* 249:16; 255:2).

Reliance on the generosity and ethical sensitivity of physicians for the care of the poor was the norm, but there were cases where Jewish communities organized medical care in a form of socialized medicine. In medieval Spain, for example, Jews played a prominent role in the state's program of socialized medicine, and in other places Jewish communities on their own hired surgeons, physicians, nurses, and midwives among their staff of salaried servants (Baron 1948, vol. 2:115, 329). The specific arrangement to fulfill this duty could vary, but both the community and individual doctors were under the obligation to heal.

In our own day these questions no longer concern the poor alone. Most people simply cannot pay for some of the new procedures, no matter how much they borrow. The question of paying for medical care in our society therefore becomes a critical issue, one that thoroughly tests our commitment to both justice and mercy. Justice requires that people get the medical care they need, regardless of their personal financial resources. Beyond that, mercy impels us to provide such care, for, as we learned from Nahmanides above, one must make sure that others have medical care as an expression of loving one's neighbor as oneself. In any case, until some way is devised to make medical care affordable and available for everyone, and until an equitable policy is enacted to determine who gets what kind of care, the case for euthanasia, even at its most cogent, is suspect, for we must question whether, under current limitations on medical care, it is indeed either just or merciful to commit suicide or help someone else die.

What would happen, though, if such social mechanisms were in place? The Jewish tradition, as interpreted by all the contemporary movements in Judaism to this point, would nevertheless forbid euthanasia as a matter of justice. As the Mishnah states: "Rabbi Elazar Hakappar used to say: . . . Against your will (or, perhaps, 'Whether you will it or not') you are formed, against your will you are born, against your will you live, against your will you die, and against your will you must in the future give an accounting and reckoning before the Sovereign of all Sovereigns, the Holy One, blessed be He" (M. *Avot* [Ethics of the Fathers] 4:22). We have God's permission and even God's commandment to engage in health care to cure sickness as long as we can, thereby staying, as it were, the decree of death potentially inherent in every illness; but ultimately our birth, our life, and our death are matters given to God and independent of our will. To commit suicide, or to help someone else do that, would be an act of human hubris, illegitimately taking a prerogative that properly belongs only to God.

The only "wiggle room" in this may arise out of the Jewish commitment to mercy. That, as we have seen, is deeply entrenched in the tradition, rooted as it is in the very character of God. It is also a strong imperative for human beings, who in this respect must model themselves after God.

Several sources offer support for such a reading of the tradition. There are, first of all, the biblical cases of suicide by Saul and Ahithophel (Saul: 1 Samuel 31:3–5; Ahithophel: 2 Samuel 17:23). The Bible tells the story of King Saul's suicide without comment, implying that his was a permitted suicide. The Talmud does not explain why, and later commentators make various suggestions, each of which would theoretically make King Saul's action a different kind of precedent. Ahithophel, on the other hand, is used as the basis for the medieval maxim that "he who commits suicide while of sound mind has no share in the World to Come."[27]

With the case of Saul in the background, however, and with compassion very much in everybody's consciousness, several exceptions to the prohibition against suicide have been gradually built into the law. One is the case of martyrdom. In light of the biblical command to sanctify God's name (reputation), the Talmud established the rule that one must choose to die rather than be forced to commit three offenses—to murder someone else, engage in incest or adultery, or bow down to idols. With regard to any other commandment, however, one must violate the commandment if necessary to save one's life, for the Torah declares that we should live by the laws, which the rabbis took to mean that we should not die by them. After announcing this principle, though, the Talmud goes on to introduce two other factors that can either broaden or narrow the times in which one must give up one's life.

If the action demanded of the Jew is in private and only for the heathen's own pleasure, then the Jew may even bow down to idols to save his life. On the other hand, if the demand is specifically to cause the Jew to violate Jewish law, or if the heathen's demand requires the Jew to transgress Jewish law in public (even if only for the heathen's pleasure), then one should not even change one's shoe strap from white to black (that is, violate even a Jewish custom) but rather choose to die in defense of Judaism.[28]

During the Middle Ages, when Jews were forced to convert to Christianity, some Jews did not wait for the Church authorities or the Christian mobs to torture and kill them if they would not convert but rather took their own lives, "and fathers slaughtered their children with their own hands." Some Jews feared that under torture they might succumb to the Christians' demands to convert, and at least some rabbis permitted such people to murder their children and to commit suicide instead (see Tosafot on B. *Avodah Zarah* 18a, s.v. *v'al y'habel 'tzmo*; Tosafot on B. *Gittin* 57b, s.v. *v'kaftzu*).

According to traditional Jewish law, a person who commits suicide for reasons other than martyrdom either is not to be buried with Jewish mourning rites and in a Jewish cemetery at all, or, according to the more lenient opinion, is to be buried in the usual burial shrouds but outside the Jewish cemetery as a clear mark to the community that suicide is forbidden.[29] There is a medieval source, however, which permits full Jewish burial of such people—although it does *not* give permission to commit suicide in the first place. In light of its leniency, one can understand that its authenticity as a responsum of the respected Rabbenu Asher (the "Rosh," c. 1250–1327) was later questioned, but others supported its authenticity. Genesis 9:5, the verse that prohibits suicide, begins with the limiting word *akh* (usually translated "but"), which Rabbenu Asher interprets to mean that there are situations in which suicide is not punished by denial of proper burial, and he uses the case of Saul as further authority for his position:

For already in *Midrash Rabbah* on the verse, "But (*akh*) for your life-blood, too, I will require a reckoning" (Genesis 9:5), the Midrash says, "You might think that even one in the plight of Saul is meant, [but] the Torah teaches us by the use of the word *akh* that the case of Saul is specifically excluded." And Saul committed suicide only because he was afraid that the Philistines would make sport of him. And do not say that only in his case, where he was fearful that he would be put to great shame, and the Philistines would boast of their defeat of Israel, and there would be a desecration of God's name, does this exception apply. No! In any case of suicide because of a multiplicity of troubles, worries, pain, or utter poverty, there is not the slightest reason to deny mourning rites. Indeed, our Sages denigrated King Zedekiah for not having killed himself rather than see his sons slain before his very eyes. And even Ahithophel, who is counted as one who will not receive a share in the world to come, is so included because he rebelled against King David, and not because he committed suicide. When then is a real case of suicide [such that Jewish burial is appropriately denied]? It is one who is an ingrate and complains even though things are good; who hates the world as do certain of the philosophers who defy the Almighty and rebel against God. But a tormented soul who can no longer endure his troubles, who indeed commits the act in order that he may prevent himself from sinning (for "trouble and poverty cause a man to violate his own conscience and the will of his Creator")—in his case there is not prohibition [to bury].[30]

Whether this text is authentically Rabbenu Asher's opinion or not, in subsequent and in current practice rabbis almost universally have ruled that a person who commits suicide must have been at least temporarily insane to do so. As a result, the person cannot legally be held liable for his or her actions and may therefore be buried within a Jewish cemetery. This does not amount to prospective approval of suicide, but it does retroactively condone it, largely as a final act of mercy for the deceased and for his or her family.[31]

A poignant ruling from the Holocaust combines these earlier sources. On October 27, 1941, all the inhabitants of the ghetto of Kovno anticipated the imminent destruction of the ghetto together with the torture and murder of all its inhabitants. At that time, a man posed a formal legal question to Rabbi Ephraim Oshry, rabbi of the Kovno community, asking whether it was permissible or even desirable to kill himself. In a long responsum in which Rabbi Oshry reviewed all the precedents cited above and more, he ultimately permits suicide

> if the person who kills himself out of fear of affliction and pain is a God-fearing man. In his case, especially, one may judge his intention favorably. Not so, however, in the case of those who have learned from the gentiles and who commit suicide because of trivial matters, and who do not believe in a God who nourishes and sustains all, or in the immortality of the soul. Therefore, in our present case, where certainly he will be horribly tortured as King Saul would have been, it appears that it would be permissible for him to commit suicide.[32]

Nevertheless, Rabbi Oshry did not want his opinion published for fear that it would undermine the commitment to life of the other Jews of the ghetto, and, indeed, other authors took pride in the small number of Eastern European Jews who committed suicide in the midst of the Nazi terror.

In the context of modern medicine's ability to sustain us long after we would have died naturally, then, and in light of what we now know about the inevitability of excruciating death from diseases such as AIDS and some forms of cancer, the mercy required by Jewish tradition may lead some to conclude that suicide in such circumstances should be permitted and perhaps even assisted. I could understand that reading of the Jewish tradition in some cases, and I sympathize enormously with the patients going through such agony; but this interpretation of the tradition remains a barely whispered one within the Jewish community, one which publicly, at any rate, is resoundingly denied. To this point, at least, contemporary Jewish authorities prefer concerted action to provide pain relief and supportive company to those who are dying. That more closely fits the Jewish understanding of both justice and mercy as applied to such cases.

An Imperative to Choose Life

Judaism's respect for life and for medicine is tempered with moral and religious values. Those values are often different from those of the fundamentalists who go under the banner of "the right to life," but the Jewish tradition is no less respectful of God's gift of life to us. Indeed, Jewish law and theology demand that we preserve good health and act as God's partners in restoring it to the sick. This is not, as it is for American ideology, a matter of individual right or a pragmatic choice so that we all can live longer and feel good; it is rather a command of God and thus a duty which we cannot elude. Therefore, in our own day, when medicine is at once so promising and so morally perplexing, these famous words from the Torah have new and deep significance:

> I call heaven and earth to witness against you this day: I have put before you life and death, blessing and curse. Choose life—if you and your offspring would live—by loving the Lord your God, heeding His commands, and holding fast to Him. (Deuteronomy 30:19–20)

NOTES

In the following notes, M. = Mishnah (edited c. 200 C.E.); J. = Jerusalem (Palestinian) Talmud (edited c. 400 C.E.); B. = Babylonian Talmud (edited c. 500 C.E.); M.T. = Maimonides' *Mishneh Torah* (completed 1177); and S.A. = Joseph Karo's *Shulhan Arukh* (completed 1565).

1. When Americans think of democracy, they generally have in mind something like the American form of government. It is important to recognize at the outset, though, that there are two general forms of democratic theory. One form,

following Jean-Jacques Rousseau, speaks of government by the *collective* will of the people, such that it is downright undemocratic to oppose or impede a government acting with the people's mandate. Popular sovereignty is therefore compatible with the starkest forms of majoritarian tyranny and the total denial of individual rights, as the aftermath of the French Revolution amply demonstrates. While such communitarian forms of "democracy" in their modern communist and socialist forms pose vexing theoretical and practical problems for Jews, the specific conflicts between American democracy and Judaism follow from the other form of democratic theory, following John Locke, which emphasizes individualism and protects minority rights through a system of checks and balances. It is that form on which this section concentrates.

2. Along with the thoughts expressed in Jeremiah 31:29–30 and Ezekiel 18:20–32, this declaration offends our sense of justice, but that is only because we are so used to thinking in individualistic terms.

3. Hillel's words are in B. *Sukkah* 53a.

4. See, for example, Deuteronomy 10:14; Psalm 24:1. See also Genesis 14:19, 22 (where the Hebrew word for "Creator" [*koneh*] also means "Possessor," and where "heaven and earth" is a merism for those and everything in between); Exodus 20:11; Leviticus 25:23, 42, 55; Deuteronomy 4:35, 39; 32:6.

5. See, for example, Maimonides' codified rules requiring proper diet, hygiene, sleep, and exercise: M.T. *Laws of Ethics (Hilkhot De'ot)*, chaps. 3–5.

6. See Bleich 1977; Freehof 1977, chap. 11; *Proceedings of the Rabbinical Assembly* 44 (1983): 182. All of the above are reprinted in Dorff and Rosett 1988:337–62.

7. Genesis 9:5; M. *Semahot* 2:2; B. *Bava Kamma* 91b; *Genesis Rabbah* 34:19 states that the ban against suicide includes not only cases where blood was shed, but also self-inflicted death through strangulation and the like; M.T. *Laws of Murder* 2:3; M.T. *Laws of Injury and Damage* 5:1; S.A. *Yoreh De'ah* 345:1–3. See also Bleich 1981, chap. 26.

8. For the legal basis for the permission and obligation to heal, see B. *Bava Kamma* 85a, 81b; B. *Sanhedrin* 73a, 84b (with Rashi's commentary there); S.A. *Yoreh De'ah* 336:1. See also *Sifrei Deuteronomy* on Deuteronomy 22:2 and *Leviticus Rabbah* 34:3. See Nahmanides 1963:43; this passage comes from Nahmanides' *Torat Ha'adam* (The Instruction of Man), *Sh'ar Sakkanah* (Section on Danger) on B. *Bava Kamma*, chap. 8, and it is cited by Joseph Karo in his commentary to the *Tur*, *Bet Yosef*, *Yoreh De'ah* 336. Nahmanides bases his argument on similar reasoning in B. *Sanhedrin* 84b.

9. B. *Shabbat* 127a; see also M. *Pe'ah* 1:1, where acts of loving kindness, such as visiting the sick, are described as deeds for which there is no prescribed measure since they are limitless in their benefit—though only, as the rabbis said, when one is sensitive to the needs of the patient so that one's visit does not become a burden and a source of suffering (see B. *Nedarim* 40a). The first two passages cited above are included at the very beginning of the daily morning service; see, for example, Harlow 1985:8–9.

10. Rabbi Nissim Gerondi (c. 1360) is the first to mention such societies, perhaps because in earlier times Jews lived in communities sufficiently small to insure that everyone would be visited even without such a formal structure to make sure that that happened. See *Encyclopedia Judaica*, s.v. "sick care, communal."

11. The rules in these last two paragraphs are summarized in Klein 1979:271–72. The classical codes deal with this primarily in M.T. *Laws of Mourning*, chap. 14, and in S.A. *Yoreh De'ah* 335. Other sources in English on Jewish practices regarding visiting the sick include Krauss 1988:123–39, Schur 1987:66–69, Abraham 1980:135–38, and *Bikkur Holim* 1992 for all the sisterhoods of Conservative congregations.

12. Noddings argues that women resolve moral questions on the grounds of caring rather than by using the moral rules that men tend to use. I must also note that, several years before Noddings's book, Milton Mayeroff wrote a book with almost the same title, claiming that caring applies to men too: "In the sense in which a man can ever be said to be at home in the world, he is at home not through dominating, or explaining, or appreciating, but through caring and being cared for" (Mayeroff 1971:2).

13. This custom is mentioned in Scherman 1986:144–45, 442–43. No explanation is given there, and the explanation I found in two published sources links it to the question the *Zohar* raises in interpreting Psalm 86:16—namely, why did David, the presumed author of the psalm, identify himself as "the son of your maidservant" rather than "son of Yeshai," his father? From this the *Zohar* concludes that when asking for God's deliverance, one identifies oneself by the name of one's mother, whose identity is beyond question. See Eisenstein 1938:220; Sperling 1957:164.

    The rationale in the folklore, though, as told to me by my father, is that when one prays for healing, one uses one's mother's name because mothers generally take care of their sick children more often than fathers do—or did! Moreover, the Hebrew term for mercy, *rahamim*, is etymologically related to the word for womb, *rehem*, and so mothers are associated linguistically in Hebrew with mercy, and that has an effect on the popular imagination. (Along these lines, though, it is interesting that *Sefer Ta'amei Ha-Minhagim* cites one source which says that to acquire God's mercy it would be better to identify the patient by his or her *father's* name. Although Sperling himself rejects that custom and quotes another source to reaffirm the custom of using the mother's name, the very existence of a source that suggests using the father's name specifically to induce God to be more merciful is a clear blow against sexism!)

14. Cf. B. *Ta'anit* 11a and Jerusalem (Palestinian) Talmud (hereafter J.) *Kiddushin* 4:12 (66d) for the rabbinic derivation from that law that abstinence is prohibited. See also M.T. *Laws of Ethics* 3:1. See also Rabbi Isaac's sarcastic question, "Are not the things prohibited in the Torah enough for you that you want to prohibit yourself other things?" in J. *Nedarim* 9:1 (41b). Voluntary asceticism was actually and repeatedly classified as a sin; see B. *Nedarim* 10a; B. *Nazir* 3a, 19a, 22a; B. *Bava Kamma* 91a; B. *Ta'anit* 11a.

15. For a moving description of how Rosenzweig's disease progressed until he could only blink his eyes, see Glatzer 1953:108–76, esp. 138–42.

16. For more on ethical wills, including medieval and modern examples, see Abrahams 1976 and Riemer and Stampfer 1983.

17. This includes even inanimate property that "belongs" to us, for God is the ultimate owner. See Deuteronomy 20:19; M. *Bava Kamma* 8:6, 7; B. *Bava Kamma* 92a, 93a; S.A. *Hoshen Mishpat* 420:1, 31.

18. Cf. RaN, *Nedarim* 40a. The Talmud records such prayers: B. *Ketubbot* 104a, B. *Bava Metzia* 84a, and B. *Ta'anit* 23a. Note that this is neither allowing a person to die nor euthanasia. In the former, people *refrain* from acting, but here people are taking the active step in beseeching God to act. On the other hand, unlike euthanasia, here it is *God* who is asked to act, not human beings who presume to act themselves.

19. I discuss these medical decisions and the methodological issues involved in making them at some length in Dorff 1991. That paper includes reference to most of the traditional and contemporary sources on these issues, and that issue of *Conservative Judaism* includes another paper by Rabbi Avram Reisner on the same issues from a somewhat different perspective (Reisner 1991). Both papers were approved by Conservative Judaism's Committee on Jewish Law and Standards as valid options within the Conservative Movement. My paper also makes reference to a number of Orthodox positions on these issues (Jakobovits, Bleich, Rosner, Waldenberg, Sinclair); Reform positions can be found in Jacob 1983:245–74 and Address 1992. To my knowledge, the Reconstructionist Movement has not taken an official stand on these issues.

In general, Orthodox Jews believe that the Torah is the literal word of God and that Jewish law is to be determined by reference to the codes and responsa of the past. Conservative Jews believe that all Jewish sources must be understood in their historical context and that Jewish law developed historically as well. Therefore, while Conservative Jews consider Jewish law binding, they are more willing than Orthodox Jews to make changes in its content in response to modern needs, but only as part of a communal decision. Reconstructionist and Reform Jews do not consider Jewish law to be binding, although many voluntarily choose to observe sections of it. The Reconstructionist Movement possesses a greater sense of community than the Reform Movement does and hence offers more encouragement to adopt the folkways of the Jewish people. Autonomy is a central value for the Reform Movement. Thus for Reform Jews, the law is at most a resource that the individual may choose to consult in making a decision; it is certainly not the authoritative command of God. These represent the positions of the rabbis of the various movements, but for the laity, family history, convenience, and friendships are at least as important in choosing an affiliation as ideology and practice are. Therefore, Jews might be members of synagogues affiliated with one movement or another even though their own personal philosophies and practices do not coincide with those of the institutions they join.

20. While the Torah is silent on this issue, sections of the latter two parts of the Hebrew Bible explicitly deny a life after death: Psalm 115:17; Job 7:6–10; 14:12 and 14; 16:22 (see also Job 10:20–22; 14:1–2; 17:13–16; 26:5–6); Ecclesiastes 3:19–22; 9:4–6 and 10; 11:8; 12:7. Daniel 12:2, coming from what is chronologically the last book in the Hebrew Bible (c. 150 B.C.E.) is the first to affirm the doctrine clearly; Isaiah 26:19, coming from Isaiah of Jerusalem (eighth century B.C.E.) also apparently affirms resurrection of the dead, but scholars construe that as a verse imported into the book of Isaiah in a much later period. On this topic generally, see *Encyclopedia Judaica*, s.v. "death."

21. Rabbi Akiba's comment on the limit of punishment in the afterlife to twelve months: M. *Eduyot* 2:10; see B. *Bava Mezia* 58b–59a; B. *Rosh Hashanah* 16b ff. for similar limits on punishment after death to twelve months; but see B. *Berakhot* 28b for a source that seems to contemplate eternal punishment. I describe these doctrines at greater length in "Choosing Life: Aspects of Judaism Affecting Organ Transplantation" (Dorff 1996). For descriptions of the rabbinic materials on this theme, see Cohen 1949:364–89 and the *Encyclopedia Judaica* s.vv. "death—in the Talmud and Midrash" and "afterlife."

22. Maller's statistics were based on a *Los Angeles Times* poll taken 14–15 December 1991 in the San Fernando section of Los Angeles. The results of that poll were reported, in part, in the Metro section of the Valley edition of the *Los Angeles Times* on 5 January 1992, but the *Times* made the full data available to Rabbi Maller, a professional sociologist, for his article in *Heritage*.

23. Abraham: Genesis 18:22–33. Jeremiah: Jeremiah 15:15–21. Job: Job 9. For a summary of the relation between God and justice in the Bible, see Dorff and Rosett 1988:110–23, and for the relation between the law and morality in rabbinic thought, see 1988:249–57. For a summary of the rabbis' theodicies, see Cohen 1949:110–20; for the rabbis' recognition that the righteous suffer and the evil prosper, see, for example, B. *Berakhot* 7a. A number of contemporary thinkers maintain their belief in God's justice by believing that God is limited in powers. Probably the most famous of these is Kushner 1981, but see also Schulweis 1984. One contemporary Jewish philosopher *does* deny God's justice—and therefore denies a theistic God; see Rubenstein 1966, chaps. 3, 13, 14.

24. For similar sentiments, including God's forbearance even with the wicked for a long period of time, see M. *Avot* 5:2; T. *Sotah* 4:1 (according to which God's attribute of mercy exceeds that of justice five-hundredfold); B. *Bava Kamma* 50b; B *Sanhedrin* 111a; B. *Yoma* 69b.

25. This is the *Ahavah Rabbah* prayer that comes just before the *Shema*, one of the two central prayers of the daily morning service. I have more or less followed the translation found in *Siddur Sim Shalom* (Harlow 1985:99) changing it in a few places to make it more literal so that the close connection enunciated between God's law and God's mercy can be even more evident to the English reader.

26. *Sifre Deuteronomy, Ekev* and B. *Sotah* 14a, as translated in *Siddur Sim Shalom* (Harlow 1985:19). The translation of the latter source leaves out the biblical texts used to prove that God does all the things it mentions.

27. As Irving J. Rosenbaum notes, this dictum is nowhere to be found in the Talmud or Midrash. Joseph ben Moses Trani (the *"Maharit,"* 1568–1639) tries to find an allusion to it in B. *Ketubbot* 103b; others try to prove it on the basis of B. *Sanhedrin* 90a, which declares that Ahithophel, who committed suicide (2 Samuel 17:23), has no share in the World to Come. Epstein (1959:102 n. 8), commenting on Genesis 9:5, suggests that this principle is implicit in that biblical verse itself; and Tukacinsky (1960:270) describes it as a self-evident logical proposition. See Rosenbaum 1976:36, 162 n. 21.

28. The biblical command to sanctify God's name publicly: Leviticus 22:32. The biblical command to live by the laws: Leviticus 18:5. The talmudic rules governing martyrdom: B. *Sanhedrin* 74a–74b. Cf. M.T. *Laws of the Foundations of the Torah*, chap. 5; S.A. *Yoreh De'ah* 157:1.

29. Maimonides and Karo prohibit full mourning rites for a suicide: M.T. *Laws of Mourning* 1:11; S.A. *Yoreh De'ah* 345:1. The custom, though, based on responsum #763 of Rabbi Solomon ben Abraham Adret (the *"Rashba,"* c. 1235–c. 1310), is to bury a suicide in the usual shrouds and in the Jewish cemetery, except that this grave is separated from the others and placed at the edge of the cemetery.

30. Rabbenu Asher, *B'somim Rosh* #345. The reference to King Zedekiah is in the *Yalkut Shimoni*'s interpretation of 2 Kings 25.

31. See Klein 1979:282–83, who cites Tosafot on B. *Gittin* 57b, s.v. *kaftzu*; *Kol Bo Shel Aveilut*, p. 319, sec. 50; *Gesher Hahayyim* 1:71-73; and *Arukh Hashulhan*, Y.D. 345:5 (all in Hebrew).

32. Rabbi Ephraim Oshry, *Teshuvot Mi-Maamakim* (Responsa from the Depths), 1:45; discussed and translated in part in Rosenbaum 1976:35–40. Rosenbaum documents Oshry's hesitation that his legal opinion be known, and he cites some of the other commentators who took pride in the small number of Jewish suicides during the Holocaust.

REFERENCES

Abraham, Abraham S. 1980. *Medical Halachah for Everyone*. New York: Feldheim.

Abrahams, Israel. 1976. *Hebrew Ethical Wills*. Philadelphia: Jewish Publication Society.

Address, Richard F. 1992. *A Time to Prepare*. Philadelphia: Union of American Hebrew Congregations.

Baron, Salo. 1948. *The Jewish Community*. 3 vols. Philadelphia: Jewish Publication Society of America.

Bikkur Holim. 1992. New York: Women's League for Conservative Judaism.

Bleich, J. David. 1977. "Smoking." *Tradition* 16, no. 4: 130–33.

———. 1981. *Judaism and Healing*. New York: KTAV.

Cohen, A. 1949. *Everyman's Talmud*. New York: Dutton.

Dorff, Elliot N. 1987. "Training Rabbis in the Land of the Free." In *The Seminary at 100*, ed. Nina Beth Cardin and David Wolf Silverman, 11–28. New York: Rabbinical Assembly and Jewish Theological Seminary of America.

———. 1989. *Mitzvah Means Commandment*. New York: United Synagogue of America.

———. 1991. "A Jewish Approach to End-Stage Medical Care." *Conservative Judaism* 43, no. 3: 3–51.

———. 1996. "Choosing Life: Aspects of Judaism Affecting Organ Transplantation." In *Organ Transplantation: Meanings and Realities*, ed. Stuart Youngner, Renée Fox, and Laurence J. O'Connell. Madison: University of Wisconsin Press.

Dorff, Elliot N., and Arthur Rosett. 1988. *A Living Tree: The Roots and Growth of Jewish Law*. New York: State University of New York Press.

Eisenstein, J. D. 1938. *Ozar Dinim u'Minhagim* (A Digest of Jewish Laws and Customs). New York: Hebrew Publishing. (Hebrew)

Epstein, Barukh Halevi. 1959. *Torah T'mimah* (Complete Torah). Tel Aviv: Am Olam. (Hebrew)

Freehof, Solomon B. 1977. *Reform Responsa for Our Time*. New York: Hebrew Union College Press.

Gilligan, Carol. 1982. *In a Different Voice: Psychological Theory and Women's Development*. Cambridge, Mass.: Harvard University Press.

Glatzer, Nahum. 1953. *Franz Rosenzweig: His Life and Works*. New York: Schocken.

Harlow, Jules, ed. 1985. *Siddur Sim Shalom: A Prayerbook for Shabbat, Festivals, and Weekdays*. New York: Rabbinical Assembly and United Synagogue of America.

Jacob, Walter, ed. 1983. *American Reform Responsa*. New York: Central Conference of American Rabbis.

Klein, Isaac. 1979. *A Guide to Jewish Religious Practice*. New York: Jewish Theological Seminary of America.

Konvitz, Milton R. 1980. *Judaism and the American Idea*. New York: Schocken.

Krauss, Pesach. 1988. *Why Me? Coping with Grief, Loss, and Change*. Toronto and New York: Bantam.

Kushner, Harold. 1981. *Why Bad Things Happen to Good People*. New York: Schocken.

Maller, Allen S. 1992. "Gigul, Dybbuks, and the Afterlife." *Heritage*, 20 March, 5.

Mayeroff, Milton. 1971. *On Caring*. New York: Harper and Row.

Nahmanides. 1963. *Kitvei Haramban* (The Writings of Nahmanides), ed. Bernard Chavel. Jerusalem: Mosad Harav Kook. (Hebrew)

Noddings, Nel. 1984. *Caring: A Feminist Approach to Ethics and Moral Education*. Berkeley and Los Angeles: University of California Press.

Reisner, Avram. 1991. "A Halakhic Ethic of Care for the Terminally Ill." *Conservative Judaism* 43, no. 3: 52–89.

Riemer, Jack, and Nathaniel Stampfer. 1983. *Ethical Wills: A Modern Jewish Treasury.* New York: Schocken.

Rosenbaum, Irving J. 1976. *The Holocaust and Halakhah.* New York: KTAV.

Rosenzweig, Franz. 1970. *The Star of Redemption.* New York: Holt, Rinehart and Winston.

Rubenstein, Richard. 1966. *After Auschwitz.* New York: Bobbs-Merrill.

Scherman, Rabbi Nosson. 1986. *The Complete Art Scroll Siddur.* Brooklyn: Messorah Publications.

Schulweis, Harold. 1984. *Evil and Morality of God.* Cincinnati: Hebrew Union College Press.

Schur, Tevi G. 1987. *Illness and Crisis: Coping the Jewish Way.* New York: National Conference of Synagogue Youth/Union of Orthodox Jewish Congregations of America.

Sperling, Abraham Isaac. 1957. *Sefer Ta'amei Ha-Minhagim U'M'korei Ha-Dinim* (The Book of the Reasons for the Customs and Sources of the Laws). Jerusalem: Eshkol. (Hebrew)

Tannen, Deborah. 1990. *You Just Don't Understand.* New York: Ballantine.

Tukacinsky, J. M. 1960. *Gesher Hahayyim* (The Bridge of Life). Jerusalem: Solomon. (Hebrew)

CHAPTER 8

Dying Well Isn't Easy: Thoughts of a
Roman Catholic Theologian on Assisted Death

Patricia Beattie Jung

For many of us dying well won't be easy, but then a good death has never been easy. In today's climate that is especially important to remember. I and many others consider ideal a death that comes with some warning and some leisure but no discomfort. It would come to an aged yet undiminished person after he or she had lived a full life, and it would be a serene, "natural" transition into new life. It is crucial that we not confuse such wishes about death with the notion of dying well or with the reality of death as we know it. A person may die well in circumstances far different from these.

Modern biomedical technologies both enhance and diminish our dying. On the one hand they may increase our capacity to die well by enabling us to bring others in on our dying. Fending off death, even if only for a short while, may give us the opportunity to turn a lonely and sudden death into a more communal and humane leave-taking. On the other hand, biomedical technologies may diminish our dying by exacerbating ancient temptations either to abandon the dying or to force unwelcome treatments on them. Over the ages people have wrestled with the ways suffering and death can unravel life; since our technological capacity to postpone death has grown, however, dying well has become increasingly difficult. These technologies necessitate an increasing number of decisions about whether we should delay death or save life, options simply not often available in the past. As these lifesaving capacities grow—and continue to grow they will—we will have to make even more of these decisions.

Certain themes surface rather consistently in moral arguments about these decisions. In this chapter I review some of the assumptions behind those themes and highlight typically Roman Catholic stances concerning them. Then I pay special attention to the way these assumptions and themes inform our care of those among us who are chronically and severely diminished and conclude by evaluating these concepts in regard to requests for assistance in committing suicide as well as for euthanasia.

Behind any analysis of suicide and requests for assistance in dying rest several potentially decisive assumptions. Ethical reflection includes not only problem solving—deliberations about the conflicts between various obligations and character traits—but problem setting as well. The latter involves raising such assumptions to conscious awareness and then critically evaluating them. Such assumptions normally constitute a framework or climate that informs both our description of the moral problem and its subsequent resolution.

Behind many Christian reflections on dying well are three moral premises worth deliberate attention, especially since in our North American context they are profoundly countercultural. Though these ways of thinking do not exhaust the assumptions Christians bring to such moral matters, they are quite influential. Faith convictions about healing and caring in light of the purpose of life, about freedom and responsibility given the ecological design of creation, and about the meaning of suffering and death help us form Christian judgments of what constitutes merciful and just decisions about life and death. Theological convictions about these issues frame moral questions both about living with diminishment and also about dying well.

Healing and Caring in Light of the Purpose of Life

Christians believe that all of creation was made for a purpose—to glorify God (Vatican Council II 1975:913). We were made to love and delight in God, each other, and all the universe, now and forever. This holy purpose was established by God and inscribed into the fabric of the universe. In order to flourish we must become what we were meant to be. We must live in accord with this ultimate structure of reality. We must cooperate with the Creator's design for the universe. Thus the purpose of our individual lives is neither self-determined nor socially constructed. Discernment of that purpose may be both personal and communal, but the end of life is not created by individual decision or social contract.

The belief that we were created to enjoy and glorify God in communion with all of creation both establishes and reinforces an obligation to love ourselves. Among Christian communions, Roman Catholics have been most consistent in articulating the intrinsic, rather than merely instrumental, character of this duty to love ourselves. It is an important component in the articulation by John Paul II of "the gospel of life" (John Paul II 1995:98, 117). Catholics have long taught that the obligations associated with charity are threefold. We have an obligation to love God, others, and ourselves.

These obligations establish a moral presumption in favor of preserving—protecting and nurturing—all of life, including our own. The duty to love oneself forms the basis for our obligation to care for our health and to seek appropriate medical assistance in that process (Pius XII 1958:395). We may not dishonor our bodies or despise bodily life without violating this obligation and denying the holy purpose for which we were created.

This duty to love oneself is the basis for both the prohibition against suicide and the right to refuse unreasonable medical treatment even when it is lifesaving. The Catholic church teaches that only those treatments that "provide benefit" are "appropriate," "proportionate," or "reasonable"; and only those treatments that do *not* "involve too grave a burden" are obligatory. Catholic bishops have been quite clear about the moral basis for this norm. The right to refuse medical treatment is not an independent right (based on liberty) but is "a corollary to the patient's right and moral responsibility to request reasonable treatment" (National Conference of Catholic Bishops [hereafter NCCB] Committee for Pro-Life Activities 1985:527). The nature of our right and responsibility to refuse unreasonable treatment will be elaborated at the close of the chapter.

The duty to love oneself also underlies the traditional moral prohibition against suicide (Sacred Congregation for the Doctrine of the Faith [hereafter CDF] 1982:510). Of course Christians recognize that though their choice is objectively wrong, many (if not most) who commit suicide may not be subjectively culpable for their decision (John Paul II 1995:30–31, 105, 120). Furthermore, even if a measure of personal responsibility may be ascribed to some who commit suicide, this sin need not be viewed as unforgivable. Indeed, it may be theologically problematic to identify anything under heaven as not being subject to God's redemptive power. Thus, even though the Catholic church continues to teach that those who commit suicide may not be given an ecclesial burial, most Catholics who commit suicide are in fact exempted from this ruling. Their exemption is based on one of two probable assumptions: either they were deranged and therefore not responsible for their decision, or they might have repented of their sin before the final moment of death.

Nevertheless, despite the qualifications of this judgment, Christians remain clear about their reasons for living and develop appropriate expectations about what that obligation may entail (Hauerwas 1977:101–16). We recognize that love for others requires that we care for the sick even when cure is not possible. We expect that such care will include visiting with, consoling, and praying for the sick. We expect care for others to be costly; we know it will demand endurance, patience, and courage. *These same expectations should accompany our notions about self-love.* Caring for oneself can also be difficult. Though often misleadingly described as instinctual, self-love is no more (or less) "natural" than love for others, with whom we are linked by creation. Both kinds of love can be difficult to sustain and balance. People sometimes need to be reminded or exhorted to love themselves. Self-love, just like other-love, can be sustained only through the work of auxiliary virtues (for example, courage), and its practice also requires communal support.

Freedom and Responsibility in the Ecological Design of Life

Most Christian traditions maintain that the universe, and all that exists therein, was created to glorify God. Life is structured toward this end. Indeed, I join many other Christian theologians in arguing that the triune relations of the godhead are expressed in the relationship between the Creator and creation and imaged within creation itself. Thus we see people as made for a kind of holy communion that reflects and mirrors relations within the Trinity.

Consequently, Christians see people not as solitary beings but as persons in community. God, our neighbors, and all that abounds on the earth itself are understood as constitutive of the self. We are interdependent: deeply connected to God, others, and the earth. So deep is our connection that it is essential to understand ourselves as part of an ecosystem. Thus John Paul II can describe notions of freedom which exalt the individual and deny the inherently relational character of freedom as perverse (John Paul II 1995:33–34). As selves we are differentiated yet "soluble" and connected. To claim that people are made for communion is to claim that they can have no authentic identity apart from it. This theme has been identified as among those central to the teachings of the Roman Catholic church in regard to medical ethics (O'Rourke and Boyle 1989:5).

One consequence of this tenet is that many contemporary Roman Catholic moral theologians do not believe that it is even possible to make exclusively self-regarding decisions. In a radical sense we are not our own. People deceive themselves if they think they can make decisions about themselves that do not profoundly impact others. "Patient self-determinations" are in this sense never really completely private.

In general, Catholic health care institutions recognize the patient as the primary, but not exclusive, decision maker regarding refusals of treatment; however, this primacy is not based on a libertarian notion that the patient has the only morally relevant voice in such matters. On the contrary, Catholic bishops view policies that ground this primacy in "right-to-privacy" arguments as dangerous, precisely because they obscure the legitimacy of other voices in such decision making and prevent the balancing of all relevant concerns (NCCB 1985:528).

The patient's best interest is not the only morally relevant factor to consider when determining what is proportionate. Pius XII noted that the resuscitation of an unconscious patient may constitute a grave burden for his or her *family* (Pius XII 1958:396, emphasis mine). In its analysis of refusals of treatment the CDF deems legitimate both the avoidance of personal disproportion and the desire not to impose excessive expense on the family or the community (CDF 1982:515). Human life is both personal and social—indeed, ecological. Decisions about appropriate treatment are not private. They are properly a matter of personal and familial judgment, of public policy and church teaching. The welfare of all of us who were created to participate in this communion—the self, neighbors, and all the earth—is morally relevant to the discernment of a responsible decision.

The Meaning of Death and Suffering

Christians may debate whether some sort of passage or transition into fulfillment (mortality per se) is a part of the Creator's original blessing.

But there is little question that the existential reality of death and the genuine threats it poses to one's personal identity, sense of community, and relationship to God are understood by Christians to be a consequence of sin (Hellwig 1978:30, 42; John Paul II 1995:13). The trauma of death is very real to us. When dying, we face the experience of being forsaken by our own body, by friends and family, and even by God. The faithful have no stake in masking the reality of death and the threat of oblivion it poses. To believe in the resurrection of the body is not to deny the power of death but to claim that ultimately death will not triumph over those united with Christ. The faithful do not deny death its power of annihilation, only its claim to victory.

For all of creation death is inexorable, and we suffer as we move toward it. In suffering we taste the loss experienced in death. Like death, suffering is best conceptualized as an identity crisis (Smith 1987). Since personal identity is in part socially constructed, so is our suffering. It is as much a function of our values as it is of physiological processes. In this sense suffering inescapably threatens both the social order and personal identity. As a result, those served by the social status quo (which includes nearly all of us to some degree) have a stake in "burying"—in isolating and putting out of sight—those persons who suffer.

Suffering may be experienced in a variety of ways. Our identities may be assaulted, or they may slowly unravel. Suffering includes various degrees of pain, other physiologically distressful symptoms (such as incontinence, breathlessness, nausea), and intermittent and progressive diminishment of cognitive and physical competencies (such as mental coherence and hearing). Although this threefold conceptual distinction may be useful, in reality suffering is not easily divisible.

For the most part pain can be clinically managed, if not eliminated, through narcotics and improved pain-management techniques. This *can be* done, though it often *is not*. In a recent study over 81 percent of the physicians and nurses surveyed confessed that they routinely undermedicated dying patients for pain. They did this in violation of explicit patient requests for better palliative care and their own better clinical judgment (Brody 1993).

Many of the other physiological symptoms associated with suffering and death—vomiting, the swelling and pressure associated with tumors, convulsions, and so forth—are not so easily managed; however, if health care professionals were to devote themselves to the task, it is reasonable to assume that the suffering linked to these symptoms could be substantially reduced. This would require a significant shift in the priorities of medical practice, extensive research, and then the prudent—case-by-case—application of the results.

There is at present little relief from the diminishment of our capacities frequently associated with debilitating accidents, chronic diseases, and terminal illnesses. With a shift in understanding the ends of medicine and extensive research, a real improvement could be made in the clinical response to such suffering. Rehabilitative medicine, if it were given greater priority, could provide patients with better ways to manage and cope with their diminishment.

In an important sense, however, the relation of medical practice to the suffering associated with diminishment will remain ambiguous. This kind of suffering can be seen as a by-product of important and valued developments in modern medical practice. Because of advances in public health and medical technology, people have longer life spans. This has resulted in an increase in the number of people living with chronic, incurable illnesses. These same factors increase the number of people whose dying could be lengthy. In fact, medicine is likely to increase the number of people facing long-term diminishment. As we develop increasingly sophisticated ways of pulling people through life-threatening crises, more of us will face severe and chronic ailments. Since treatments for the most part fall far short of being cures, health care actually increases both the percentage of us who will face significant diminishment and the length of time we are likely to do so.

Modern medicine has given rise to higher expectations on the part of health care professionals and patients alike, but the reality is not altogether wonderful. As one recent newspaper headline put it, "a physician's best hope may be a patient's worst nightmare." So while people remain afraid of dying, they have become even more afraid of having to endure destructive pain and live in endless suffering (Callahan 1991). John Paul II notes that these fears surface in "a cultural climate which fails to perceive any meaning or value in suffering," so people are sorely tempted to resolve the problems posed by suffering by eliminating not only the dying but the incurably ill as well (John Paul II 1995:26–27).

Suffering as a School for Communion

In contrast to the climate fostered by this "culture of death," the church teaches that suffering, especially in the form of diminishment, can sometimes be educative or a "factor of possible personal growth" (John Paul II 1995:41). Suffering may result in stripping the self of sinful tendencies. In facing death we may finally let go of "all the baggage which constitutes and masks our poverty" (Keefe 1981:261). Suffering can expose as trivial much to which we have been idolatrously devoted. In this sense suffering can be a transformative time of grace, both spiritual and moral. Indeed, our religious heritage affirms that the hour of death may be the "teachable moment" par excellence. This is partly what is at stake in the traditional reluctance to permit a deprivation of (or even a significant reduction in) the consciousness of the dying without due cause. Of course while the value of pain relief must be weighed carefully against the loss of communion and insight (CDF 1982:514), forgoing pain relief is recognized as morally "heroic" or beyond the call of ordinary duty (John Paul II 1995:118–19).

Because our culture structurally reinforces radical individualism, we see much that challenges autonomy as being painful. Though their illnesses are not often literally contagious, those who suffer are frequently viewed as dangerous. Their dependence and need reveal our notion of individual strength to be an illusion. They disclose everyone's interdependence. Those who suffer serve both as pupils and as teachers in the school of suffering. For many of us, learning to receive care graciously will be more difficult than learning to give care. Coming to terms with our limits and accepting our finitude can be a very difficult life task. It is hard to face the permanent or the progressive loss of our capacity for independent living, particularly in a culture that stresses self-reliance and individualism. In this respect diminishment may serve an important pedagogical function for both the individual and the community.

We ought not, however, romanticize suffering. Suffering can not only force detachment from what is trivial and isolating; it can also separate us from the humanizing roles and relations that bear witness to the blissful communion for which we were made. Decomposition does indeed accompany death; decomposition is not communion. Suffering can break spirits, crush relationships, and brutalize communities. While all suffering may be educative, that into which it schools us may not always be humanizing.

It is important to remember that "the facts" about suffering do not speak for themselves. The meaning of suffering is significantly determined by the convictions the sufferer brings to the experience. Suffering can "teach" important lessons. People must learn both to give and to receive care. Monika Hellwig and Drew Christianson were among the first contemporary Roman Catholic moral theologians to call for the development of a "theology of dependence" (Hellwig 1978:14–15; Christianson 1980). Even though this offers an important corrective to certain proclivities in our culture, I think such a theology will prove inadequate as the theological foundation for our moral decision making.

What makes life wearisome is precisely the diminishment of the capacity for the interdependence that marks full communion. This is precisely what scares many of us about diminishment and death. Because radical dependence on others expresses a diminishment in our capacity for participation, reciprocity, and mutuality, it is just as problematic as an atomistic, isolated existence. Neither images of dependence nor images of independence adequately represent that interdependent communion for which many Christians believe people were created.

Responsibilities of the Sick and Suffering

Our culture tends to view the sick as not having responsibilities to others. In contrast, Christian convictions may seem quite hard-hearted. Christianity has never considered those who suffer as altogether free of responsibility. Christianity teaches that it is appropriate to ascribe ongoing, if altered, responsibilities to those among us who suffer. Indeed, part of what it means to care for those who struggle with diminishment is to help them recognize their continuing obligations in our community.

At the very most some of us have special obligations as we face diminishment and death. We may be called upon to participate in drug trials and other experimental protocols. We may be called upon to lobby for better long-term care facilities or to speak up for the civil rights of those similarly disabled. We may discern in our dying a call to care for and encourage those with earlier stages of the disease that will prove fatal to us. In other words, some of us may find a personal vocation, a calling, in the circumstances of our illness or suffering.

At the very least we have some obligation to try to die in a way that promotes trust and peace among those who survive us (Hauerwas 1977:110–11). According to the mainstream of Christian moral tradition suicide does not do this. It is important to recognize this because some decisions to abate lifesaving treatments may be suicidal. (Of course, not every such decision is.) Suicide violates not only the duty to love the self but also the obligation to love others. The Catholic church teaches that suicide is an offense against one's neighbor and that it contributes to the breakdown of community and society as a whole (CDF 1982). This is vividly expressed in the tendency of one suicide to raise the risk of others.

On the one hand, many who commit suicide seem not even to be aware of others. They are self-absorbed, shrouded (already) in their pain. On the other hand, their decision is simultaneously an indictment and rejection of the love of others. To the family and friends of the deceased, some suicides say loudly and clearly: "You are not enough! You are not worth living for!" Often those who have survived the suicides of their beloved suffer. A part of them is killed too. Indeed, many (if not most) who have suffered the loss of a loved one through suicide are eventually treated for symptoms typical of post-traumatic stress disorders.

Just because an act of suicide is understandable, premeditated, or bloodless does not mean that it is any less an act of violence. It may gravely harm those left behind. Indeed, such rational suicides may prove especially harmful to the community, precisely because they are so cold-blooded and tidy. More ostensibly hostile and gory suicides can be interpreted more easily by the survivors as the act of a desperate moment, like a crime of passion. At any rate, Christian moral tradition establishes that the burden of proof rests on those who claim that their suicide would do no harm to the community.

Suffering as Sacramental

Between the minimal duty to die in a way that promotes peace among those who survive and the heroic contributions some will make come a distinctive set of obligations implicit in the life of Christian discipleship. (As is evidenced at the conclusion of this chapter, in some cases "simply" being willing to wait patiently for death may be more heroic than is commonly thought.) Christians understand themselves to be called *always and everywhere* to bear witness to Christ. Even in sickness the

Christian should witness to the transforming effect of the life, death, and resurrection of Jesus Christ on human life (Fiorenza and Galvin 1991:255).

In "Sharing Christ's Passion," Mary Therese Lysaught (1992) points out that this sacramental witness has been expected of Christians even in the context of their suffering and on the occasion of their death. In such contexts Christians may reveal to others God's power to take from death its sting. When Christians anoint the sick we remind ourselves that not even sickness and death can shatter the communion we share in Christ. By signing them with oil the Church invites those who suffer (and those who care for the sick) to become for all the world living, incarnate signs of the work of God in Christ Crucified.

God's grace can inform and be made visible in our suffering and diminishment. When linked to and made a sign of Christ's suffering and death, illness can become a vehicle for proclaiming God's healing, redemptive grace. It is most regrettable that liturgies for anointing the sick speak of restoring people to their "former health" (Talley 1981:248). (Of course, such healing is sometimes both possible and desirable. My point is that healing in these restorative or resuscitative senses is a gift distinct from the sacrament.) When Christians anoint the sick we sign our *new* life in Christ; we do not annul the reality of our "suffering unto death" but signal the defeat of its bitterness. In this sacrament in a most personal and bodily way, those among us who are sick are consecrated to Christ—that is, linked to the real presence of God among us. Those who are dying become incarnate signs of God's good news about suffering and death. Just as our lives may be made a prayer, so too one may make of dying a prayer. Those who suffer may orchestrate or preside over their diminishment and even come to celebrate its ultimate defeat in Christ.

Liturgical activity has served as a source of doctrinal wisdom from the earliest days of the Church. (Of course the relationship between such rituals and tradition is dialogical.) Though their lessons are not always heeded, liturgies can be a source of wisdom about the moral life as well (Downey 1987; Grassi 1985; Hellwig 1976; Searle 1980; Sedgwick 1987; Willimon 1983). Unlike arguments that can be constructed on the basis of rules and principles, sacramental ethics (like those based on narratives) establish frameworks within which certain practices—like awaiting death patiently—may be said to cohere (or not).

When diminishment and death are part of the liturgies in accord with which one lives, as they are for Christians, then suffering does not necessarily result in the deconstruction of one's world. The sacraments provide a ritual context within which the faithful experience all of life's crises, including illness. These rites are the framework through which Christians are empowered to respond sacramentally to diminishment and death. In this sense the sacraments prepare Christians for suffering. This may enable some of us not to unravel completely before suffering but instead to find their truest identity confirmed and their faith reinforced by it.

Through our faith in God's steadfast presence in and power over diminishment and death, Christians bear witness to the gospel. St. Paul argues that Jesus is made visible to the community in and through mortal bodies as they suffer affliction (2 Corinthians 4:7–12). Pain, distress, diminishment, and death simply happen. All of us respond to this brutal fact of life out of our faith convictions. Generally speaking we recognize that the way we care (or do not care) for others who suffer expresses our ultimate beliefs. My point is that the way we suffer (especially the way we suffer diminishment) also witnesses to our ultimate convictions.

Much might be said about this "Way of the Cross." I would highlight four aspects of God's gracious work among us that may be distinctively embodied by those who are sick and dying. I intend this list to be not exhaustive but merely suggestive of ways God's grace may be experienced in suffering and death. God's grace comes as an unmerited and free gift and a vocation to be lived out.

First, so passionate is God's love for us that, in order to be with us, God accepted and bore diminishment and death. So, too, we are called to love each other so much that ultimately we live with diminishment and accept death for the sake of this gospel.

Second, Jesus did not travel the road to Jerusalem alone. He invited the disciples to accompany him. He asked them to wait and pray with him in the garden. He did not isolate himself, deny his needs, or push others away. This openness to the care of others left him vulnerable. His companions fell asleep. He was deserted. So, too, we are to invite others into our suffering, and thereby live with the risks and reality of abandonment.

Third, Jesus comforted others in his suffering unto death. This comforting took many forms. Jesus brought people together. He connected his mother and the beloved disciple while on his cross (John 19:25–27). Jesus also practiced forgiveness—forgiving the thief at his side (Luke 23:43), his persecutors, and the disciples he predicted would abandon him (Luke 23:34). Presumably Jesus forgave God as well (Luke 23:46). Lysaught argues that for Christians "suffering becomes an occasion for practicing forgiveness—of our own bodies, of others who remind us of the precarious contingency of our existence, of those who leave through suffering and death, of God" (Lysaught 1992:303). As we are enabled, so we are called.

This brings us to the fourth way those who are diminished and dying among us may bear a unique witness to Christ. The Son remained faithful to the Father even as he lamented his experience of being forsaken by the Father. In our diminishment (as in our dying) Christians are called to be such living signs of Christ Crucified. We are enabled to face, not deny, death—to descend into it, because we trust that we will be raised up "on eagle's wings."

As is the case throughout life, in suffering Christians are called to embody God's passion for communion with all of creation. This led Christ to a new creation by way of the cross. It is not easy for those who suffer to hold fast to a Christian construction of diminishment and death. Thankfully, we receive as a gift from God that which we are called to embody. The work of initiating and sustaining such a sacramental witness in suffering may (and often does) fall on the Church.

That Christians rely on each other for help in living graciously with diminishment and in dying well (as they have in making of the rest of their life a faithful witness) comes as no surprise. Christians know they can be faithful in life *only* together. (In the practice of infant baptism, for example, some in the community act on behalf of others, doing for them what they cannot as infants do for themselves. Such intervention in the name of others imitates God's own incarnate way of loving, of doing for us in Christ what we could not do.) The point is that all sacramental activity is inherently communal. Those who are sick can be protected from abandonment and overtreatment, and thereby nurtured into more faithful ways of living with diminishment and dying. At the same time those suffering unto death can illumine for their caregivers the truth that nothing can ultimately defeat the communion God has established in Christ among us.

Just and Merciful Health Care Decisions

These three premises—about healing and caring in light of the ultimate purpose of life, about freedom and responsibility in the ecological design of life, and about the meaning of death and suffering—form a framework for the way many Christians view their health care decisions. They establish the parameters within which one may live and die well. What count as merciful and just decisions about how to care for the irreversibly dying and the chronically and severely diminished must be congruent with these convictions.

Care of the Irreversibly Dying

It is considered permissible to abate, that is, to refuse, withhold, or withdraw, death-delaying treatments in two contexts. First, one ought to cease or not initiate treatments whenever such treatments are judged useless. When it will not be effective in prolonging life for a significant period, treatment ought to be stopped and the patient allowed to die. Clearly the notion of medical futility is not a completely value-free concept, but the improbability of clinical success constitutes the physiological basis for the notion.

Most Roman Catholic biomedical ethicists would argue that the abatement of futile treatments is permissible but not required. I would argue that a full appreciation of and respect for our traditions about freedom and responsibility given the ecological design of life will draw the Church to the conclusion that there is no obligation to provide medically futile treatments, even when they are requested by patients or their surrogates. Indeed, concern for the commonweal as expressed in the effective stewardship and just distribution of resources obliges us not to fulfill such wasteful requests. In fact I believe that this is the (unstated) conclusion to which the corpus of the Church's teachings points.

Second, one may choose to cease treatments or not to initiate treatments—even when the effect of such a decision will be to bring on or hasten death—whenever these treatments impose burdens out of proportion to their benefits. Though the abatement of excessively burdensome treatment is generally understood to be permissible and is frequently requested, it is not common. In a recent study more than half of the health care professionals surveyed confessed that they overtreated their dying patients with excessively burdensome therapy (Brody 1993).

A treatment is excessively burdensome whenever the price paid for its brief delay of death—its monetary and communal costs, medical and spiritual risks, interpersonal strains and further physiological trauma and aggravation—is disproportionate to the palliative, spiritual, interpersonal, or communal benefits that can be reasonably expected. In one sense it does not matter whether the treatments in question are the high-tech interventions associated with an intensive care unit or a simple course of antibiotics. Both may be "extraordinary" for this patient in this circumstance.

Let me be especially clear about this one point: when a choice to abate death-delaying treatments is justified, that does not mean we may simply forsake or abandon the dying. We remain obliged to provide them with steadfast, supportive care while they await death.

Care of the Chronically and Severely Diminished

While abating futile treatments may be appropriate for patients in a dying state, it may not be for those who are chronically and severely diminished. Reflecting on a long tradition, Catholic moral theologian John Mahoney notes that the traditional distinction between killing and letting die enabled medical personnel to abate futile treatments "for patients identified as in the dying state" (Mahoney 1992:677). One cannot simply rip this distinction out of its original context and apply it to the care of the chronically and severely diminished. There is a difference between letting someone who is dying die and letting someone who is living die. For those whose condition is not terminal, none of the life-support treatments to be abated can be said to be clinically futile.

The only relevant question is whether it is permissible to abate such lifesaving treatment when the burdens of those treatments outweigh their benefits. Let us think about a relatively simple example. Though not irreversibly fatal, an accident or disease process may leave a person incapable of even simple relations with others. When a person's capacity for relationship has been virtually *destroyed*, not merely diminished, the burdens associated with lifesaving treatments *may* outweigh their benefits. The Catholic bishops of Washington, Oregon, and Texas, for example, suggest that the medical provision of nutrition and hydration to those who are irreversibly comatose *may* be extraordinary. They acknowledge, of course, that there is no moral consensus among teachers of the Church on this point, and John Paul II cautions that personal dignity cannot be simply "equated with the capacity for viable and explicit, or at least perceptible, communication" (John Paul II 1995:33).

One problem with this type of case, of course, is that it is not always easy to make this diagnosis. For some the loss of the capacity for relationship is a gradual decline, rooted in an irreversible and relentless illness like Alzheimer's. For others the loss of capacity for relationship may be temporary—for example, the side effect of certain medications or treatments. In still other cases like comas that are drug- or trauma-induced, the loss may be potentially but not certainly reversible. A few persons thought to have been in persistent vegetative states have "awakened" and returned to normal life. Such reversals are highly unlikely after three months, but medicine never operates with certainties. Nevertheless, when the front lobes of the brain have begun to deteriorate, the potential for relationship this side of resurrected life is virtually nil.

What about cases where the person's capacity for relationship is *diminished* rather than destroyed? Here we enter very murky waters indeed. Though I am not prepared to argue that all refusals of lifesaving treatment in such situations are wrong, in most the burdens associated with lifesaving treatments do not outweigh their benefits. For example, studies indicate that patients with cervical-level spinal cord injuries and the health care professionals who attend them frequently underestimate the quality of life that can be achieved through rehabilitation (Patterson et al. 1993). Whether based on misinformation or more rational grounds, a choice to abate lifesaving treatments by such patients *may* be suicidal.

Indeed, there may not be a meaningful distinction between refusals of lifesaving treatment and suicide, except for the intention of the agent. It can be cogently argued that a suicide occurs if and only if (and whenever) a person *intentionally* terminates his or her own life, no matter what the causal route to death. Consider, for example, a generally healthy person who has a potentially terminal condition but who might easily avoid dying for literally a lifetime by taking a cheap and painless medication; if that person refuses such reasonable treatment in order to induce death, that person has committed suicide from a moral point of view. Notice that, although the causal route to death was indirect and passive, the person's purpose was *not* the avoidance of futile or disproportionately burdensome treatment. The intention was obviously to die. I believe the moral significance of a person's *intention* is what is underscored in the moral tradition surrounding this matter.

Admittedly there is some confusion in this regard. In its "Declaration on Euthanasia," the Sacred Congregation for the Doctrine of the Faith defined *euthanasia* as "an action or an omission which *of itself* or by intention causes death, in order that all suffering may in this way be eliminated" (CDF 1982:516, emphasis mine).

This would imply that euthanasia (and suicide as well) can be defined in terms of both method and intention. This is a conclusion drawn by many theologians (see, for example, Keenan and Sheehan 1992). Yet it has long been recognized that some pain-management techniques may compromise respiration and actively hasten death. This secondary effect has been viewed as permissible when the person's intention was to control pain, not induce death. Therefore, although not yet incorporated into its traditional formulations of the heart of the matter, the Catholic church's teachings point to the decisive nature of the agent's intentions. At this juncture it is important to note that whether the concept of intention can carry all the moral freight I have ascribed to it is a matter of significant debate among ethicists (Beauchamp and Childress 1989:127–34).

The facile distinction that some ethicists make between passive and active forms of suicide may be morally quite hazardous. Many people jump to the false conclusion that while active forms of suicide are generally immoral (though certainly forgivable and often even understandable), passive refusals of treatment or "omissions" are generally morally acceptable. In contrast, the Catholic church teaches that the duties to love oneself and others establish a strong moral presumption against both active forms of suicide and refusals and omissions of life-saving treatments. The very invisibility of most decisions to abate treatment may make them more dangerous from a moral point of view. They do not elicit the moral scrutiny typical of more overt, conspicuous requests for assistance in death (Battin 1991).

The Moral Significance of Awaiting Death

If it may sometimes be legitimate to abate death-delaying treatment, and sometimes even lifesaving treatment, the question arises: why await death? May it not be legitimate for people to commit suicide, with or without assistance from health care professionals? Even though cases where pain is clinically unmanageable are very rare, many patients do suffer extreme pain while awaiting death. Furthermore, they are overtreated, and their death illegitimately delayed. Such practices amount to patient abuse, which is inexcusable. The solution does not reside, however, in institutionalizing mercy killing. Instead, we need to structure into our health care institutions programs that reinforce on an organizational level the attitudinal changes regarding overtreatment and pain management already present on a personal level in most health care professionals.

Insofar as we are able, we have an obligation to protect those who are diminished and dying in our midst from both neglect and overtreatment. We have the obligation to provide appropriate (that is, not disproportionately burdensome) care for those who are diminished and to provide for the comfort, hygiene, and dignity of those who are dying. Such care takes a great deal of personal strength and moral stamina, and it will sorely tax our communal resources. Such caregiving is far from glamorous. It is costly and homely.

Coincidentally, insofar as we are diminished and dying, we have obligations to the community. We have the obligation to learn to receive care graciously. Perhaps through our diminishment and dying we will be enabled to contribute in a special way to the care of others. Finally, there is for Christians the call to bear witness to Christ's suffering with us in the present. The fulfillment of these obligations requires, minimally, that we await death with patience and strength.

Living in this way with diminishment calls for bravery. Dying in this way takes courage. Awaiting death for many entails suffering. That this suffering can be meaningful—that it may serve a pedagogical function and a sacramental, evangelical purpose—may explain why Christians are charged to await death. And yet to show such patience to be religiously meaningful is not to establish it as morally required under all circumstances.

Unanswered Questions

Like all other professionals, moral theologians face occupational hazards. We may be tempted to define ourselves too rigidly as social prophets whose primary job it is to challenge the ways of the world. Of course, to be such a gadfly is most certainly part of our calling. (For that I am grateful, since much of what I have argued in this chapter is profoundly countercultural.) But we must always remember that such prophecy carries with it the tendency to oversimplify and to take positions that may blind us to the moral ambiguity of some situations (Mahoney 1992:665–66).

If we are to move from prophecy toward wisdom in such matters, our teachings must recognize and wrestle with the fact that life's burdens are not equitably distributed among us. Living is clearly more burdensome for some than for others. Living may indeed always take courage, but for some it may require a kind of bravery that goes beyond any imaginable call of duty. In some cases it may be morally heroic merely to keep on living.

In light of these brute facts, the question arises: how much suffering can people be expected to endure? Awaiting death will undoubtedly test the patience of most of us. For some of the diminished among us, the awaited moment of death may be a lifetime away. Are there any limits to the patience that can be required of us?

When pneumonia visits, in many cases we let the sick succumb to their good friend. Not all those who pray to die are fortunate enough to have such a visitor.

REFERENCES

Battin, Margaret P. 1991. "Euthanasia: The Way We Do It, The Way They Do It." *Journal of Pain and Symptom Management* 6, no. 5 (July): 212–19.

Beauchamp, Tom L., and James F. Childress. 1989. *Principles of Biomedical Ethics.* New York: Oxford University Press.

Brody, Jane E. 1993. "Doctors Admit Ignoring Dying Patients' Wishes." *New York Times,* 14 January, A18.

Callahan, Daniel. 1991. "Aid in Dying: The Social Dimensions." *Commonweal* 118 (9 August): 476–80.

Christianson, Drew. 1980. "The Elderly and Their Families: The Problems of Dependence." *New Catholic World* 223:100–104.

Downey, Michael. 1987. *Clothed in Christ.* New York: Crossroad.

Fiorenza, Francis Schüssler, and John P. Galvin, eds. 1991. *Systematic Theology: Roman Catholic Perspectives.* Minneapolis: Fortress Press.

Grassi, Joseph A. 1985. *Broken Bread and Broken Bodies: The Lord's Supper and World Hunger.* Maryknoll, N.Y.: Orbis Books.

Hauerwas, Stanley. 1977. *Truthfulness and Tragedy: Further Investigations into Christian Ethics.* Notre Dame, Ind.: University of Notre Dame Press.

Hellwig, Monika K. 1976. *The Eucharist and the Hunger of the World.* New York: Paulist Press.

———. 1978. *What Are They Saying about Death and Christian Hope?* New York: Paulist Press.

John Paul II. 1995. *The Gospel of Life: On the Value and Inviolability of Human Life.* Washington, D.C.: United States Catholic Conference.

Keefe, Donald J. 1981. "Death as Worship." In *The Sacraments: Readings in Contemporary Sacramental Theology,* ed. Michael J. Taylor, 253–64. New York: Alba House.

Keenan, James F., and Myles Sheehan. 1992. "Life Supports." *Church* (Winter): 10–17.

Lysaught, Mary Therese. 1992. "Sharing Christ's Passion: A Critique of the Role of Suffering in the Discourse of Biomedical Ethics from the Perspective of the Theological Practice of Anointing of the Sick." Ph.D. diss., Duke University.

Mahoney, John. 1992. "The Challenge of Moral Distinctions." *Theological Studies* 53:663–82.

National Conference of Catholic Bishops (NCCB) Committee for Pro-Life Activities. 1985. "Guidelines for Legislation on Life-Sustaining Treatment" (10 November 1984). *Origins* 14, no. 32 (24 January): 526–28.

O'Rourke, Kevin D., and Philip Boyle, eds. 1989. *Medical Ethics: Sources of Catholic Teachings*. St. Louis, Mo.: Catholic Health Association of the United States.

Patterson, David R., Cindy Miller-Perrin, Thomas McCormick, and Leonard Hudson. 1993. "When Life Support Is Questioned Early in the Care of Patients with Cervical-level Quadriplegia." *New England Journal of Medicine* 328 (18 February): 506–9.

Pius XII. 1958. "The Prolongation of Life" (24 November 1957). *The Pope Speaks* 4, no. 4 (spring): 395–96.

Sacred Congregation for the Doctrine of the Faith (CDF). 1982. "Declaration on Euthanasia" (5 May 1980). *Vatican Council II*, 2:510–16.

Searle, Mark, ed. 1980. *Liturgy and Social Justice*. Collegeville, Minn.: Liturgical Press.

Sedgwick, Timothy F. 1987. *Sacramental Ethics: Paschal Identity and the Christian Life*. Philadelphia: Fortress Press.

Smith, David H. 1987. "Suffering, Medicine, and Christian Theology." In *On Moral Medicine: Theological Perspectives in Medical Ethics*, ed. Stephen E. Lammers and Allen Verhey, 255–61. Grand Rapids, Mich.: Wm. B. Eerdmans.

Talley, Thomas. 1981. "Healing: Sacrament or Charism?" In *The Sacraments: Readings in Contemporary Sacramental Theology*, ed. Michael J. Taylor, 241–52. New York: Alba House.

Vatican Council II. 1975. "Pastoral Constitution on the Church in the Modern World" (7 December 1965). *Vatican Council II*, 1:913.

Willimon, William H. 1983. *The Service of God: How Worship and Ethics Are Related*. Nashville: Abingdon Press.

CHAPTER 9

Anna, Ambiguity, and the Promise:
A Lutheran Theologian Reflects on Assisted Death

James M. Childs, Jr.

I was an inexperienced seminarian discovering my limits, perhaps for the first time, consciously, in my young life. It was my clinical term, and I was assigned to pastoral care duties in the state psychiatric hospital. The patient I remember best was a woman I will call Anna, not for the sake of anonymity only but because I actually cannot remember her name. I shall not forget her face, however. It was long and thin, to go with her body. It had all the deep lines and crevices one would expect in someone well into her eighties, punctuated by clouded, sightless eyes.

Anna had had a long history of being in and out of the psychiatric hospital. Each time she was returned to her family, something happened to reactivate her severe manic-depressive state. Her last period of living at home had ended abruptly when she discovered that termites had eaten a hole in the floor behind the couch. The discovery sent her into an emotional tailspin from which she did not recover. Now, having out-lived most of her family, but not her illness, she was in the hospital for the duration. And the duration was becoming increasingly unendurable. Blind, alone, and suffering assorted physical ailments of advanced age, Anna was consigned to that ward in the hospital for those who had a combination of mental and physical illness. It was the closest thing to bedlam I had ever experienced.

She spoke to me of her suffering, of lying in bed in the darkness of her own visual and emotional night, hearing the constant screams and groans of those around her. In the grip of fear, misery, and loneliness, she cried easily and often.

Yet in her darkness the light of faith still burned, and this she could see clearly. There was no doubt in her mind that Jesus knew her sufferings and that God loved her and had a home for her. So we sat together each week, the cries of others all around us, and I listened to her refrain of relentless inner pain. I held her hand, and we prayed for death to come quickly and soon. And we thanked God for the promise of new life.

For a long time I worried about my time with Anna. I fretted that I had so little to offer her and that somehow it was theologically wrong to pray for death. Of course, as I myself realized, these worries were the intrusion of self-concern upon the practice of ministry. I had become concerned about my own performance rather than being a conduit for God's performance of grace and healing. And, for a while, I let that be the primary lesson of my encounter with Anna. As I entered upon this study, however, I recalled Anna's situation. I thought of it anew in the light of our concerns over the moral status of assisted suicide and euthanasia for those who want help dying when their agonies are too great to bear, and I realized that much more could be learned from Anna's story.

It will be helpful to reflect upon Anna even though her experience does not illustrate the kinds of circumstances that normally evoke advocacy for assisted suicide or euthanasia. Anna's case draws us into fundamental theological questions about death and dying without the urgency of savage pain and imminent death and without the complications of legal and procedural ambiguity over whether certain actions and decisions are best described as passive or active. Those conditions certainly can raise ultimate questions in dramatic ways, but they can also distract us. Anna's story enables us to take a conceptual step back from the most extreme cases to reflect upon fundamental insights and principles that can then be tested in cases where people are at the outer limits of human endurance.

I also think that there are points at which we can identify with Anna and thereby gain greater empathy and understanding in relation to those who want help in dying. I hope to show that Anna can help us get in touch with our own sense of despair, even *within faith*, and thus provide us with an opportunity to explore how life in faith may shed light on the issues we face.

These issues are not, of course, just decisions regarding euthanasia or assisted suicide: they also raise the question of how we establish moral authority in our time. I feel a need to linger a moment with that question so that, when we return to Anna and start down the path of theological reflection, we may have a better understanding of the cultural context in which we travel and our destination within that context.

Moral Authority: Apologetics without Apology

A number of reasons have been offered to explain the current high degree of public interest in and growing acceptance of active voluntary euthanasia and assisted suicide. Among the most frequently cited factors are the emphasis upon autonomy in contemporary culture and the growing conviction that medical science has gone too far in its efforts to prolong and manage life. Taken together, these two factors point us in the direction of the serious and increasingly well recognized problem of moral authority.

First, advocacy for individual autonomy and the kind of individualism that is rampant in our society are mutually reinforcing. Autonomy when blended with individualism easily leads to the conviction that we may each do with our own life precisely what we please. Such an outlook thrives in a pluralistic society like our own, where there appears to be little or no moral consensus. A few constraints may hinge on our outstanding obligations to other parties, but once those obligations are resolved, we are completely free to proceed as we would like in the disposition of our life (Engelhardt 1989:7–9).

Second, the conviction that medical science has gone too far in prolonging and managing life not only reflects the terror of many in our society but also pushes us to admit some of the disappointment we feel in our Enlightenment faith in reason and the empirical sciences to conquer our problems and settle issues of value and principle. This shortfall in the Enlightenment hope is embodied, I think, in the ambiguity of medical science's life-prolonging power and the quandary it often creates for rational analysis of moral choice.

The subjectivity of individualism and the uncertainty created by medical science are exacerbated by the relativism that has undermined the degree of moral consensus that the accepted authority of religious institutions once helped to provide, even in a diverse society. Religious authority for ethics has been weakened in our society by secularization, pluralism, and an account of reality based on constant evolutionary change rather than constancy in the order of things. In this context of historical, cultural, scientific, and social relativism, unbridled individualism and freedom of choice seem to make perfect sense.

At the same time, there is an apparent concern and even longing for some constraints, some renewal of moral consensus and authority. A heightened autonomy from authoritarian moral traditions may spell freedom, but what defines responsibility? Does the testimony of faith communities on issues of life and death, good and evil, still have any promise for effectively and persuasively projecting a horizon of moral definition within which to identify basic principles that give coherence to human action and self-understanding? Many believe that the secular pluralism characteristic of our society militates against the formative influence of religion, at least at the level of public policy (Brock 1992:14); however, as a Christian and a theologian, I think that religious insight can still have a formative influence on the ethos of our society and even a positive influence on the formation of its public policy. I do not mean by this claim that Christian theology will hold sway or convert others outside its faith. As my later remarks on public dialogue should make clear, I think that Christians, as they sit down with people of other religious and cultural traditions, have a particular contribution to make in the process of identifying values that can be held in common. Moreover, certain features of Christianity's theological heritage in the Reformation equip it well for public dialogue.

Christian theology is no stranger to the tension and ambiguity that lie at the heart of our present ethical struggle, a struggle that seems to present a new version of the age-old problem of the absolute and the relative. In one way or another, key themes in Christian theology deal both with this tension and with the problem of anchoring moral authority in a sea of relativism. Let me try to illustrate.

Luther's radical view that we are saved by grace alone, through faith, without the works of the law, logically requires that we acknowledge the equally radical nature of sin. Furthermore, though we may speak of the complete and present reality of our justification in Christ and of growth in faith and love that expresses our sanctification, the consummation of our justification and sanctification is an eschatological promise. Radical grace and radical sin coexist. We are an already/not-yet people. Therefore, life is defined by the constant interplay of law and gospel, judgment and grace. This inner and almost paradoxical tension of life is expressed in the corollary formula *simul justus et peccator* (at the same time justified and sinner). If we are to affirm the efficacy of God's justifying grace and still acknowledge the irrepressible and continuing reality of human sin, even for Christians, then we have to acknowledge the reality and coinherence of opposites to which the *simul* points us. Much of our contemporary struggle to recover moral authority even as we lapse into relativity might well be analyzed as a case of losing our grip on the paradox: We have tried to domesticate the transcendent and have thereby lost our proper relation to it. We underestimate both the reality of sin and the necessity of grace.

Paul Tillich has developed this insight in his helpful and well-known notion of the Protestant Principle. The Protestant Principle, for Tillich, was a hedge against the demonic absolutization of that which is relative, the elevation to infinite authority of that which is finite. As a corollary of our conviction that we are saved by grace alone, the Protestant Principle held in effect that nothing but the promise of that grace can be absolutized. All claims to authority are relative to that standard and are rightly criticized when they claim too much. Thus, to absolutize the moral claims of authoritarian institutions (both religious and secular) is to fail to recognize that salvation by grace alone means no institution of a historical, fallen world can have that kind of authority. By the same token, to elevate the autonomy of the individual as the ultimate authority in moral terms is to ignore the perduring reality of human sin and to reject the gift of grace and its divine giver. This leads to profanation, a world without transcendence or a sense of the unconditional, a world without the foundations of moral authority (Tillich 1957:170ff.; 1963:98–106).

In contemporary theology the heightened appreciation of the historical nature of all reality has led to a recovery of biblical eschatology with its orientation to the future. We are now led by this perspective to speak of the proleptic structure of all things, of a future fulfillment, already revealed, projected, and assured by the Christ at Easter, but not yet fully realized in our continuing daily existence. In other words, our vision of the ultimate good is present to us while yet being future; it calls to us and directs us, but we can only anticipate it in limited ways under the condition of diverse particularity and our fallen existence (Childs 1978:131ff.).

The paradox of the *simul*, the Protestant Principle in its critique of both heteronomy and autonomy, and the already/not-yet tension of proleptic eschatology in contemporary thought are all branches on the same theological family tree. They provide a theological account of human experience that illumines our struggles to find the universal in diverse particularities, to find the infinite under the conditions of finitude, and, as always, to find some vision and hope for the good in an evil world where reason alone cannot dissolve the radical ambiguity of a life that includes suffering and death. Yet our theological constructs provide more than an interpretive key for life in a finite and often tragic world. In the tensions they express is the promise of God in Christ that points beyond the struggles to hope, a hope that offers a vision of the ultimate good for which we then can strive in anticipation under the penultimate conditions of historical life.

This combination of realism and hope equips us well for public dialogue in today's world; we have the self-critical capacity needed for the give-and-take and a promise that connects with human experience and fills the particularities of a pluralistic world with the stuff of universal hope. Dialogue requires a combination of recognition that one does not have a corner on the truth and steadfastness concerning the vital center of one's faith.

Another reason for believing that theology can contribute to the recovery of moral parameters is the potential for dialogue logically inherent in our pluralistic state of affairs. It is an axiom of contemporary social analysis that we are all locked into the particularity of our social location, cultural conditioning, and the special features of our personal history and formation. Our society is a conglomeration of people and groups of people possessing different outlooks and modes of thought that are corollaries of the particular circumstances of our formation.

One feature of this state of affairs is that it threatens us with a new and more profound basis for relativism in values, meaning, and truth.

Another feature, however, is that once we recognize the reality of the particularity of all thought forms and cultural expressions, we have leveled the playing field and are better prepared for a public dialogue in which representatives of religious traditions can speak apologetically without apology—that is, in the explicit terms of their own faith traditions. One thinks of the dialogical proposals of Michael Perry in *Love and Power*, the reflections on public theology in books like Ronald Thiemann's *Constructing a Public Theology*, and the call for a global ethic in Hans Küng's *Global Responsibility*. Of course, faith traditions that choose to be dogmatic and overbearing are poor candidates for such a dialogical process of seeking moral consensus. Those, however, that participate in the kind of critical perspective evidenced in the Protestant Principle are well equipped for dialogue.

To probe and outline thoroughly the needed dialogical structure and the specific ways in which it might bear upon the issues of euthanasia and assisted suicide are beyond the scope of this chapter. My task here is to explore the Christian witness we bring to that public dialogue. To achieve this goal, I want to address some fundamental theological themes related to the ethical issues of euthanasia and assisted suicide and, in so doing, resume our conversation with Anna.

Suffering and Dying

Christianity takes dying and suffering seriously. What happens in and to our physical self matters, and it matters greatly. The hope and the promise of the Christian gospel is not the immortality of the soul but the resurrection of the body. In this it reflects the materiality of its heritage in the Hebrew Scriptures and in the faith of the people of Israel.

Christianity connects suffering and death with sin, not as punishment for sin but in the understanding that sin is a condition, a state of affairs, in which we are alienated from God, who is the source of wholeness and life.

Indeed, the effects of that alienation pervade the whole of reality so that we may speak theologically of the fallenness of our world and the brokenness of our existence. And we can speak experientially of being mired in a dysfunctional and conflictual existence in which even nature seems cruel and quixotic and in which tragedy, our own and that which we share with the human community, seems to stalk us at every turn. As Helmut Thielicke puts it, "so long as we are here below, we are implicated in innumerable, suprapersonal webs of guilt . . . we are actors in a thousand plays which we individually have not staged, which we might wish would never be enacted, but in which we have to appear and play our parts" (Thielicke 1966:436).

I believe, then, that we can connect with Anna's suffering and with her as a person at those times when our own heightened sense of human sin puts us most keenly in touch with the suffering and despair born of that sinful condition. Knowing that we share with Anna the pain of a fallen existence in a fallen world enables us to be *with* her—and to go beyond sympathy to empathy and understanding.

For me Anna raises the question, what does it mean when, in the midst of suffering, a Christian wants to die? In a very real sense we are able to identify with her and with that question at moments of intense personal encounter with the terrible reality of sin: the shameful deeds that haunt us or the shame of our inaction, the pain and guilt of broken relationships we seem powerless to heal, the failures that threaten our very life, the experience of dreadful loss, the times we feel helpless in the tight grip of the demonic. The torments of these experiences are like those that Anna endured: the noises of bedlam accosting us in the darkness of our soul. And we want to die. Desperately, we want to die, for there seems to be no release from such torment.

We want to die to the sin that plagues us. We know as a proposition of faith that we have died to sin once and for all in our baptism, but we feel the visceral truth of that theological abstraction when we are in touch with the torments of life gone amok, and we want, quite simply, to die. Whatever remorse and shame we may feel about a specific sin on such an occasion, it is but a window to the larger reality of human brokenness, the fallen reality we inhabit and that we ultimately share with Anna.

The witness of the cross in Christian understanding is that it is a mirror held up to the human condition. It reflects back to us the reality of sin and the suffering and death it begets—both the malevolence and willful cruelties of human behavior represented by those who crucified the Christ and by the thieves who hung at his side and the victimization of those who, like the innocent Christ, are simply overtaken by the tortured, systemic dysfunction of life and its institutions.

For although God redeems our suffering, and although suffering may be the occasion for spiritual growth and discovery, there is nothing innately ennobling about it. For Anna to pray for death and to project a mysterious blend of despair and hope is to echo in some respects Jesus himself and the event of the cross: He struggled with impending suffering and death in Gethsemane, yet he accepted it; he spoke words of grace to thieves and persecutors alike, betraying an intimacy with the Father, and yet he cried out, "My God, why have you forsaken me?"

Perhaps the mystery of Anna's blend of despair and hope, like that blend in Jesus on the cross, is a signpost to the mystery of the cross as a symbol of both despair and hope; a sign of anguish and healing; a sign of the tragedy of sin, suffering, and death, and a sign of redemption and new life; a sign of our alienation from God and a sign of God taking upon God's self our suffering and death; a sign of estrangement and a sign of forgiveness and reconciliation.

So we sat together each week, Anna and I, the cries of others all around us, and I listened to her refrain of relentless inner pain. I held her hand, and we prayed for death to come quickly, and we thanked God for the promise of new life. Despairing though she was at this end stage of a long and joyless life, her prayer in all its desperation was still one of hope. And we too, in our cries of confession, utter desperate cries for release. In the word of God's forgiveness, with the sign of the cross, death comes swiftly, and life begins again.

Freedom and Responsibility

In the Bible and in the history of Christian thought, a key locus for understanding what it is to be human is the doctrine of the image of God. Tracing the biblical teaching that human beings are created in the image of God and the development of that idea in Christian tradition is a lengthy process (Childs 1978). For present purposes I will simply summarize key points of this teaching as interpreted in the Christian tradition.

1. The creation account in Genesis 1 tells us that humanity is a special creation. It is distinguished from all other living things by having an immediate relationship with God. This relationship we might well describe as personal. Humanity is "on speaking terms" with God, as George Forrell once put it. In the command to represent God in the care of the earth (Genesis 1:27) we see reflected the marks of personhood: freedom and responsibility. Responsibility is inconceivable without freedom, and freedom is inconceivable without responsibility.

2. However, humanity is not God but the *image of God*. Our being is dependent upon God. We are not to find the meaning of our existence or the fulfillment of our existence in either nature or ourselves. To be God for oneself or to find the ultimate in other things is to rebel not only against God but also against our own true selves by stepping outside the intimate personal relationship with God that constitutes our very being. This betrayal of God and ourselves is the meaning of the Fall story and the notion that underlies the all-encompassing sin of idolatry.

3. Although in sin we are alienated from our true being as image of God, God means to perfect us in all that the image implies through the redeeming work of Jesus Christ. Indeed, our perfection in the image of God is a promise of the resurrection when God's promise for the future is realized in all its fullness. (Childs 1992:94–95)

It is clear from even this brief account of the doctrine of the image of God that there are strong biblical and theological warrants for respecting the autonomy of individuals as a principle of moral obligation. That is to say, freedom and responsibility, which are the heart of autonomy, are also the heart of that personhood in relationship with God which is the essence of our existence in the image of God.

Yet even a staunch defender of autonomy in the arena of medicine, James Childress, has also cautioned that a Christian account of autonomy will need to recognize that autonomy is limited by the fact that people are both finite and sinful. Not only is our vision limited by the particularities of our finitude, but it is also easily distorted by the egocentricity of our sinful nature and its penchant for selfishness and insensitivity to the needs of others. In short, Childress recognizes the point made above that the biblical doctrine of sin tells us we are alienated from our true nature as image of God. Consequently, the principle of autonomy must constantly be placed under the criticism of a New Testament norm of love (Childress 1986), which is an antidote to unbridled independence and a reminder that we are constituted by community with God and each other.

Being in conflict with ourselves and finding ourselves in a world of conflict make freedom and responsibility a burden, to say the least. For many, it is a terror. The never-ending struggle to create structures of decision making that will add certainty (or perhaps self-justification) to freedom and responsibility is a testimony to this enduring problem of the human spirit.

It is integral to the promise of the Christian gospel that in Christ there is new freedom and new possibility for responsibility in that freedom. The Christian ethic is an expression of the freedom of the gospel. We do not love to please God; we love because it has pleased God to love us.

Martin Luther's well-known treatise *On Christian Liberty* captures the dynamic of freedom in the gospel and new possibilities for responsibility in that freedom in a most remarkable and memorable way. The premise of Luther's piece is the seeming paradox that the Christian is a perfectly free "lord" of all, servant to none, and, at the same time, a perfectly dutiful servant to all (Luther 1957:343ff.). The point of the treatise is that the assurance of our forgiveness and salvation—our justification—in Jesus Christ by faith and grace alone sets us free from the condemnation of the law. In this we are perfectly free and judged by no one. We are therefore free to bind ourselves, with an uncoerced love, to our neighbor in service. Being free from fear for ourselves, we are freed for service to others. This freedom to be bound is a new possibility for responsibility in life under the gospel promise. Rather than rising up simply to accuse us or make demands of us, the precepts of the love that Jesus teaches rise up as possibilities that we are free to pursue.

To Luther's vision I would add the additional biblical vision that the promise of the reign of God, revealed in Christ, is a promise for the fulfillment of those values that love seeks in freedom and responsibility. When in freedom and responsible love we seek to affirm life and protect it, we do so in the knowledge that life in all its fullness is the promise of God's ultimate reign. When we seek justice and equality among people, we do so in the confidence that in the fullness of God's promised dominion, there is neither slave nor free, Jew nor Greek, male nor female, but all are one in Christ. To summarize this understanding of the Christian ethic, then, the impulse of responsibility in love is born in the freedom of the gospel, and the values for which it strives are fulfilled in the free gift of the promised reign of God. The exercise of responsibility in the freedom of the gospel, striving for the values that God promises, is a testimony to the hope that is within us.

Concerning decisions at the end of life, the freedom to be bound may, in some circumstances, be a choice to endure suffering responsibly in order to honor our life and, in so doing, to honor life itself. The nuances of meaning for such a decision and its implications for others would, of course, differ significantly from case to case. A young man of my acquaintance, dying of cancer, chose to spend his last days at home with only minimal pain medication so he could remain in full conscious contact with his wife and children until the end. The multiple levels of long-lasting meaning in that choice will take a generation to discover. By contrast, one who affirms life while quietly dying alone in the hospital may touch only a passing few as she takes these last steps in a spiritual pilgrimage.

The extent to which one chooses to be bound to the value of life purely out of love and freedom will differ from case to case as well. Is the person who weighs life against death engaged in the kind of high-minded struggle St. Paul recounts as he thinks about continuing his work or going to be with Christ in death (Philippians 1)? Or is the choice for life the result of fear or the absence of help? Perhaps it is a choice by default, the inaction that comes with indecisions. I suspect that in most circumstances our decisions are forged by a variety of influences and constraints, internal as well as external. Certainly Luther recognized that the life of responsible love and Christian liberty, a sign of the new person in Christ, was always in conflict with the old person.

The ambiguity of the self, in its constantly conflicted state, is paralleled by the ambiguity of a conflictual world, which often presents us with the sort of terrible choices between competing evils that are so often the subject of ethical reflection. The freedom of the Christian in the promise of the gospel, then, is also the freedom to risk in the face of radical ambiguity. This, I take it, was Luther's meaning when he penned those famous words in his letter to Melanchthon, *Pecca fortiter, sed fortius fide et gaude in Christo* (Sin boldly, but believe and rejoice in Christ more boldly still). He did not, of course, mean that the freedom to risk was a cavalier matter, that freedom from condemnation meant freedom to sin. He meant, as theologian Dietrich Bonhoeffer has pointed out, that when all is said and done, we cannot extricate ourselves from the prevailing reality of life in a sinful world; however, we are free to boldly risk such decisions nonetheless.

As related to decisions at the end of life, the freedom to risk, responsibly, may mean a choice to end suffering and life itself, to honor life in that way, to honor divine mercy, and to embrace the promise of everlasting life. As William F. May observes in his essay in this volume, there are even some circumstances, however rare, in which the courage to kill mercifully is required. Bioethicist Kenneth Vaux, while carefully qualifying his remarks, nonetheless concludes that certain agonies of fatal disease call for the compassion our faith demands and justify euthanasia (Vaux 1989:21).

The freedom to be bound, to honor life even in the midst of suffering, is a hedge against egoism, against the arrogant absolutization of autonomy. It reminds us that we are dependent beings, *image* of God, not God. The freedom to risk making an end to suffering and life is a hedge against the absolutization of temporal, bodily existence and the glorification of human virtue through the glorification of useless suffering. I am reminded of theological ethicist Harmon Smith's wonderful paraphrase of Jesus' words, "A person does not live by life alone" (Smith 1970:125). Giving virtually unconditional value to either autonomy or bodily existence leads to idolatry. To say this, I hasten to add, is to set theological parameters for our ethical reflection; it certainly does not entail approval of euthanasia.

Let us return to Anna. Anna in her way embraced both sides of Luther's paradox. She was free to pray for death in the spirit of gospel freedom, not absolutizing her bodily existence. But she was free to be bound to respect for the life that was in herself by simply awaiting God's deliverance, not absolutizing her self-determination. It may be argued that ending her life was not a choice she really had. To be sure, Anna's choices were spiritual choices, not courses of action, but they were no less real. Moreover, there is a range of cases—usually described as "allowing to die" cases, often including "double-effect" decisions to medicate for the relief of suffering even when such treatment shortens life—in which an attempt is also made to affirm the paradoxical dimension of freedom and responsibility; responsibly and freely deciding to uphold and honor life, however diminished, and yet free not to absolutize physical life or make a virtue of suffering; free to seek or provide release.

Certainly we see many examples of persons who simply accept, affirm, and live their lives despite being reduced to debilitated conditions that many of us would consider unendurable.

Just as certainly we know of cases that take us beyond the best efforts of the most insightful casuistry, where nothing remains except the promise of our freedom to sin boldly. I am put in mind of a friend's recent story about a colleague of his who had gone home to die from the cancer that was eating away his body. As the end drew near, the family called my friend's wife, a registered nurse, to come and sit with them, for the last hours were proving to be terrible. This man's agonies of pain during his final hours simply overpowered the multiple-strength doses of morphine that the doctor had prescribed to relieve the pain. After death finally came, my friend's wife returned home and confided her firm conviction that, had she had something by which to end his life then and there, she would have done so. At times we are driven beyond the certainty of a logical resolution to a different level of certainty, one born of compassion and set free by the gospel.

Though Anna was not in savage pain, little of her life that I could fathom or imagine made sense. I wanted her death as ardently as she herself did. And yet the witness of her faith brought a dignity to that life which has made a lasting impression upon me and doubtless upon others, leaving me to affirm the ambiguity of her circumstance as she seems tacitly to have done in the expression of her faith.

Again, the increasing public debate about autonomy in our choices at the end of life is heightened by the growing conviction that medicine has gone too far in its effort to prolong life. As Daniel Callahan has observed, interest in euthanasia is often spurred by fear of what medicine might do to us (Callahan 1989:4, 6). To assert our autonomy, then, is to assert our right to control the conditions of our dying and to curb the pretenses of medical science. There is, of course, an irony in all of this. We want to control the medical science and technology that we created to bring disease and death under control. We want to be emancipated from the power of a technology designed to free us from the power of disease and death. Freedom continually turns into bondage and requires new efforts at freedom. The freedom of the Christian, as we have been discussing it, is in a profound sense freedom from freedom itself—that is, freedom from the bondage of having continually to free ourselves by ourselves, the freedom to be the *image* of God, and to let God be God.

Mercy and Justice

The Bible connects mercy and justice in a way that is important to our concern.

First of all, mercy is an expression of God's forgiving and God's desire to be reunited with us by ending our estrangement. Divine forgiveness expresses the same compassion of God that we meet in the Hebrew Scriptures. The richly nuanced concept *chesed*, loving-kindness, encompasses God's deliverance of the people from suffering and captivity, the bounty of nature that God provides for the fullness of life, and God's intervention in history to renew continually the covenant with Israel and with all humankind.

The understanding of forgiving love as mercy is clearly a dominant motif in the New Testament. Unmerited forgiveness of sin is at the heart of God's merciful promise of salvation (Ephesians 2:4, Titus 3:5, Hebrews 4:16, 1 Peter 1:3, Jude 21). As forgiveness restores life, wholeness, and community in the reign of God, so God's mercy extends to the suffering and needs of the whole person. Jesus' works of healing and feeding and his teaching of God's mercy are ample testimony to that truth. In Mark's account of the healing of the paralytic (Mark 2), Jesus makes the closest possible connection between healing and forgiving and relates both to the divine power and intention that he claims for himself. In the mercy of God, healing, life, wholeness, relief of suffering, and the forgiveness of sin are deeply interrelated. Thus, in the Greek *eleos*, as in the Hebrew *chesed*, is combined compassionate forgiveness and compassionate concern for the needs of the whole person and for all manner of human suffering. This comprehensive understanding of mercy is the foundation for seeking justice in biblical terms (Crosby 1988:163).

The biblical understanding of justice is not an abstract set of principles and laws, designed to provide a canon of fairness for society or an intricate expression of various rights, either natural or conferred. Principles and laws are certainly necessary, but they are fulfilled only when they are infused with the compassion of mercy. Thus Jesus confronts the Pharisees in Matthew 9:13: "Go and learn what this means, 'I desire mercy, not sacrifice.'" Strict adherence to religious codes, analogous to strict adherence to civil law or some account of justice, is shallow righteousness, lukewarm justice, if it lacks the warm blood of mercy and compassion (Childs 1992:64).

The biblical understanding that justice must be fueled by mercy in an often cruel and tragic world is illustrated by the jubilee tradition in the Old Testament and the appropriation of that tradition in the New Testament. The Old Testament tradition of the jubilee year is discussed in Leviticus 25. There we find that, at every fiftieth year, liberty is to be proclaimed throughout the nation and all those who have been dispossessed for their debts to be forgiven their debts and restored to their land and to their families. This jubilee decree appears to have its background in sabbath-year provisions, which also included the forgiveness of debt, the release from slavery imposed by unpaid debts, and the restoration of land and family (Childs 1992:64).

Both biblical scholars and ethicists have seen in the jubilee tradition an image of biblical justice as liberation or deliverance (Ringe 1985:16–32; Lebacqz 1987:122–35). The provisions of the jubilee, which bear little resemblance to any accepted practices of economic justice, demonstrate that the Bible regards justice from the vantage point of those in need rather than from the perspective of distributive and retributive principles of obligation. The jubilee tradition combines forgiveness of debt with concern to end suffering, meet human needs, and restore human community.

The closely knit meanings of mercy that underlie justice in the jubilee tradition are embraced by Jesus in Luke 4 when he chooses Isaiah 61:1–2, which echoes the jubilee tradition, to help define his person and work as the Messiah.

We who have received mercy are called upon to show mercy. The words of the prophet Micah are well known to us: "He has told you, O mortal, what is good; and what does the Lord require of you but to do justice, and to love kindness, and to walk humbly with your God?" (Micah 6:8, NRSV). And, of course, Luke's gospel enjoins us to be merciful as God is merciful (6:36). Indeed, the Beatitudes, which pronounce a blessing upon the merciful (Matthew 5:7), suggest that we are not only commanded to imitate the mercy of God but empowered to do so as well. As Robert Guelich has pointed out, the word conventionally translated as "blessed" might better be rendered as "congratulations." The implication of this observation is that something is being conferred rather than demanded (Guelich 1982:67). So we say, congratulations, you can be merciful, for God has given you the grace to be so.

In connection with our concerns over assisted suicide and euthanasia, the biblical linkage between mercy and justice and the call of the faithful to be merciful suggests to me this question: Is our sense of justice fueled by mercy?

One of the many nuances of meaning for *justice* is the upholding of what is right. In the minds of many people, upholding what is right in matters of euthanasia has meant prohibition against assisted suicide and euthanasia. Yet the Bible warns us that justice without mercy can easily become a cruel exercise in self-justification. In telling the story of Anna, I mentioned fretting about my own role and effectiveness in my ministry to her. My compassionate care for Anna was deflected, at least to a significant degree, by my preoccupation with "doing the right thing," both professionally and theologically. Preoccupation with one's own rectitude can too easily become a concern with self-justification and lead one to lose sight of the profoundest meaning of the gospel—that it is God alone who justifies. I missed giving something to Anna, I suspect, because I worried that I was giving so little or giving the wrong thing. Justice without mercy, upholding the right thing purely for its own sake and without compassion for the people affected, betrays an absence of the kind of freedom in the gospel that makes compassion possible.

I am reminded of Harriet Goetz's reflections on the way in which one's adherence to an absolute standard may be called into question:

> I deeply admire those Christians who are attempting to live the seamless garment ethic—to be utterly consistent in their pro-life values, allowing no wrinkles or tears in that holy garment. But as I look into a face distorted with pain, I would have to question whether I was more concerned with my seamless garment than another's suffering. There is a line in a novel by Penelope Lively that makes this point: "Tell the man on the guillotine that the action lies elsewhere." Likewise, tell the man on his bed of pain that the action is really to be found in my system of ethics or in hospital procedure manuals or in the law of the land. The dying one might think otherwise. (Goetz 1989:620–21)

One suspects that what Goetz calls for in some circumstances of dire suffering is a kind of jubilee. That is, when justice is fueled by mercy, compassionate efforts to relieve suffering may need to triumph over strict adherence to legal and moral sanctions for the preservation of life.

To be sure, just as the jubilee tradition can hardly form the basis for social policy in matters of economic justice, so considerations of mercy alone will not suffice to establish just policies regarding euthanasia and assisted suicide in an ambiguous world.

Certainly the Lutheran tradition, from which I come, has drawn distinctions between the exercise of personal love and compassion, on the one hand, and the formulation of law and the establishment of justice, on the other. This is Luther's two-realms distinction. Patterns of law and justice under the civil use of divine law need to be established and rigorously upheld to prevent evil and reward good. This is an expression of God's left-hand mode of ruling, and God entrusts it to the appropriate authorities. In their personal lives Christians uphold that law but go beyond it in the spirit of Christlike love for the neighbor. This is the manifestation of God's right-hand mode of ruling in the hearts of believers through the gospel of Jesus Christ.

I will not rehearse the history of the various distortions and dualisms that have come out of Luther's two-kingdoms concept. It has often led to a separation of love (mercy) and justice. This separation has tended to frustrate the influence of love on the development of justice (Childs 1978:30–31). Suffice it to say for the present that the separation of love from justice is not entailed, not even in Luther's thought per se. On the contrary, love and the manifestation of love in mercy shapes, judges, and informs justice and the law. Justice is a principle of love. It is an avenue through which love expresses its care and concern for all people. Love is richer than justice and is more than justice, in the same way that mercy transcends the law of the land in the jubilee. The law is necessary, as Luther saw, to preserve life and the common good in an evil world. At the same time, he also saw, along with Luke in the Book of Acts, that we must, when forced to choose, obey God rather than human ordinances (Luther 1962:111). Therefore, while we need to make and sustain laws that preserve life in appropriate ways, we also need to bring them continually under the judgment and influence of mercy and love. To absolutize the law in separation from mercy and love would betray the Reformation insight that the only thing absolute is the mercy of God.

Anna never spoke of suicide. We cannot know what she might have thought or said about the discussion in these essays in light of her own situation. Sanctioning assisted suicide was not even an issue for the society of her day, let alone for persons of her piety. We do know, however, that she had the mercy of God's promise to sustain her in her faith and the ministry of those who brought her that word. For her, it seems, that was sufficient comfort, even though she wanted desperately the release of death. For some that is not sufficient comfort when the ravages of pain and dying press upon them. Where is the mercy of God for them? This is the kind of insistent question people like Harriet Goetz keep raising. In the name of God's mercy, how do we correlate our obligations to preserve life and to relieve suffering? Attempting a final and definitive answer to that question is dangerous. To stop asking it is more dangerous still.

Much more can be said concerning justice and mercy, especially in connection with a just system of health care delivery and its relation to assisted suicide and euthanasia. We will probe this connection as we reflect now on our final thematic pair, recognizing that *caring* especially is closely akin to the mercy that animates biblical justice.

Healing and Caring

Theologically speaking, healing is related to salvation. In the New Testament we see that Jesus' works of healing are connected to his saving mission.

To heal is to knit together and make whole. That is what the love of God in Christ does in a world of estrangement and alienation. Paul Tillich has taught us that the demonic tears the very fabric of reality and that the love of God, which we are called to show as well, has as its object the reunification of the separated (Tillich 1963:136–38). This reunification, this healing, is perceived at every level of existence. It begins with the saving work of the Christ whereby God in Christ reconciles the estranged world to God's own self (2 Corinthians 5:19).

It spills over into reunification of persons and communities that are at enmity with one another through the ministry of reconciliation. Powered by God's grace, we are called to heal the breaches so that the anticipatory, eschatological community can truly be described as the body of Christ. In that body all, in their individual diversity, are knit together in an organic unity; they live under the abiding admonition to be what they are and to maintain the unity of the Spirit in the bond of peace (Ephesians 4:3). With the command to love our enemies, all barriers to reconciliation are removed in principle and in hope.

The reunification of the separated, the healing of divisions, is true also within persons themselves. Again, it is Paul who speaks of division and tension in the self that is at war with itself: "for I do not do the good that I want but the evil I do not want is what I do. . . . Who will rescue me from this body of death?" (Romans 7:19, 24). Paul speaks of the spiritual reality of a life troubled by the struggle between the old person and the new, between the already and the not-yet. But he also connects the struggle with sin to death and the body, reinforcing the connection between the forgiving love of God and a holistic sense of healing.

The peace of God that passes all understanding, the peace pronounced and conferred upon the disciples by the risen Christ, is the gospel message that in him God's *shalom*, wholeness, is fulfilled.

Anna's life was ravaged by divisions within, not only the more common spiritual conflicts we all have but the profound lesions inflicted by her mental and physical disease and the way in which conditions cut her off from authentic community. Thus, it seemed important to hold her hand and simply be there. Ultimately, though brokenness and death are theologically related, for Anna, in light of the promise, only death would bring healing. In the meantime, the promise of the healing that Christ accomplished kept final despair at bay while she awaited that welcome passage. Perhaps even the touch of an anxious young man was a conduit of healing grace, trifling and ambiguous though it was in many ways.

By connecting healing with the love of God and the neighbor love to which it gives birth, we have already moved into the realm of caring. In so doing, I want to recall remarks about justice and mercy that are siblings to these thoughts on caring.

Justice fueled by mercy will distribute and administer the goods of health care not only "according to need" as opposed to "merit" or "ability to pay," for example, but also according to need in terms of the needs of people being served rather than the needs of the institutions serving them. This, it seems to me, is a way of expressing a key feature of justice, *participation*, the inclusion of those most affected in the determination of the institutions and policies affecting them (in this sense, justice affirms autonomy over paternalism). The health care system will thus be truly caring in dedication to health or healing rather than to system.

Could Anna have been better cared for? Would it have mattered? I'm in no position to hand down indictments, but I suspect the answer to both is yes. In part, her depression was the illness, but in part it was the endless days of being utterly alone while surrounded by a cacophony of strange sounds from troubled people.

Yet the kind of caring required for Anna's healing is a tall order to fill. In *Prisoners of Men's Dreams*, Suzanne Gordon examines how the feminist dream of humanizing the workplace has fared as more and more women have made gains in business and professional life. Her answer: not very well. Instead, it is the women who are being transformed in large numbers. Why? To a great extent, this happens because we have created a society in which, at least among the fortunate, our ambitions and expectations create demands that crowd out the space and the aptitude to care. A new vision is needed to liberate both women and men for caring (Gordon 1991:274–75, 286–87). Clearly, the Christian community has a powerful vision of caring and the freedom to care in the manifold meanings of the gospel promise we have been exploring. It is ours to share. And for caregivers who need help and comfort to manage the task, the promise is there as well.

In the Beatitudes Jesus announces the possibility of mourning as a virtue of love. The capacity for mourning, more than simply grief over loss, is a gift of grace, the gift of being attuned to human suffering and the ability to be genuinely *with* those who suffer just as the Christ, in his incarnation, is Immanuel, "God with us." The aptitude for this profound empathy stands in contrast to our natural tendency to recoil from those who are dying or suffering terribly. It is an expression of love's readiness to accept everyone in need without qualification and without regard to the attractiveness of the other. It is a virtue that recalls for us Paul Ramsey's admonition to care for the dying, to keep company with them in their last moments of life (Ramsey 1970:114).

From the Christian perspective, healing and caring are expressions of that love born of the gospel promise, the love that knits together as, indeed, the love of Christ has knit us together, with God, within ourselves, and with one another. Such healing and caring love certainly give support to movements like hospice. It is in tune with the observation (made by Ann Dudley Goldblatt elsewhere in this volume and by others) that the legalization of euthanasia and assisted suicide is unjust in the absence of universal health care.

Had she had a more caring, healing community, Anna might still have wished for death, but she might have done so with greater serenity. This is true of countless others in more severe suffering at the end stages of life. Insofar as we affirm the responsibility for life as a personal, moral obligation to ourselves, the community has some responsibility to do all that it can to help us fulfill that obligation. Beyond providing needed health care and community for the suffering and dying, we need to concern ourselves with such basic issues as pain management. Ethicist Stephen Post connects our poor record in addressing the medical science of pain management with our society's more general tendency to undervalue caring and the endurance it requires (Post 1991:35–36).

Through caring we witness penultimate healings that make real and keep alive the promise of ultimate healing in the resurrection in God's dominion. I experienced something of that in the death of my own mother. After a time of growing apart, I came to her in the hospital where she was suffering from cancer. I walked the corridor with her and expressed my love and concern for her well-being. That night she said to my father, "He must really love me. Did you see how concerned he was?" The next day she died as I held her hand and recalled aloud the promises of the baptismal liturgy, the recollection of her baptism into the death and resurrection of Jesus Christ. The healing of our relationship prepared the way for her ultimate healing. There are many such stories.

I have argued for the possibility of an effective Christian witness in a pluralistic society, and I have tried to uncover some of the resources of the faith for that witness. Assisted suicide and euthanasia were once "settled questions" in public opinion, among medical professionals, and within communities of faith. The question of legalization was not even voiced. Obviously, this is no longer the case. Yet, in a real sense, for those who speak out of the Christian faith, very little has changed. Our commitment to the sanctity of life remains the same. Our recognition that ultimately life is dependent upon God for its origin and its hope also remains the same. What has changed is a growing desire for autonomy in our society and a whole set of new circumstances that prolong suffering and dying as a by-product of the advance of medical science. But the experience of these changes only serves to deepen our abiding sense of the tragedy and ambiguity of life and to drive us ever deeper into the liberating realization of our dependence upon the grace of God in Jesus Christ. In that freedom of the promise we are delivered from bondage to arrogant forms of autonomy and the judgment they finally bring upon us. We are free to be formed by the grace of God in uncoerced virtues that are stronger than self-will: courage and love.

REFERENCES

Brock, Dan W. 1992. "Voluntary Active Euthanasia." *Hastings Center Report* 22 (March–April): 10–22.

Callahan, Daniel. 1989. "Can We Return Death to Disease?" *Hastings Center Report* 19, no. 1, Special Supplement (January–February): 4–6.

Childress, James F. 1986. "Autonomy." In *Westminster Dictionary of Christian Ethics*, ed. James F. Childress and John Macquarrie. Philadelphia: Westminster Press.

Childs, James M., Jr. 1978. *Christian Anthropology and Ethics*. Philadelphia: Fortress Press.

———. 1992. *Faith, Formation, and Decision*. Minneapolis: Fortress Press.

Crosby, Michael H. 1988. *House of Disciples*. Maryknoll, N.Y.: Orbis Books.

Engelhardt, H. Tristram, Jr. 1989. "Fashioning an Ethic for Life and Death in a Post-Modern Society." *Hastings Center Report* 19, no. 1, Special Supplement (January–February): 7–9.

Goetz, Harriet. 1989. "Euthanasia: A Bedside View." *Christian Century*, 22–28 June, 619–22.

Gordon, Suzanne. 1991. *Prisoners of Men's Dreams*. Boston: Little, Brown.

Guelich, Robert A. 1982. *The Sermon on the Mount*. Waco, Tex.: Word Books.

Küng, Hans. 1991. *Global Responsibility*. New York: Crossroad.

Lebacqz, Karen. 1987. *Justice in an Unjust World*. Minneapolis: Augsburg Press.

Luther, Martin. 1957. "Freedom of a Christian," trans. W. A. Lambert and rev. Harold J. Grimm. In vol. 31 of *Luther's Works*. Philadelphia: Muhlenberg Press.

———. 1962. "Temporal Authority: To What Extent It Should Be Obeyed," trans. J. J. Schindel and rev. Walther I. Brandt. In vol. 45 of *Luther's Works*. Philadelphia: Muhlenberg Press.

Perry, Michael J. 1991. *Love and Power*. New York and Oxford: Oxford University Press.

Post, Stephen G. 1991. "American Culture and Euthanasia." *Health Progress* (December): 32–38.

Ramsey, Paul. 1970. *The Patient as Person*. New Haven: Yale University Press.

Ringe, Sharon. 1985. *Jesus, Liberation, and the Biblical Jubilee*. Philadelphia: Fortress Press.

Smith, Harmon L. 1970. *Ethics and the New Medicine*. Nashville: Abingdon Press.

Thielicke, Helmut. 1966. *Theological Ethics*, vol. 1. Ed. William H. Lazareth. Philadelphia: Fortress Press.

Thiemann, Ronald F. 1991. *Constructing a Public Theology*. Louisville, Ky.: Westminster/John Knox Press.

Tillich, Paul. 1957. "The Protestant Principle and the Proletarian Situation." In *The Protestant Era*, abridged ed., trans. James Luther Adams, 161–81. Chicago: University of Chicago Press.

————. 1963. *Systematic Theology*. Chicago: University of Chicago Press. (See especially vol. 3.)

Vaux, Kenneth. 1989. "The Theologic Ethics of Euthanasia." *Hastings Center Report* 19, no. 1, Special Supplement (January–February): 19–22.

CHAPTER 10

Assisted Suicide and Euthanasia: A Biblical and Reformed Perspective

Allen Verhey

I am an evangelical, according to a letter from the Park Ridge Center. Now, I am usually happy to be called an evangelical, for I take the term to identify me as one who longs to think and to live my life in the light and power of the gospel, the good news, the evangel.

But different people take the term to mean different things—and sometimes things I am not happy to be called. Some, for example, take the term to mean a fundamentalist with manners. And some associate the term with bumper sticker warnings of imminent rapture. Set aside such stereotypes, however, and the term remains a slippery one. Different people use it in different ways, and not altogether coherently.

I am also a Calvinist, a Protestant formed and informed by the Reformed, or Presbyterian, tradition. It says so in the same letter. And I am usually happy to be called a Calvinist, for I take the term to identify me as one who longs to form and to transform the whole of culture in the light and power of that same gospel.[1]

But different people take the term *Calvinist* to mean different things, too, and sometimes things that I would rather not be identified with. Some, for example, take the term to mean a capitalist with piety. And some infer that I must be a hard determinist. A close reading of

Calvin might set aside such stereotypes, but even so, this term, too, remains a little slippery.

Evangelical and *Calvinist*—the terms are fluid, but so are the terms that I have been invited to consider from my particular Christian tradition and community. Justice and mercy, suffering and dying, healing and caring, freedom and responsibility—these, too, are slippery terms. These, too, are used in different ways, and not altogether coherently. The meanings shift when the terms are embedded in different accounts of the fundamental meaning of human life and its flourishing, and they shift again when that embeddedness is denied.

I will attempt to provide an evangelical and Reformed understanding of these notions and of their relevance to the questions raised by assisted suicide and euthanasia, and I will attempt to contrast such an understanding with other accounts of the meaning of these terms and of their implications. Permit me to begin, however, in a way familiar and fundamental to anyone formed by the sort of evangelical and Reformed communities that formed me: by attending to Scripture. The text is Matthew 27:3–10, the story of Judas's suicide:

> When Judas, his betrayer, saw that he was condemned, he repented and brought back the thirty pieces of silver to the chief priests and the elders, saying, "I have sinned in betraying innocent blood." They said, "What is that to us? See to it yourself." And throwing down the pieces of silver in the temple, he departed; and he went and hanged himself. But the chief priests, taking the pieces of silver, said, "It is not lawful to put them into the treasury, since they are blood money." So they took counsel, and bought with them the potter's field, to bury strangers in. Therefore that field has been called the Field of Blood to this day. Then was fulfilled what had been spoken by the prophet Jeremiah, saying, "And they took the thirty pieces of silver, the price of him on whom a price had been set by some of the sons of Israel, and they gave them for the potter's field, as the Lord directed me."

It is, you will agree, a curious story, and one that has caused no little embarrassment.

The story has been embarrassing to those evangelicals who have insisted on the so-called inerrancy of Scripture, for a quite different story is told of Judas's death in Acts 1:18–19. There, for example, there is no hint of suicide. But I am not interested today in Scripture's contribution to the work of historical reconstruction. I am interested, rather, in Scripture's contribution to moral formation. Evangelical and Reformed communities have always sought to be "people of the book."

The passage is also embarrassing to the one who takes Scripture to be, if not a manipulable oracle, at least a timeless moral code and who expects to find in it a moral rule that articulates and substantiates a conviction widely shared in evangelical and Reformed communities, that is, that suicide is a sin prohibited by Scripture. It is not there, not here in Matthew 27, not anywhere.[2] Some people (but no evangelical that I know of) have read the silence of Scripture as if in such silence Scripture either whispered an implicit approval or shouted a divine indifference to suicide.[3] Such readings may be accused of the same fault of which some evangelicals are often accused: assuming that Scripture intends to provide a manipulable oracle or a timeless code for the moral life.

The story is also a little embarrassing because Christians have sometimes read it—along with other parts of Matthew's story of the passion—"against the Jews." An anti-Semitic reading of Matthew's gospel is simple but wrong. The community that Matthew instructed and defended was a Christian community that included Gentiles but which was still largely Jewish. Moreover, the community was instructed to treasure its Jewish heritage and to be faithful to it. To read Matthew's story "against the Jews" is not to read it faithfully or to remember faithfully the Jesus whose story he told. Indeed, it is clear that Jesus is "handed over" by one of his own, by one of those who followed him, by one who belongs (allowing the anachronism) to the church. There is no faithful reading of the text without discipline, without humility, without the readiness to read Scripture not only "for ourselves" but "against our-selves" (Bonhoeffer 1985:185, 308–25),[4] over against our own lives, in judgment upon them and not just in self-serving defense of them, over against even our own conventional reading of biblical texts, subverting our efforts to use Scripture to boast about our own righteousness.

Beyond the specific minor embarrassments associated with this passage, it should be admitted candidly that the attempt to read Scripture as if it were relevant to twentieth-century issues in medical ethics is itself a little embarrassing. The problems are obvious enough: there is the silence of Scripture, the strangeness of Scripture, the diver-sity of Scripture, and the undeniable fact that appeals to Scripture have sometimes done a great deal of harm. Moreover, modern medicine seems a thoroughly secular enterprise. And contemporary medical ethics—concerned as it frequently is with narrowly focused quandaries and questions of regulation in a religiously pluralistic society—seems to require (and surely prefers) arguments that are not tied to a particular community's memory.

Nevertheless, that sort of embarrassment is an acceptable risk to one who is evangelical and Reformed. For to be such means that one longs to live the story one loves to hear, longs to live (and give birth and suffer and die, and care for those giving birth, suffering, and dying final-ly) in ways that are formed, reformed, and transformed by the gospel. This longing is not served by ignoring the resources of the tradition or by silencing the peculiar voices of Scripture. Scripture, the evangelical and Reformed communities insist, is not merely an archaic relic in an age of science and reason; it still evokes loyalties, still forms character and conduct into dispositions and deeds "worthy of the gospel," and it still calls for the transformation of the world. And testimony to Scripture's account of the moral life as "good news" still belongs to the task of an evangelical and Reformed ethic. Even if that ethic cannot pro-vide a foundation for such an account in the impartial, rational, and uni-versal principles of the culture of liberalism, it need not and may not suppose that such an account will not be recognizable as good—and as good news—in a world God made. The Calvinist is confident that the human sense of dependence, gratitude, remorse, hope, and responsibility still looks for and finds confirmation and fulfillment in the story of Scripture and in lives formed by it.[5]

Enough of these introductory remarks. Enough has been said, I hope, to make it clear that reading Scripture faithfully—and "performing" it creatively, to use the apt phrase of Nicholas Lash (1986:37–46)—will require discernment. Discernment is the virtue of being able to recognize "fittingness." In reading Scripture, discernment is the ability to recognize the plot of the whole story, to see the wholeness of Scripture, and to order the interpretation of any part toward that whole. And in reading Scripture as "profitable . . . for training in righteousness" (2 Timothy 3:16), discernment is the ability to plot our lives to "fit" the whole of Scripture, to order every part of our lives—including the endings of them—toward that whole. The questions, then, for evangelical and Reformed communities become whether certain notions of justice and mercy, suffering and dying, healing and caring, freedom and responsibility fit the story of Scripture, and whether assisted suicide and euthanasia cohere with the story we long to live as the story of our lives and deaths.

The Story of Judas—and of Jesus

It is time to return to the story of Judas. But if what I have just said is right, then we may only return to the story of Judas as a part of the whole. It is not by itself, after all, the story that should form our lives, our character and conduct, but it is, as part of the whole, a story that belongs to Christian reflection about the moral life and a good death. The story of Judas's suicide is part of the story Matthew tells in memory of Jesus, but at the beginning of that story Matthew points us back to creation, and at the end of it Matthew points us forward "to the close of the age" (Matthew 28:20). The whole story, according to Matthew, moves from creation to final fulfillment by the grace of God made known and made real in Jesus.

The Gospel of St. Matthew deliberately evokes Jewish remembrance of the stories of Genesis in its opening line: "This is the book of the generations of Jesus the Messiah, son of David, son of Abraham."[6] And when Matthew makes both a refrain and a central theological category of "fulfillment,"[7] it is no less the Torah than the Prophets that is fulfilled rather than broken, and no less Genesis than Exodus. In Jesus of Nazareth the story of creation is brought to its fruition. Judas, in betraying Jesus, betrays the God who "in the beginning" signaled the good gifts of life and flourishing with breath and with a blessing. And his suicide is of one piece with such a betrayal.

Creation, of course, is only the beginning of the story. It continues with the story of human sin. It is a dreadful mystery, but this much is clear: the fault was not in God and not in nature. The fault was in a human choice. Somehow human freedom was not received as a gift but asserted against the one who gave it and called to humanity in the midst of it. Freely humanity refused to depend on God, on whom their freedom depended as its source and destiny. Humanity attempted to seize what could only be received from the gracious hand of God. Its grasping at freedom in the demand to be "autonomous," to be a law to themselves, brought not freedom but bondage, a voluntary bondage to the powers of sin and death that usurp God's rule and resist God's cause. In its wake came death and a curse.

The story of human sin did not end with Adam's fall but continued in Cain's murder of Abel and in what Matthew calls the flow of "all the righteous blood shed on earth, from the blood of righteous Abel to the blood of Zechariah" (Matthew 23:35).[8] And that blood continued to flow, of course, when Herod slaughtered the innocent children of Bethlehem (Matthew 2:16–18).[9] Finally, Judas repeats the same old story of human sin, "betraying innocent blood." And by his betrayal he subjects both himself and Jesus to the powers of sin and death. It is not shocking that death and woe follow the deed (compare Matthew 26:24); his suicide fits the story.

Human sin is not the end of the story, either, however. Sin and death are not the first words about our world, nor the last words. Human sin might have smashed a cosmos back to chaos, but God sustained it and restrained the effects of sin upon it. God called to humanity in the midst of bondage, and that call provided once again and ever again the source and destiny of human freedom. There is the story of wrath and judgment, of course, of God destroying the world with a flood. But God renews the divine intentions of life and flourishing and freedom. The signs of it are a rainbow and God's own sanction against shedding the blood of one made in God's "own image" (Genesis 9:6; compare Matthew 26:52b).

Then God created a people, a peculiar people, a people set apart from others in order to be a blessing to "all the families of the earth" (Genesis 12:3). Among this people there were storytellers and lawgivers and priests and prophets and sages who struggled to find words fit for remembrance and apt for instruction in righteousness, for training against the powers of sin and death. The storytellers celebrated life, and the lawgivers set among the laws a command, "You shall not kill" (Exodus 20:13). The prophets both spoke God's word against the shedding of innocent blood and risked their lives for the sake of God's cause and covenant. And sages formed and tested wisdom by experience. They knew that the innocent sometimes suffer. They knew as well as any prophet that piety is not always prudent. And they knew "a living dog is better than a dead lion" (Ecclesiastes 9:4). It is little wonder that the people formed and reformed by these stories and by this law, by these words prophetic or sage, have toasted life (*l'hayyim*) and celebrated human flourishing, even while they endured both martyrdom and suffering for the sake of fidelity. It is little wonder that the Talmud prohibited suicide or that contemporary Jewish communities continue to prohibit it.[10]

Among this people there was Jesus of Nazareth, whose story Matthew tells as a story of fulfillment and whose story Christians celebrate as a story of promise. Jesus came announcing that the good future of God, the "kingdom of God," the end of the rule of sin and death, was "at hand" (Matthew 4:17), and he made that future present by his words of blessing and his works of healing. Like the prophets, Jesus was ready to suffer and die. He did not "choose" death or suffering, not for himself and not for any other, but he was ready voluntarily to endure both for the sake of God's cause in a world not yet under the unchallenged rule of God.

Suffer and die he does—on a Roman cross. And there he makes the human cry of lament his own while sharing the certainty of a hearing at the end of it (Matthew 27:46; compare Psalm 22:1, 29–31). He was "handed over" by Judas to the priests, by the priests to Pilate, by Pilate to suffering and death. And when the powers of death and doom had done their damnedest, God raised him up, defeating the powers of sin and death, vindicating Jesus as Lord and Christ, and assuring God's own good future when "death shall be no more; neither shall there be mourning nor crying nor pain any more" (Revelation 21:4). Since that day the symbol of God's intention has been not only breath and a rainbow, not only a commandment, but an empty tomb. And since that day the sign of God's presence "to the close of the age" has been a cross.

The story of Jesus' passion is remembered by each of the evangelists. Indeed, the gospels decisively tie the memories of Jesus as healer and teacher to the remembrance of the cross. There is no remembering Jesus that neglects the story of his suffering and death.

Matthew's story of the passion of Jesus, like Mark's, shows Jesus being rejected, betrayed, deserted, denied, condemned, mocked, and killed. The Jewish chief priests and elders play a role in Jesus' suffering, but so does Pilate. Both renege on their responsibilities to protect the innocent (and both use the same words to do it, "See to it yourself"; Matthew 27:4, 24). The crowds who cry out for Jesus to be crucified

play a role in the story of Jesus' suffering, but so do the disciples of
Jesus, who "deserted him and fled" (26:56). And among those disciples
Judas and Peter play perhaps the largest roles of all. The two seem to be
deliberately paired by Matthew: at the supper, at the arrest, and at the
ends of their respective stories. Their ends are described in parallel
terms: Peter "went out and wept bitterly" (26:75), and Judas "went and
hanged himself" (27:5). And that is the last the reader of Matthew's
gospel hears of either of them.

Matthew does not pause to provide a moral judgment about the
suicide of Judas. He does not have to. The Jewish tradition he cherish-
es would leave little doubt about the appropriate judgment on the act.
Matthew simply reports it as part of Judas's story, and it "fits" that story.

It seems his destiny in a way. Jesus says at supper, "Woe to that one
by whom the Son of Man is betrayed! It would have been better for
that one not to have been born" (Matthew 26:24). Such words of woe
make known God's future judgment as surely as words of blessing make
present God's future triumph.[11] Matthew is quite uninterested in the
question of Judas's "freedom" when he chooses to kill himself, quite
unconcerned about whether in this discrete action Judas exercises a
rational autonomy. The crucial choice had been made some time
before, and now he seems almost fated to die at his own hand. The end
of the story of Judas in Matthew's gospel is a tragic one.

It may be helpful to follow Matthew's lead and to set Peter's weeping alongside Judas's suicide. These are not pretty scenes. Breathless
from his sobbing, Peter gasps for air and for his spirit. He is a broken
man, a crushed rock. And Judas hangs, his face, too, contorted, his body
bent. Perhaps he gasps for air and for his spirit hanging from that rope.
He, too, is a broken man, a crushed spirit.

Peter's weeping and Judas's suicide are sad stories, the tragic endings of stories of denial and betrayal. It is not given to us to penetrate
into the motives for Peter's denial or Judas's betrayal. But these are sad
stories of good men who could not or would not understand that Jesus

is the Christ as the suffering one and that to be his disciple is to share in his suffering. These are tragedies, stories of good men with flawed vision.[12] They thought the world the sort of place where suffering could be avoided. They learned too late that it is not so. They learned too late that in a world like this one, it's not a question of whether to suffer or not, but whom we will suffer with and what we will suffer for.

These are sad stories, tragedies, because they speak of good men who lack not only understanding but the virtues required of discipleship. Peter lacked courage. He wanted to follow a way that led to Palm Sunday, but not a path that led all the way to Good Friday. God forbid that such a thing should happen to Jesus—or to him! It would make discipleship too costly. Discipleship would require heroism. Surely the way ought to lead to success, to triumph, not to suffering and death.

Judas lacked not courage but patience. Unlike Peter he may have been ready to die for the sake of God's triumph, but he was also ready to kill. He had given his life to this cause; he had committed himself to the triumph of God against all the self-serving pettiness of rulers like Pilate and the self-serving piety of religious people who collaborated with his ilk. Perhaps the betrayal was, as some have suggested, a desperate attempt to provoke a confrontation between this Jesus who would not fight the necessary battle and the rulers who held the power. Judas was ready to seize what could only be received. He was ready to do evil that the good might come. He was unwilling to endure patiently, unwilling to depend on the gracious sovereignty of God, unwilling to wait for God to vindicate Jesus and God's own cause. He was ready and eager to take matters into his own hands. He would take responsibility for seeing that things turned out right.

These are sad stories, finally, because Peter and Judas suffer. Peter suffers now from his earlier attempt to avoid suffering. It's a tragedy, the story of a good man who would save his life and, in the effort, lost it, the story of a man who learned too late that the only way to save his life was to give it up. He suffers now because in denying Jesus, he has denied his own identity; he has denied himself. He has said "I am not me" when he said "I am not a follower of Jesus." He chose not to suffer with Jesus and thus with all who suffer. He chose not to suffer for the sake of God's cause in the world or for his own integrity. So he ended up suffering anyway, but alone and pointlessly, with no one and for the illusion of a world right now in which there is no suffering.

And Judas suffers too, of course. When he saw that Jesus was condemned, did he lose the little hope left that he could provoke the confrontation with the powers that would invoke legions of angels? Such hopelessness is killing sad. When he saw Jesus condemned, did his loyalty to Jesus and his loyalty to God's good future seem caught in an irreconcilable conflict? Such a threat to one's integrity is killing sad. When he saw Jesus condemned, did the life he had lived in discipleship seem pointless and the life he had yet to live seem senseless? Such purposelessness is killing sad. The very tragedy of Judas ought to keep us from judging him too quickly or too severely. Surely in that killing sadness, a piece of halakah, a rule against suicide, however carefully crafted, might not be enough to prevent his suicide. What he needed was grace, not law.

Of course, Matthew's congregation knew it was not the end of the story for Peter. It knew that Peter had finally learned well what he had learned so slowly and that he had died a martyr's death at the hands of Nero's lackeys. It knew that Peter's weeping was repentance and that the one who raised Jesus from the dead also raised Peter from his tears and called him once more to follow Jesus. It's a good story. In their fear, they had good company! In their failures, they had a rock! With hope and confidence they could endure suffering and even death, knowing that this life is not the highest of all goods, that "just because it belongs to God, [a] man may be forbidden to will its continuation at all costs. He may be ordered to risk and expose it to varying degrees of danger. . . . Wanting to live on at all costs can then be only an elemental, sinful, and rebellious desire. . . . It may be that he must offer himself" (Barth 1961:401).

But Matthew's congregation knew no other end for Judas than ignominy. It knew no future for Judas, no story of this sad man being lifted up, like Peter, to a new life. It is not that Judas failed to repent. Indeed, Matthew explicitly says that Judas repented and puts the words of repentance on his very lips: "I have sinned by betraying innocent blood." But even in his repentance, Judas rejected the gracious sovereignty of God, the sovereign graciousness of God. He would be his own judge; he would take even his own judgment into his own hands. Death is due, for innocent blood has been spilled, but Judas is unwilling to let God be the judge, to wait patiently for the judgment. In his choice to kill himself he continues the same impatient refusal to live in the confidence of God's sovereignty that led to his betrayal.

Even the story of Judas, however, is not without hope. Matthew tells it as a story of fulfillment. As the prophet Zechariah was treated contemptuously, so was Jesus. As the prophet's services were derisively priced at thirty pieces of silver, the legal indemnity of a gored slave (Exodus 21:32), so were Jesus'. Matthew quotes a version of Zechariah 11:12–13, but he cites it as from Jeremiah. The words of Zechariah are words of judgment and woe, but by the reference to Jeremiah, Matthew provides a midrashic clue that the last word is not judgment but blessing. Jeremiah, too, had bought a field with silver pieces, and he buried the deed in a potter's jar (Jeremiah 32). In the midst of the judgment and woe of Jerusalem's destruction, Jeremiah's purchase was a prophetic signal of hope. In the midst of hopelessness, Jeremiah reminded people of God's faithfulness to the identity God had established in deeds of covenant and words of promise. One could be carefree in the face of death and destruction. Only let each one be faithful to the identity established for God's people in those deeds of covenant and words of promise. Let each one trust God and live with courage and with patience.

A good storyteller does not need to pause at the end to explain the relevance of the story. It is a good story I am telling, but I am not a very good teller of the story. Let me, therefore, simply state the conclusion: Although there is no explicit condemnation of suicide in Scripture, there does not have to be, for it states, if indirectly, much more powerfully than simple prohibition, why suicide, assisted suicide, and euthanasia are forbidden. They do not fit the story of God's grace and faithful human response. They cohere rather with the story of betrayal and denial. In what follows I hope to show that certain notions of justice and mercy, of suffering and dying, of healing and caring, of freedom and responsibility cohere with this story and that others do not. And I hope to show that, where others have used these notions to reach a conclusion in favor of assisted suicide, they are probably drawing on other stories than the one my tradition has taught me to love and told me to live.

Justice and Mercy

"Do justice!" "Love mercy!" Who can argue with these imperatives? Surely not one who has been formed by Scripture, for the prophet Micah gives such commands by way of summarizing what the Lord requires (Micah 6:8). But we may well ask whether we still mean the same things by *justice* and *mercy*. The terms are slippery, and they shift in meaning as the background for intelligibility shifts. And as the meanings shift, so do the applications to the issues of assisted suicide and euthanasia.

In our pluralistic culture we sometimes use the terms as though they were freestanding, independent of any embeddedness in particular stories. As a result we sometimes have and use minimal notions of justice and mercy.

A minimal notion of justice insists on respect for the autonomy of each person, demands the protection of individual rights, and attempts to guarantee a space for each one to act in ways that suit one's preferences as long as such actions do not violate the autonomy of another. Such a notion of justice, of course, has its own tradition, its own story. It fits the story of Enlightenment liberalism.

The strengths of such a justice should not be denied. In a heterogenous society like ours, where people with different cultural and religious identities are forced to live with one another (and enriched by their interaction), such a justice can provide a context for conversation and a challenge to the arbitrary dominance of one perspective or person over another.

But the weakness of such a notion of justice should also not be overlooked. Its fundamental weakness is its minimalism, which shows up in a variety of ways. Such a notion does not tell us what goods to seek, only certain constraints to exercise in seeking them. Moreover, it is attentive finally to only one constraint, the prohibition against violating another's freedom. Such a notion of justice tends to reduce the significance of covenantal relationships (husband-wife, parent-child, doctor-patient) to matters of contract. And, by its emphasis on the procedural question, on the question "Who should decide?" it pushes to the margins of public discourse the substantive moral questions of conduct and character, the questions "What should be decided?" and "What should the one who decides be?" This minimalism does not make it wrong, but if its minimalism is not acknowledged, it distorts and subverts the moral life (and the moral death). It is true, for example, that nonconsensual sex is wrong—but there is more to say about a good sexual life, and if we deny that there is more to say, then we distort and subvert a good sexual life. And it is true that my wife and I sometimes resort to the language of contract, to the "rights" and "duties" that belong to our contract, but if that were the only language we had for our relationship, then we would distort and subvert the covenant of marriage.

This minimal notion of justice underlies many contemporary claims for the moral legitimacy of suicide. Suicide, after all, is (at least sometimes) an autonomous act: chosen, preferred by a free individual. Guaranteeing to each one a space to act in ways that suit one's preferences requires making a space for decisions to commit suicide. What matters publicly, after all, is simply that there be such a space, not how it is filled. And such a notion of justice also backs claims for the legitimacy of assistance with suicide and euthanasia, for the single-minded attention to consent as a constraint seems to prohibit only "nonconsensual killing."

It is true, of course, that nonconsensual killing is wrong—but there is more to say about our relationships with the suffering and dying, and if we deny that there is more to say, then we subvert and destroy the possibility of covenantal relationships with the suffering and dying.

Our culture is prepared to acknowledge that something more than justice is required in these relationships and to name that something more "mercy." But it has, I think, a minimal notion of mercy, too. Our culture acknowledges as morally appropriate the emotive response to another's suffering that we call mercy, the response that moves us to action when we see suffering.[13] The problem with the minimal notions of mercy and compassion, however, is that, while they tell us to do something, they do not tell us what to do. Such a mercy can justify almost anything. Such a notion of mercy supports contemporary claims about the legitimacy of assisted suicide and euthanasia, which at least qualify as "doing something" to put a stop to suffering. Such acts are sometimes described (and justified) in terms of their motive as "mercy killing."

The minimal notions of justice and mercy, then, seem to justify assisted suicide and euthanasia. Assisted suicide and euthanasia, after all, are chosen by autonomous individuals, and they end the suffering of one who hurts. How can one argue with the validity of the inferences that justify assisted suicide and euthanasia?

One might point out that, if we begin to regard killing as a work of mercy, it will be hard not to be merciful (and deadly) toward those who have lost or never achieved a capacity for autonomy. One might point out that, if we begin to regard being killed as a right, it will be difficult to limit the space for the exercise of that right to those cases where the suffering is severe and beyond human remedy.

Or one might ask whether such minimal notions are finally adequate to the moral life. None of us is as independent and autonomous as the minimal notion of justice pretends, nor should we want to be. And when compassion kills, when the desire to help becomes confused with the desire to obliterate, then "taking care of strangers" has a sinister double meaning that should make us morally cautious (Burt 1979:v–vii).

Or one might provide a different context for the intelligibility of these notions and, so, a different way to understand these concepts and their implications. Do justice. Love mercy. Yes, but when the prophet gave such instruction, he connected it with a third instruction, "Walk humbly with God!" And he presented the whole as the requirement of God, as the response of faith and faithfulness to the God who creates and judges and renews and calls a people to covenant. Justice and mercy embedded in such a story are not minimal requirements.

They are first of all characteristics of God. The justice of God is God's own faithfulness to covenant, God's fidelity to the intentions with which God formed the world and a people. And God's mercy is God's grace, God's persistence to bless and God's presence to suffering. God's mercy intends, despite the powers of sin and death, even now a little space for joy and rest and finally the triumph of *shalom*. And "to the close of the age" God's mercy shares the pain while the creation groans and the tears while any creature weeps.

Justice and mercy are also, of course, characteristics of those who would be faithful to God, who would walk humbly with God. They are the shape of response to God and to all things in ways appropriate to the relations of all things to God. Such justice tells us something of the goods to seek, life and human flourishing among them. Such justice exercises some constraints besides respect for the sometimes arbitrary preferences of another, constraints that include the prohibition against the destruction of an embodied image of God. Such justice will nurture covenantal relations, not reduce them to contractual or instrumental relationships. It will defend the weak and advocate for the powerless against the powers that resist God's cause. Such mercy will persist in blessing "the least of these" (Matthew 25:40, 45) and will be present to them in the midst of hurt and harm. It will visit the sick (Matthew 25:36, 43), not abandon or eliminate them. Indeed, it will discover in "the least of these" and in their vulnerability the very image of Christ (Matthew 25:40, 45). To walk *humbly* with God will acknowledge that there are limits to our powers—and so to our responsibilities. We are not God; our powers are not messianic; they provide no escape finally from human mortality or from the human vulnerability to suffering. Even while we work for God's cause, we wait and watch for it.

Such justice and mercy fit the story of Scripture, but such justice and mercy do not fit assisted suicide and euthanasia.

The story of Judas as a part of the whole suggests an evangelical and Reformed reply to suicide and "consensual killing." They are wrong; they fit the story of betrayal, the story of a refusal to leave salvation and judgment in the hand of God, the story of the refusal to depend on the grace of God. And in our context, unlike Matthew's context, it is important and necessary to say that they are wrong. The rule of such a justice will prohibit eliminating the sufferer in the name of eliminating suffering. Even so, the mercy formed by such a story will not be satisfied with simply shouting that prohibition. While it refuses to obliterate the sufferer, it also refuses to abandon the sufferer; it will seek to remedy the suffering, and it will be prepared to leave the final judgment and the final salvation to God.

A prohibition, even one formed out of Scripture's story, will almost certainly not be sufficient as a response to the despair which prompts suicide or to our culture (Barth 1961:406). Given the sort of world it is, a world not yet God's good future, there are many people who quite reasonably despair. Their bodies are broken, or their spirits are crushed; their circumstances seem hopeless, or their dignity seems lost; and the One who bears down on them no longer seems to sustain them. A law, a rule, a cogent philosophical or religious argument may not dissuade them from suicide (Gustafson 1984:201–7). Indeed, a prohibition may only increase the fascination with the forbidden—and in some cases identify a final form of rebellion and betrayal against the One on whom they depend but whom they have come to distrust.

What is required in such cases is not law but a powerful and creative word of grace. That word may be mute, of course, a voiceless presence communicating a readiness to hear and to share the sorrow still voiceless, too. Or the word may find voice (as the sufferer does) to be raised in com-plaintive lament. Or the word may prompt the courage Peter learned so late and the patience Judas never did learn. The word of grace may be a deed (like *dabar*), a little thing that expresses faithfulness in our relations to others, some little signal that one is permitted to live, not obliged to live, even while it gives no permission to kill. It may be some token that one is also permitted to die, not obligated to die, even while it gives no permission to live on at all costs. The word of grace will sometimes take the form of the rule itself, to say no to the request of assistance in suicide, for deeply confused with such requests are tests of perceptions that others would prefer that they be dead. What is required is a word of joy that is capable of acknowledging the reality of their sadness, a word of hope that is capable of recognizing the limits on their real options. What is required is gospel, the good news that the human senses of dependence, remorse, and hope meet a God who can be trusted, even in the midst of suffering and dying. I do not mean to suggest that what is required is a homily, surely not a glib assurance that all is well, or the cheap advice that one engage in a little positive thinking. I mean a faithfulness that keeps company with the suffering and dying and with God, a faithfulness that walks humbly with God and humbly in the imaginations and affections (as well as the cognitions) of those in despair. I mean at the very least to commend hospice care as "fitting" to the story.

Even so, given the sort of world it is, even such words and deeds may not be enough to call a person from despair and suicide, and the tragedy of their lives and deaths should keep us from judging them (or ourselves) too quickly and too harshly. And sometimes we need mercy when we render judgment, even just judgment, on one who has mournfully assisted another in suicide. Justice requires a verdict of guilty, but mercy might suggest not a different verdict but a suspension of the sentence in tragic circumstances.

Suffering and Dying

For Christians the significance of suffering and dying is determined by the story of Scripture, stories of creation and fall and redemption, stories of a cross and of an empty tomb. To be sure, the significance is complex; there is a certain dialectic in the dispositions toward suffering and dying in the story of Scripture.

On the one hand, life and its flourishing belong to the creative and redemptive cause of God. The signs of it are breath and a blessing, a rainbow and God's own sanction, a commandment and, finally, an empty tomb. Therefore, life and its flourishing will be recognized and celebrated as goods, as goods against which we may not turn without turning against the cause of God. They are to be received with thanksgiving and used with gratitude. Acts that aim at death and suffering do not fit this story, do not cohere with devotion to the cause of God or with gratitude for the gifts of God. To intend death is to join Cain in his evil and Judas in his betrayal.

On the other hand, life and its flourishing are not the ultimate goods. They are not "second gods" (see Barth 1961:392). Jesus walked a path steadily and courageously that led to his suffering and to his death. Therefore, Christians may not live as though either survival or ease were the law of their being. To do so is to join Peter in his denial. Sometimes life must be risked, let go, given up. And sometimes suffering must be risked or shared for the sake of God's cause in the world. The refusal ever to let die and the attempt to eliminate suffering altogether are not signals of faithfulness but of idolatry. And if life and its flourishing are not the ultimate goods, neither are death and suffering the ultimate evils. They need not be feared finally, for death and suffering are not as strong as the promise of God. One need not use all one's resources against them. One need only act with integrity in the face of them. Matthew says as much when he reminds his readers of Peter's story and Jeremiah's message of hope.

This dialectic is captured in the distinctions between killing and allowing to die and between choosing suffering and patiently bearing it. The moral significance of those distinctions, of course, is being challenged—and may be difficult to defend when the story in which they are embedded is denied or ignored.[14]

The moral distinctions are hard to defend, for example, in the context of a utilitarian calculus, where the only relevant consideration is outcome, results, consequences. If the consequences are the same, it is hard to see in a utilitarian calculus why the moral evaluation of mercifully allowing one to die and mercifully killing someone ought to be different. Moreover, if the standard for assessing the consequences is the maximization of preference satisfaction, and if anyone (whether arbitrarily or reasonably) prefers death to life in his or her particular circumstances, then it is not hard to see the moral obligation to kill the suicidal (or to inflict pain on the masochist).

The distinctions seem more at home—at least initially—in the context of the sort of moral minimalism that focuses on rights and their correlative duties. In this context, for example, one can distinguish between negative and positive rights, between rights to noninterference and rights to assistance. So one can distinguish the right to life as a negative right not to be killed from the right to life as a positive right to assistance in preserving one's life. And one can also distinguish the right to die as a negative right not to have one's dying interfered with from the right to die as a positive right to assistance in one's dying. Since rights to noninterference are usually regarded as imposing much more stringent correlative duties than rights to assistance, and since the negative right to life imposes a duty not to kill, one could at least argue that, therefore, there can be no positive right to die and no duty to assist in suicide that would be imposed by such a right. But the distinction quickly loses any force against the background of such moral minimalism. Not only does the right to die seem to extend to suicide, it would also seem to extend to assistance in suicide if a contract had been freely entered. Since the right to life, like any right, is a legitimate claim, and since one may refuse autonomously to make the legitimate claims that are one's own to make, if I refuse to claim my negative right to life, then it is hard to see why killing me would be a violation of that right. So, consensual killing looks morally indistinguishable from consensual allowing to die in this context, too.

The distinction does, however, fit the story of Scripture and the notions of suffering and dying formed by it. The martyrs knew the story well, and they "bore witness" to it by choosing neither death nor suffering but by being ready to endure either for the sake of God's cause in the world and their own integrity. Their comfort was that they were not their own but belonged to God, the giver of life, from whom not even death could separate them. And their comfort was their courage.[15] In more mundane and commonplace ways, many Christian patients still display the same comfort and the same courage, still bear witness by their readiness to die but not to kill, by refusing both offers of assisted suicide and offers of treatment that may prolong their days but only by rendering those days (or months or years) less apt for their tasks of reconciliation with enemies or fellowship with friends or simply enjoyment with the family.

Because there was breath and a blessing, because there was a rainbow and a commandment, because there was an empty tomb, Christians will not choose death, will not intend death. But because the one who was raised had suffered and died, Christians will acknowledge that there may be goods more weighty than their own survival or ease, goods and duties that determine how they should live, even while they are dying.

There is more at stake here than the distinctions between choosing death and accepting death, between intending suffering and enduring it. At stake is an eschatological realism in response to suffering and dying that can protect both religion and medicine from their temptations to triumphalism. The gospels tied the memory of Jesus as the risen one to the cross. No memory of Jesus may neglect or ignore the cross. We live—and suffer and die—under the sign of it. It is not yet, still not yet, the age of God's unchallenged sovereignty.

Apart from the story of the cross the church is always at risk of distorting the gospel into a Pollyannaish triumphalism and then of self-deceptively ignoring or denying the sad truth about our world or the sad truth about some medical patient. But the church is not the only group that needs to remember that we live under the sign of the cross.

Our culture is always at risk of trumpeting the good news of some medical breakthrough and then ignoring the sad truth that there is no medical technology to rescue the human condition from mortality or vulnerability to suffering. Apart from this eschatological realism our culture is at risk of extravagant (and idolatrous) expectations of medicine, tempted to regard the physician as a medical wizard whose magic will deliver us from death and suffering.

Jesus has been raised, the "first fruits of those who have fallen asleep" (1 Corinthians 15:20), but we live under the sign of the cross, and the good future of God is not yet fully come. Yet, to those who suffer, although the story of Jesus is a glad story indeed, it does not deny the sad truth about our world. It does not announce here and now an end to our pains or an avoidance of our death, but it does provide an unshakable assurance that we do not suffer alone, that we are not and will not be abandoned, that Jesus suffers with us, that God cares. The glad story of Jesus is indeed a hard reminder that in a world like this one, however righteous or repentant we are, we cannot expect to be spared pain, sorrow, or death. Certainly health and life are goods that I may and must seek, but they are not the greatest goods, and if "a disci-

ple is not above his teacher" (Matthew 10:24), then one's own survival
and one's own ease may not become the law of one's own being. In our
sad stories we keep good company. That's a part of the good news—and
this, that beyond the cross is the resurrection, the triumph of God over
death and harm (Bouma et al. 1989:138).

The stories of Jesus are good news to the sufferer and a call to
those who would follow Jesus to heal and to care.

Healing and Caring

According to the Reformed tradition, medicine is a calling, a vocation.
The notion of a vocation served initially to vest the work of physicians
with a new dignity, a dignity not less than the vocation to a "religious"
life. It emancipated the work of physicians (and others) from the control of priestly power. At the same time it vested the work of physicians
with a new direction, for the life and work of the physician were themselves regarded as "religious," as a response to God and, indeed, as a
form of discipleship. When Calvinists named medicine a calling, they
asserted that medicine, too, could serve the cause of God. They situated the practice of medical skills and knowledge within the story of
Scripture and its demands of faithfulness.

In that story Jesus came preaching that the kingdom of God was at
hand and already making its power felt in his words of blessing and his
works of healing, and in that story Jesus suffered and died. He called the
disciples to follow him, to preach and to heal (Matthew 10:5–15), and to
take up the cross (16:24). The Christian community is called to heal just
as surely as it is called to proclaim "good news," and it is called to be
present to those who suffer just as surely as it is called to heal and to
preach. It is to be a healing and caring community. The Christian community may not surrender this calling to medicine, but part of its calling is to be the support (and reform) of medicine. Physicians who own
their work as a calling, as a form of discipleship, will not dismiss the special skills and training, the special competence, of medicine. But neither

will they dismiss the story of Scripture as the story they long to live *per vocationem*.[16]

There is today in the debate about assisted suicide and euthanasia a struggle for the identity of the profession of medicine. It is not a novel struggle, or a new debate, for that matter, but the meaning of the profession is at stake.

In ancient Greece physicians defined their role in terms of restoring health and easing pain. They saw the good of health and their powerlessness against death. When patients were mortally ill, "overmastered by their diseases,"[17] these physicians refrained from efforts to cure them—and sometimes killed them. To relieve the suffering of the dying these physicians counted among the tools of their trade poisons and other techniques to produce a painless death.

The famous Hippocratic oath, of course, stood against such practice: "I will neither give a deadly drug to anybody if asked for it, nor will I make a suggestion to this effect."[18] The oath was a minority report, but this effort to reform the practice of medicine was remarkably successful. It shaped the conduct and character of medicine for centuries. Because the goods intrinsic to medicine were to heal the sick, to protect and nurture health, to relieve pain, limits could be imposed on the use of skills within the practice. The skills were not to be used to serve alien ends, and the destruction of human life was regarded as an alien and conflicting end. But while they would not kill, there was not yet any sense of an obligation to prolong the life of those overcome by their illness.[19]

The physician's perspective was to shift again, however, with the development of a new vision and new powers. Francis Bacon saw a "third end" for medicine, the preservation of life, and he regarded this goal as the "most noble of all." He rejected the traditional resignation in the face of those "overmastered by their disease"; he complained that "the pronouncing of these diseases incurable gives a legal sanction, as it were, to neglect and inattention and exempts ignorance from discredit"

(1970:487–89). Bacon's recommendation was innovative for its time, and it came to shape the medical community and identity as powerfully as the once innovative oath had. Physicians were enlisted on the side of life, fighting a messy but heroic battle against death. Their courage was their refusal to call any disease incurable. Their weapons were forged in study and research. Their allies were the university and its laboratories.[20]

Among the effects of this shift, of course, was the ability to cure a number of diseases that once overwhelmed the sick. For that, of course, we must be thankful. But we must rue other effects. Ironically, Bacon's complaint about the neglect and inattention and ignorance that were sanctioned by the former medicine can be turned against the medicine Bacon inspired.

Where neglect is identified with a decision no longer to attempt to cure, there medical care and the project of healing are reduced to cure. Where attention to patients is identified with the effort to cure them, there attentiveness to patients is reduced to attentiveness to their pathologies. Where "knowledge is power," regarded as power over nature and celebrated as bringing human well-being in its train, there care for patients is reduced to treating their bodies as manipulable nature in an effort to cure them. The ironic result is that this view of medicine sanctions another kind of ignorance, ignorance of the identities of patients, of the particular stories they tell, the individual aims they cherish, and of their communities. And when such ignorance is sanctioned, the physician will be ill-prepared to understand and respond to the particular ways in which patients suffer, in which they experience their condition as a threat to their embodied integrity.[21] Care motivated the search for a cure, of course, but the search for a cure pushed care to the margins.

Notice, moreover, that where knowledge is power over nature and where such power is assumed to bring human well-being in its train, there the fault that runs through the world and through our lives is located in nature, not—as in Scripture's story—in the mystery of human freedom. Nature is regarded as the threat to human flourishing, and that nature, at least human nature, includes mortality and a certain vulnerability to suffering. Knowledge exercised as technological power is regarded as the source of human well-being; therefore, nature, including human nature, can be and must be mastered and manipulated for the sake of human flourishing.

I do not claim that all physicians shared this vision or this project, but I do claim that the Baconian vision shaped the practice of medicine.[22] The Baconian account of medicine had great success, but the limits of that success are told in sad stories of lingering dying, tragic stories of physicians who see only diseases and lose sight of the human realities of their patients, sad stories of patients suffering not only from certain pathologies but from the treatments for them. Today the Baconian account of the physician's role is under attack. The identity of the physician is being revisioned and refashioned in our age. That provides both opportunity and danger.

One option for medicine shares Bacon's confidence in knowledge as power over nature and the assumption that the threat to human well-being is located in nature, but this new option shifts attention to a still more noble end, the elimination of suffering. The task now is to eliminate suffering, even if one has to eliminate the sufferer to do it. The great enemy is no longer death but suffering. The physician turns now to new technologies (except, of course, that the technology itself is as old as hemlock) in an effort to master human nature's vulnerability to suffering. Knowledge is still power over nature, including human nature, and its mastery includes not only keeping people alive but killing them.

A second option for medicine is more modest about the well-being that comes in the train of technology, and agnostic about any good that belongs to medicine as a practice. In this revisioning the physician has certain skills and tools that he or she may offer in the marketplace, contracting to do the bidding of the one who pays. The identity of physician is that of an entrepreneur. Well-being still comes in the train of such knowledge, but only by reducing well-being to the satisfaction of the sometimes arbitrary preferences of medical consumers and contractors. And if the consumer prefers death, a contract can be made, and caveat emptor!

There is a third option for revisioning the identity of a physician: the option of seeing medicine as a vocation, a calling, a form of discipleship. Such a medicine situates the practice and its skills within the story of Scripture and its demands of faithfulness. It sees itself as a response to God, as a form of service to the cause of God, while it waits and hopes and aches for God's final triumph and trusts in a God who is always and already present to those who hurt.

Such a medicine will be less tempted to triumphalism, to the expectation of a technical solution to human mortality and vulnerability to suffering. It will not deny the not-yet character of our existence and of our medicine, not to itself and not to its patients. It will not claim to inaugurate God's good future for a patient. On the contrary, such a medicine will sustain and nurture truthfulness about our finitude, about the limits imposed by our mortality. It will sustain and nurture humility, the readiness to acknowledge that we are not gods and that our powers are not messianic.

Such a medicine will also sustain and nurture gratitude for the gifts of life and health and for the opportunities within its limitations— sometimes to cure, sometimes to heal, sometimes to save a life, sometimes to remove someone's pain, sometimes to help a person cope with suffering, sometimes to relieve the bitterness of someone's tears, and at least to wipe those tears away with tenderness.

Such a medicine will acknowledge that death and suffering are real and that they are real evils, but, because Jesus suffered, died, and was raised, it will not regard death or suffering as ultimate evils. In response to God such a medicine can nurture and sustain care, even for those it cannot cure. It will acknowledge in "the least of these" the very image of the Lord who calls them to serve. It will be ready as a Simon of Cyrene (Matthew 27:32) to help bear the cross another bears, a stranger called, compelled, and blessed to be present to the suffering one and so to Jesus.[23] Such a medicine can be present to the suffering and dying without panic, without the anxious effort to substitute for an absent God. Such a medicine can nurture and sustain a more carefree care.

In-response-to-God medicine will be suspicious of the reduction of the embodied image-bearer either to mere biological organism or to mere capacities for choice; it will nurture and sustain respect for and attentiveness to the integrity of embodied persons made in God's image. Finally, such a medicine will sustain and nurture the sense of God's forgiveness in the midst of moral ambiguity and so the courage to make the ambiguous choice in the confidence of God's grace and future.

The stories of Jesus do not fit the story sometimes told by medical practitioners to patients (and sometimes told by patients to medical practitioners) that death is the ultimate enemy and the worst evil, to be put off by any means. And if people sometimes then blame physicians for keeping them alive beyond all reason, the stories of Jesus and his cross do not fit the story told by Jack Kevorkian and the Hemlock Society that suffering is the ultimate evil and life the great enemy, and that a good doctor is a good killer. The stories of Jesus teach physicians to delight in their tools as gifts of God, to celebrate scientific advances for the powers they give to intervene in the sad stories patients tell with and of their bodies. But these stories also correct those who have mistaken technology for the savior, who rely on technology to remedy the human condition or to sustain either their patients or their care for them in the face of their suffering and dying. If God is God, and if God is the sort of God of whom the story is told, then medicine as a vocation will be disposed to cure when possible, ready to care always, ready to let go of a patient to death and to God when care requires it, but never ready to kill.

Freedom and Responsibility

"Maximize freedom!" Who can argue with such advice? Surely not one formed by Scripture, for human freedom is a gift of God and part of God's cause. "For freedom has Christ set us free" (Galatians 5:1). But one may ask, of course, what freedom means. "Be responsible!" Who would suggest that one be anything else? But the term is empty until we identify to whom and for what we are responsible. Freedom and responsibility are often celebrated, but these remain slippery terms, dependent on their moral context for their significance.

The story of Judas that Matthew told invites a chastened account of both. Matthew was evidently not interested in the issue of whether the suicide of Judas was a free and autonomous choice. It seemed almost fated. The crucial choice had been made some time before, in the decision to betray Jesus, and his tragic end fit the story of his betrayal and seemed almost to be determined by it. In his choice to betray Jesus, Judas chose not just a discrete action but a self, a life and a death. There might yet have been a turn from the sad course he had set himself upon, but it would have required a faithful response to the grace of God. By the grace of God, after all, Peter had turned from his cowardice and tears to a life of heroic discipleship. But Judas was unable or unwilling to make such a response; his sense of limitless responsibility made it difficult for him to receive anything as a gift, including the grace of God. He could not even leave judgment to the hand of God. He could not or would not be patient, dependent upon the grace of God. He could regard a limited responsibility only as irresponsibility.

The Reformed tradition has celebrated and cherished both freedom and responsibility, but it has also continued to be suspicious of them in ways schooled by such a story. The enthusiasm for freedom has been chastened by the recognition that human freedom is intimately related both to the determinate features of human existence and to the grace of God. And responsibility has always been construed finally as answer, response, accountability to God. Such responsibility reaches to every part of life, for a faithful response to God renders us also responsible for relating to all people and all things in ways appropriate to the relations of all people and all things to God (Gustafson 1981:158, 227; Gustafson 1984:146, 275). But such responsibility remains a creaturely and limited responsibility, since it is God who will make things turn out right in the end, in the eschaton. Because human freedom is a part of God's creation and cause, responsibility to God will include the protection of and respect for freedom, but because it is response to God, it will not celebrate as justification or intend as good the vision of autonomous and self-interested persons who are as strangers to one another, protected from one another by their individual rights. Since human life and its flourishing are the gift of God and the intention of God, responsibility to God will include the protection of and respect for life, but because human responsibility is response to God (and not a substitute for God), it will not bear the burden of a divine and limitless responsibility to eliminate death or suffering.

The Reformed tradition has consistently preferred an Augustinian account of human freedom to a Pelagian account. Pelagius had described human freedom as the capacity of a neutral agent to make choices unconstrained and uncoerced, to contemplate options without internal or external restraints. Equipoised between good and evil, undetermined even by their own previous choices, neutral selves can will what they will. Augustine and the Reformed tradition saw nothing to cherish or respect in such an account of freedom. In Augustine's view there are no neutral selves, no indeterminate agents who face choices unformed by the past; one's choices form the determinate features of the future and of the self.

The Reformed tradition, therefore, has always appreciated the significance of the determinate features of human existence. Particular human beings and their choices are formed by their natural endowments (including, we may say now, their genetic endowments), their natural communities, their culture, their past choices, and the choices of others with respect to them. These determinate features of human existence limit human freedom and human responsibility. But they also enable it. There is no human freedom that does not marshal endowments, weigh the claims of particular communities, interpret their culture, assess past choices, and respond to actions upon them. Human beings do all that, of course, not from some disinterested point in transcendence over all that, but engaged in and with the determinate features of their existence. Freedom in this context is the capacity of a self to establish a self, an identity, to form a whole of the disparate and determinate features of one's life; here the evidence of freedom is not arbitrariness but consistency and predictability. The exercise of freedom determines not just a discrete action, cut off from the past and the future, but the whole of one's life.

The two traditions also differ, of course, in their accounts of the relation between God's grace and human freedom. For the Pelagian the human being is and must be free even with respect to the relation to God. The neutral agent must face that choice, too, without constraint. For the Augustinian there is no freedom that does not have God as its source and destiny. The contradiction is not between the sovereign grace of God and human freedom but between human freedom and human sin. In sin the human being both affirms freedom by choice and denies freedom by a choice that denies the source and destiny of freedom. It is a contradiction captured in the phrase "voluntary bondage." In that contradiction the world could have been smashed back to chaos, but God graciously called and calls human beings to turn and to return. And in that call the grace of God is again the source of human freedom, and fellowship with God is again the destiny of human freedom. In the Reformed account, God is always at work graciously renewing human freedom, providing new opportunities for new selves. Of course, that is always mediated through the mundane stuff of life, but in our choices we are always finally responding to God and to the call of God.

The Reformed tradition will be an advocate of freedom, then, but it will also insist that a choice is not right simply because it is freely made. The Reformed tradition reminds us that our choices, including our social choices, including even the presumably innocent choice to "maximize freedom," express and form the determinate features of our life and of our common life. In the name of freedom we may ironically increase our bondage.

The point can be illustrated with respect to technology. Technology is frequently introduced as a way to increase our options, as a way to maximize our freedom. But it can become part of the determinate features of existence; it can quickly become socially enforced. The automobile was introduced as an option, an alternative to the horse, but it is now socially enforced. The horse remains, I suppose, a "recreational vehicle," but don't try to ride one home on the interstate. The technology that surrounds our dying was introduced to give doctors and patients options in the face of disease and death, but such "options" have become socially enforced; at least one sometimes hears, "We have no choice!" Now it is possible, of course, to claim that cars and CPR are the path of progress, but then the argument has shifted from the celebration of options and the maximizing of freedom to something else, to the meaning of progress. The point is simply this: we need to ask not just whether the social legitimation of suicide, assisted suicide, and euthanasia serves freedom by increasing our options but also whether it will be moral progress if and when what is introduced as a new option becomes socially (even if not legally) enforced.

Moreover, even if a particular option does not become socially enforced, simply providing the option, simply "maximizing freedom" by giving social legitimation to certain choices, can and does affect the determinate features of our life and our common life. Our choices, even to regard certain things as choices, form selves, and our social choices, even to increase options, form our common life.

Consider, for example, the life of a night clerk at the convenience store (Velleman 1992:671). One determinate feature of her existence is frequently identified on the front door: "The night clerk cannot open the safe." To maximize the freedom of the night clerk, one might give her the option of opening the safe. But to increase her options in this way would change the determinate features of her life, and not happily—or innocently: not happily because, given the vulnerability of a night clerk, to change the determinate features of her life in that way would lessen her security; and not innocently because, under cover of maximizing options, we would be forming ourselves to regard the vulnerability of others as a matter of moral indifference.

The sick and suffering are vulnerable, too, and a policy innovation to increase their options will change the determinate features of their existence, and not necessarily happily or innocently. That giving them the choice can be described as maximizing freedom is not a sufficient justification for such policy innovations, if simply having the choice renders the sick and suffering still more vulnerable. To the vulnerability of the sick and suffering we will return, but first note that choices to increase options sometimes eliminate options.

Choices, including presumably innocent social choices to maximize freedom by increasing options, shape our life and our common life. They affect the determinate features of our existence, and they may eliminate certain options in the name of increasing freedom. David Velleman provides a nice illustration of this.

I invite you to dinner. The invitation is presented as an option, of course. But by increasing your options, I have effectively eliminated what you may suddenly recognize as the option you would prefer, the option you had a moment ago but have no longer, the option of *both* not spending three hours with me *and* not having me know that (and why) you would rather not. The invitation increases your options, but it also eliminates an option. It gives you a choice between those two but eliminates the option of having both. Suppose you choose not to go. You have good reasons. But notice that you still might prefer not to have had this new option. Notice that you no longer have the option you might like best. And notice that you have to justify your choice (Velleman 1992:672).

When we provide social legitimation of the option of suicide, we may increase options, but we also effectively eliminate an option, namely, staying alive without having to justify one's existence. That happens to be an option that the Reformed tradition would choose if it could, an option the Reformed tradition would like to protect and preserve, for it fits with the story of life as a gift. Given the new option in the name of maximizing freedom, one may choose, of course, not to be killed, but the person who makes that choice is now responsible for it, accountable for living, and he or she can be asked to justify that choice.

With this point we return to the issue of the vulnerability of the sick and suffering, for this burden of justification can add to the burden of suffering. The requirement that we account for our existence becomes part of the determinate features of that existence and a part of the context for making the choice it is now ours to make. The very giving of the choice can thus create some pressure to make a particular choice.

The vulnerable will be subject not just to the pressure of malicious thugs and con artists, not just to the pressure of relatives who may be better off financially or emotionally if the vulnerable were to die, not only to the pressure of "compassionate" friends who would like to see the suffering stop, but also to the pressure of their own sense of obligation to justify their existence. And they respond to that pressure by drawing on resources determined in part (and undermined in part) by the social choice to provide the option of assisted suicide as a way of maximizing freedom.[24]

The point is not a subtle one. It gets lost, I think, only when we overestimate our autonomy and independence; it gets lost when we lose a sense of our dependence and interdependence. Our self-concept is always confused with our interpretation of how others think and feel about us. The suicide threat is, after all, sometimes a call for help, an inquiry whether anyone really cares. To reply to such an inquiry by giving the option can all too easily be read as an answer to that inquiry, and it can diminish the resources a person has for choosing still to live. And if that is true in individual cases, it is also true culturally. Providing the choice of assisted suicide to the vulnerable, to the dependent, to those who are no longer in control is recommended, no doubt, as a way to increase their options, to enable them to assert their independence and to take control. It expresses a culture and forms attitudes that value autonomy, independence, and control. The effect of maximizing freedom in this way may be to make it more difficult for the sick and suffering, the dependent and those who seem not in control, to refuse the option of death, harder to justify their existence. This social innovation in the name of increasing options not only eliminates the option of receiving life as a given, it also shapes the way the options will be perceived when life is a choice.

Giving people the option of dueling is an instructive parallel (Velleman 1992:676). We no longer give people that option. That is moral progress, I think. Of course, people still have the option, but we do not provide social legitimation for it. My point is not to express disapproval of dueling but rather to observe the relation between determinate features of a culture, the options it provides, and the pressure on choices that members of that culture make. The social choice to provide the option of dueling expressed a determinate culture, one obsessed with honor. And that very feature of the culture was part of the determinate context within which persons made their choices, making it more difficult not to throw down or to pick up the gauntlet. Our culture may be obsessed with individual autonomy. It would express (and reinforce) that feature of the common life by offering dependent people a choice, offering them an option that extends self-control. But the reason we have for giving the option may well make it more difficult for people not to just give up and choose assisted suicide.

If we choose to give this option of assisted suicide, we are choosing not just a discrete piece of social policy but a pattern for our life together that asks the weak and the sick to justify their existence. To refuse freely to give that option is to choose a pattern for our life where life is received as a given even when it is not cherished as a gift, where being dependent on others and on God is accepted as our common situation. If such is to be the pattern for our life together, then our responsibility will not be limited to leaving our neighbors alone; it will extend to learning to care for each other in the midst of suffering. Our responsibility will surely include respect for a neighbor's capacities for agency, but it will also include attentiveness to the neighbor when the neighbor's embodied integrity is threatened. That attentiveness will own responsibilities for being present, for being faithful, for being helpful, but it will not own responsibility for providing an escape from human mortality or from human vulnerability to suffering. Our responsibility is limited by the simple fact that we are not gods nor our powers messianic. Unlimited responsibility fits Judas's refusal to depend on God. The final salvation belongs to God. We need not substitute for God; we need not anxiously shoulder the responsibility of making everything turn out right.

Our responsibility is not just to repeat the prohibition of suicide. And our judgment must never be too quick or too harsh. The final judgment, too, belongs to God. But we are responsible to be faithful, to live the story we love to tell, not to betray that story or the one of whom it is told; we are responsible, that is, to speak some word of grace, even if that word is silent presence or a com-plaintive cry. The person who is contemplating suicide needs grace, not options.

NOTES

1. See the characterization of Calvinism as "world-formative Christianity" in Wolterstorff 1983:3–22.

2. The Bible contains stories of five or six suicides (Abimelech in Judges 9:50–56; Saul in 1 Samuel 35:1–5 and 2 Samuel 1:5–16; Ahithophel in 2 Samuel 17:23; Zimri in 1 Kings 16:18–19; possibly Samson in Judges 16:23–31; and Judas) and one story of a suicide prevented (the jailor at Philippi in Acts 16:25–29), and in none of them is there an explicit condemnation or prohibition of suicide.

3. See, e.g., Williams 1957:254–55, and Battin 1982:72–89. On such readings Augustine is usually given the credit (or the blame) for the Christian tradition's condemnation of suicide. See further Amundsen 1989.

4. I have attended to the methodological questions involved in reading Scripture as relevant to medical ethics in Verhey 1992b and 1994. I will not here again describe or defend those methodological proposals, but I do hope that the use of Scripture here will display the methodology there proposed.

5. This account of what Calvin called the *sensus divinitatis* is dependent on Gustafson's account of a "natural piety" (1981:129–136).

6. Matthew 1:1; this is my translation in an effort to bring out the parallels to the refrain of Genesis, e.g., Genesis 2:4, 5:1, and so forth. Unless otherwise noted, biblical references are to the Revised Standard Version.

7. E.g., Matthew 1:22; 2:14, 17, 23; 3:15; 4:14; 5:17.

8. Abel and Zechariah, son of Jehoiada, were the first and last murdered people mentioned in the Hebrew Scriptures (Genesis 4:8 and 2 Chronicles 24:20–22). Matthew's passage strongly foreshadows the death of Jesus, of course, and when he identifies Zechariah (mistakenly but deliberately) as the "son of Berachiah," he refers the reader to the prophet Zechariah quoted in Matthew 27:9–10.

9. The passage is found only in Matthew's gospel.

10. See Elliot Dorff's chapter in this volume and see Brody 1989.

11. Moreover, Jesus' admonition at his arrest that those "who take the sword shall perish by the sword" (Matthew 26:53) echoes God's own sanction in Genesis 9:6 ("Whoever sheds the blood of man, by man shall his blood be shed") and foreshadows Judas's death.

12. Perhaps we are being too generous with Judas, but nothing in Matthew corroborates John's view that Judas was a thief, that he had been corrupted by greed. Well, almost nothing. It is true that Matthew changes the account in Mark so that Judas asks what he will be given if he betrays Jesus. That can be read as though Judas's motive were pecuniary, but it is much more likely that Matthew makes this change in order to establish more cogently the "fulfillment" of Zechariah 11:12–13. Judas was and remains for Matthew one of the twelve.

13. Oliver O'Donovan makes this point compellingly (1984:10–12). Compassion, he says, is "the virtue of being moved to action by the sight of suffering," but it "presupposes that an answer has already been found to the question 'What needs to be done?'" (p. 11). In the context of our culture's confidence in technology, compassion will simply arm itself with superior technique, relying not on wisdom but on artifice against suffering (p. 12). See also Verhey 1992a.

14. See Meilaender 1976 and Wennberg 1989:150–56. I do not mean to rest the distinction between allowing to die and killing on the distinction between omission and commission, and I surely do not mean to suggest that the distinction provides a formula for resolving hard questions. There are clearly some cases of omission that can only be described as intending the death of the patient—for example, the failure to treat Baby Doe's esophageal atresia. And there are some cases that are hard to classify as allowing to die or as killing. (For instance, Wennberg cites a case in which a diabetic with painful and terminal cancer stops taking his insulin; did the diabetic allow himself to die or did he kill himself? [1989:136–42].) Still, "there is a theologically significant difference between *shaping* one's dying and *creating* one's dying" (Wennberg 1989:137), between intending death and foreseeing it, between choosing death and choosing how to live while one is dying.

15. Consider besides the martyrs the first question and answer of the Heidelberg Catechism: "Q. What is your only comfort in life and death? A. That I am not my own but belong—body and soul, in life and in death—to my faithful Savior Jesus Christ. . . . Because I belong to him, Christ by his Holy Spirit assures me of eternal life and makes me whole-heartedly willing and ready from now on to live for him."

16. Troeltsch (1931:610) makes the distinction between the Lutheran account of vocation and the Calvinist account of vocation in this way: For Luther, Christians were called *to* a particular work and were to exercise Christian faith *in vocatione*. That left the particular work regarded in a traditional way. For Calvin, Christians were to serve the cause of God *through* their vocation, to exercise Christian faith *per vocationem*. That required the particular work to be transformed, ordered to the mission of God.

17. As the Hippocratic treatise "The Art" would put it somewhat later (Reiser et al. 1977:6).

18. Ludwig Edelstein's translation, in Burns 1977:14.

19. On the Hippocratic oath see Cameron 1991, Kass 1985:224–26, and Lammers and Verhey 1987:72–96.

20. See William F. May's accounts of the "fighter" and the "technician" (1983:63–106).

21. See Eric Cassell's lament about the inattentiveness of medicine to suffering (1991).

22. It must be admitted that the Baconian vision of science and medicine was shared and nurtured by Puritan scientists and physicians. See Webster

(1976:246–92). The optimistic—indeed millennial—expectations of Bacon and the Puritans turned triumphalist with their success. Bacon's call for knowledge to be practical, tested by experience and experiment, and apt for the restoration of dominion over nature to human hands and, so, for progress toward human well-being, was heard as a religious vocation by the Puritans, but ironically it led to a different conception of God, a designer God who, having fashioned a world, politely withdrew, leaving the world to the hands of human freedom and reason. The different conception of God led inevitably to a certain indifference to the God so conceived.

23. I owe this image to Dr. Andy Von Eschenbach, who used it at a physician-clergy breakfast at the Institute of Religion to describe his own sense of calling to be a physician.

24. Kass 1990:41; cf. also Wennberg's powerful account of "negative fallout arguments" (1989:187–92).

REFERENCES

Amundsen, Darrel W. 1989. "Suicide and Early Christian Values." In *Suicide and Euthanasia: Historical and Contemporary Themes*, ed. Baruch A. Brody, 77–153. Dordrecht: Kluwer Academic Publishers.

Bacon, Francis. 1970. *De Augmentis Scientiarum: The Philosophical Works of Francis Bacon*, ed. J. M. Robertson. New York: Books for Libraries Press.

Barth, Karl. 1961. *Church Dogmatics*. Vol. 3, pt. 4, trans. A. T. Mackay et al. Edinburgh: T. and T. Clark.

Battin, M. P. 1982. *Ethical Issues in Suicide*. Englewood Cliffs, N.J.: Prentice Hall.

Bonhoeffer, Dietrich. 1985. *No Rusty Swords*, trans. E. H. Robinson and John Bowden. New York: Harper and Row.

Bouma, Hessel, III, Douglas Diekema, Edward Langerak, Theodore Rottman, and Allen Verhey. 1989. *Christian Faith, Health, and Medical Practice*. Grand Rapids, Mich.: Wm. B. Eerdmans.

Brody, Baruch A. 1989. "A Historical Introduction to Jewish Casuistry on Suicide and Euthanasia." In *Suicide and Euthanasia: Historical and Contemporary Themes*, ed. Baruch A. Brody, 39–75. Dordrecht: Kluwer Academic Publishers.

Burns, Charles, ed. 1977. *Legacies in Ethics and Medicine*. New York: Science History Publications.

Burt, Robert A. 1979. *Taking Care of Strangers: The Rule of Law in Doctor-Patient Relations*. New York: Free Press.

Cameron, Nigel M. de S. 1991. *The New Medicine*. Wheaton, Ill.: Crossway Books.

Cassell, Eric J. 1991. "Recognizing Suffering." *Hastings Center Report* 21 (May–June): 24–31.

Gustafson, James M. 1981. *Ethics from a Theocentric Perspective*. Vol. 1, *Theology and Ethics*. Chicago: University of Chicago Press.

———. 1984. *Ethics from a Theocentric Perspective*. Vol. 2, *Ethics and Theology*. Chicago: University of Chicago Press.

Kass, Leon. 1985. *Toward a More Natural Science: Biology and Human Affairs*. New York: Free Press.

———. 1990. "Death with Dignity and the Sanctity of Life." *Commentary* 89 (March): 33–43.

Lammers, Stephen, and Allen Verhey, eds. 1987. *On Moral Medicine: Theological Perspectives in Medical Ethics*. Grand Rapids, Mich.: Wm. B. Eerdmans.

Lash, Nicholas. 1986. *Theology on the Way to Emmaus*. London: SCM Press.

May, William F. 1983. *The Physician's Covenant: Images of the Healer in Medical Ethics*. Philadelphia: Westminster Press.

Meilaender, Gilbert. 1976. "The Distinction between Killing and Allowing to Die." *Theological Studies* (September): 467–70.

O'Donovan, Oliver. 1984. *Begotten or Made?* Oxford: Oxford University Press.

Reiser, Stanley, Arthur Dyck, and William Curran, eds. 1977. *Ethics and Medicine: Historical Perspectives and Contemporary Concerns*. Cambridge, Mass.: MIT Press.

Troeltsch, Ernst. 1931. *The Social Teaching of the Christian Churches*. Vol 2., trans. Olive Wyon. New York: Macmillan.

Velleman, J. David. 1992. "Against the Right to Die." *Journal of Medicine and Philosophy* 17 (December): 665–81.

Verhey, Allen. 1992a. "Compassion: Beyond the Standard Account." *Second Opinion* 18, no. 2 (October): 99–102.

———. 1992b. *The Practices of Piety and the Practice of Medicine: Prayer, Scripture, and Medical Ethics*. Grand Rapids, Mich.: Calvin College and Seminary, The Stob Lectures Endowment.

———. 1994. "Scripture and Medical Ethics: Psalm 51:10, the Jarvik 7, and Psalm 50:9." In *Religious Methods and Resources in Bioethics*, ed. Paul Camenisch, 261–88. Dordrecht: Kluwer Academic Publishers.

Webster, Charles. 1976. *The Great Instauration: Science, Medicine and Reform, 1626–1660*. New York: Holmes & Meier.

Wennberg, Robert N. 1989. *Terminal Choices: Euthanasia, Suicide, and the Right to Die*. Grand Rapids, Mich.: Wm. B. Eerdmans.

Williams, G. 1957. *The Sanctity of Life and the Criminal Law*. New York: Alfred A. Knopf.

Wolterstorff, Nicholas. 1983. *Until Justice and Peace Embrace*. Grand Rapids, Mich.: Wm. B. Eerdmans.

CHAPTER 11

Claiming a Death of Our Own:
Perspectives from the Wesleyan Tradition

Lonnie D. Kliever

I first began thinking seriously about active euthanasia in 1982 in connection with my work as a research consultant and humanities advisor for a documentary film about a burn patient's wish to die (*Dax's Case* 1984). In the summer of 1973, Donald "Dax" Cowart was critically injured in a propane pipeline explosion that burned more than 60 percent of his body. For more than a year, Cowart underwent repeated surgical procedures and daily treatment of the most extraordinarily painful kind. Throughout treatment, he demanded to be allowed to die. His accident left him totally blind, permanently disfigured, and severely disabled. To this day, though he lives in reasonable comfort and enjoys financial security, Dax maintains that he should have been allowed to die. Indeed, he describes himself as a victim rather than a beneficiary of medical science.

During my work on the film *Dax's Case* and a subsequent volume of essays by the same name, I was among the few collaborators on both projects who did *not* believe that Dax Cowart should have been assisted in dying or even allowed to die (Kliever 1989). Dax's insistent demands to die had been explained away by his physicians and family alike as protests against pain and as efforts to gain control—virtual temper tantrums born of physical and psychological helplessness. My background research for the film, which included reviews of hospital records and extensive interviews with all the principals, convinced me that Dax was indeed deeply ambivalent about his wish to die. That ambivalence was most visible during a brief stay at the Texas Institute for Rehabilitation and Research, where his refusal to receive treatment was finally honored. Within two or three days, his wounds became infected and he was near death. Dax then agreed, albeit at the persuasion of his mother and lawyer, to be transferred to the burn unit of John Sealy Hospital in Galveston where he could receive critical care. That same ambivalence about living or dying was reflected in his ongoing battles with his physicians during his treatment in Galveston and in several half-hearted suicide attempts following his discharge from the hospital.

In the years following the release of the film and the publication of the book, I participated in a number of programs and panels on *Dax's Case*. Each viewing of the film or discussion of the book was a jolting reminder to me of the unspeakable agony that Dax endured and of my profound sympathy for his wish to die. But I resolutely maintained the view that Dax should not have been allowed or assisted to die. Not only was I convinced that Dax was deeply ambivalent about his own death, but there were no legal or moral guidelines at the time that would have sanctioned either allowing to die or euthanasia. Even if such precedents had been in place, Dax was not suffering a terminal illness or an irreversible coma. For that reason, his doctors believed that withholding treatment from him would have been tantamount to assisted suicide, which was a felony in Texas at the time. A lawyer whom Dax contacted through a family member concurred in that interpretation of Texas law. Moreover, I was convinced on philosophical grounds that suicide by its very nature could never be a rational and responsible action.

But I began to rethink my views on euthanasia a year ago while preparing a paper for a conference on chronic illness and disability at the Institute for the Medical Humanities of the University of Texas Medical

Branch at Galveston (Kliever 1995). Once again, the Cowart case was my focus for a consideration of the problems of crushing pain, permanent impairment, and severe disfigurement. What I learned from approaching *Dax's Case* as a "narrative of illness" rather than as a "right-to-die film" was the inseparability of pain and grief in all human suffering. Human suffering cannot be split into uncommunicating categories labeled physical and mental, or outer and inner. These dimensions of human suffering are inseparably bound together. As such, suffering is always an assault on human meaning and purpose as well as a barrier to communication and communion. Moreover, when taken to the very limits, human suffering can completely shatter one's sense of self and world. Because Dax had undergone that kind of suffering, his demands to die were certainly understandable. The person he had been no longer existed, and the person that he might become was beyond his imagination.

While this reconsideration of *Dax's Case* did not convince me that Dax should have been allowed or assisted to die, it did help me to see that chronic illness and impairment, to say nothing of terminal illness and degenerative disorders, can reduce a person's sense of bodily integrity and personal dignity to a point where human life as such is more a burden than a blessing. That realization brought me face to face with the question of whether voluntary death could be both rational and responsible—that is, a course of action that neither violates sound judgment nor breaks faith with the human community.[1]

Given this challenge to my views on euthanasia, I welcomed the opportunity to participate in the Park Ridge Center's project "Choosing Death in America: The Challenge to Religious Beliefs and Practices." I was especially eager to explore questions of euthanasia in relation to *religious* belief and practice, for two seemingly contrary reasons. On the one hand, the current discussion of euthanasia is couched almost entirely in secular terms. Biomedical ethics for the most part remains pluralistic, libertarian, and individualistic. Moral arguments for the "right to die" are based on philosophical appeals to autonomy and constitutional appeals to privacy. But such appeals to liberty and privacy provide no moral grounds for physician-assisted or physician-performed euthanasia. The right to assistance in dying cannot be derived from the right to be left alone. On the other hand, our dominant religious traditions that stress human freedom and social solidarity are historically opposed to euthanasia. Although recent studies have shown that the Bible does not speak definitively on suicide, both church and synagogue came to regard suicide as self-murder and therefore as forbidden if not unforgivable (Clemons 1990). Suicide is seen as a premature abandonment of the struggle against death and an implicit betrayal of the human community. So we are left with a dilemma of sorts: our civil traditions permit voluntary death as a *private* action; our religious traditions condemn voluntary death as a *selfish* action. Our civic traditions do not provide social support to those who choose death. Our religious traditions do not provide spiritual solace to those who choose death. But if *religious* warrants for euthanasia can be found, both of these problems are resolved. We would have a medical ethics that provides social support and grants spiritual permission to choose death under certain circumstances. In addition, some of the bitter acrimony surrounding the abortion debate could be avoided.

This chapter is a search for such religious warrants. I use the word *search* advisedly because one looks in vain for unambiguous sanctions of voluntary death in the biblical tradition. The most one can hope for is a defense of euthanasia that is consistent with broadly defined biblical views on death and dying. But rather than appealing to a personal reconstruction of the biblical tradition, I will draw on one confessional expression of biblical faith to lend theological concreteness to my reflections, namely the Wesleyan tradition. Although I am not a Methodist theologian, I have chosen to work with the Wesleyan heritage because it is a mediating Christian tradition of sorts.[2] John Wesley brought together the spiritual and the physical, the religious and the ethical, the ancient and the modern, the customary and the scientific in a remarkable way. One need not be a Methodist to gain some appreciation of Wesley's vision of wholeness or to learn from his road map of the journey toward wholeness in life and in death.

Appropriating the Wesleyan Heritage

The Wesleyan heritage offers a coherent religious and moral vantage point for raising new questions about euthanasia that go beyond the current narrow debates over the "right to die" and the "sanctity of life." But, as philosopher Hans-Georg Gadamer has argued, such an appeal to a classic text or historic tradition works in both directions (Gadamer 1975:263–64). On the one hand, we bring our own set of questions and assumptions to such a text or tradition, and its sheer otherness challenges us to think again. On the other hand, the materials from the past will yield new insights and meanings to our fresh interrogation. Neither our assumptions by themselves nor the text or tradition by itself, but rather the interaction between the two, determines the outcome of that encounter. From the side of the Wesleyan tradition, that interaction will raise serious questions about narrow philosophical defenses of euthanasia. From the side of the contemporary situation, that same interaction may raise serious questions about dogmatic religious prohibitions against euthanasia.

This interplay between the classical heritage and the contemporary situation is fully consistent with what Methodist theologian Albert Outler called the "Wesleyan quadrilateral" (Holifield 1986:6–7). The quadrilateral was constituted by the four theological criteria to which Wesley appealed as a Christian thinker. The primary source of theological reflection was *Scripture*, the written testimony to God's self-disclosures in human history. The second source was *tradition*, the collective wisdom of earlier Christian communities. The third source was *experience*, the personal and communal appropriation of God's saving grace. The final source was *reason*, the studied effort to avoid self-contradiction and unnecessary conflicts with scientific and empirical facts.

In this scheme of things, the truth of Scripture, tradition, and experience transcends the reach of reason, but it does not contradict the truths of reason.

Wesley's own response to slavery exemplifies a transformative encounter between past tradition and present situation (Wesley 1958–59a:59–79). Slavery was a practice that prevailed among the ancient Jews, Greeks, Romans, and Germans, and it was transmitted by them to the various kingdoms and states that arose out of the Roman Empire. Although slavery declined in almost all parts of Europe during the Middle Ages, it was revived in the colonial empires of the European superpowers that later girdled the globe. As such, slavery was sanctioned by both the legal and religious traditions of these Christian empires. But Wesley was appalled by the very concept of slavery, never mind the brutalities of slave traffic and slave treatment. In rejecting slavery, Wesley argues that natural justice and mercy, to say nothing of the revealed law and love of God, take precedence over any civil law or religious custom that violates the liberty and dignity of a human being. Any person who can acknowledge another person's human nature and feel another person's human pain knows that slavery is wrong. Wesley's argument against slavery marshaled extensive empirical evidence of the slave's human nature and human pain. The *facts* of slavery viewed in light of the *values* of justice and mercy compelled a change of mind about the practice of slavery, notwithstanding the prevailing legal canons and religious customs sanctioning slavery. In other words, Wesley was a firm believer that "new occasions teach new duties" (Lowell 1939:263).

Of course, an impressive array of Methodist theologians and ethicists has already examined the Wesleyan tradition and concluded that euthanasia is almost always wrong. For example, James Laney argues that suicide as an escape from terminal illness or prolonged pain is always a premature abandonment of the struggle against death and is an implicit betrayal of the human community. "Suicide is inescapably unethical not only because it is a taking of life, but because it is invariably social. Suicide cannot help but be a negative condemnation of the whole of life, and thus of the relations of those who live on after" (Laney 1969:250). Stanley Hauerwas goes further by insisting that suicide represents a failure of faith: "Our unwillingness to kill ourselves even under pain is an affirmation that the trust that has sustained us in health is also the trust that sustains us in illness and distress; that our existence is a fight ultimately bounded by a hope that gives us a way to go on" (Hauerwas 1977:111). To be sure, most ethicists formed by the Wesleyan tradition do allow for the withdrawing or withholding of treatment that artificially prolongs biological life. The moment comes when care for the dying means caring for them through their dying rather than battling against their dying. Indeed, Paul Ramsey goes so far as to suggest that hastening the dying of those who are overmastered by pain or inaccessible to human care may be permissible as an act of mercy (Ramsey 1970:111). But such rare exceptions to the general rule against direct inducement of death do not invalidate the rule. Neither Wesley nor most of his theological heirs approve of euthanasia.

But the Wesleyan theological heritage may well yield a different solution to the dilemma of euthanasia when looked at from a different vantage point. New studies of suicide restore the distinction between pathological and rational suicide and question the dichotomy between suicide and martyrdom (Droge and Tabor 1992; Dworkin 1993). New analyses of suffering question the separation of physical and mental pain and connect suffering and dying on a continuum of loss. New reflections on the distinction between allowing to die and euthanasia raise questions about the hidden dangers and implicit cruelty of allowing to die. New attention to the meaning and means of care for the dying raises questions about the refusal to hasten the dying of those who want to die. How might these new ways of thinking about suffering and dying be deepened by the Wesleyan heritage? How might the Wesleyan heritage be broadened in the light of these new responses to end-of-life issues?

Can a dialogue between this historic tradition and the contemporary situation yield religious warrants for assisting those who choose to die in order to end their lives with bodily integrity and personal dignity?

Re-visioning the Wesleyan Tradition

Wesley was deeply interested in questions of health and medicine.[3] Indeed, he was more involved in the theory and practice of medicine than was any other major figure in Christian history. His own medical guidebook, *Primitive Physick*, which was published in 1747, went through thirty-eight English editions and twenty-four American editions by 1880. This book contained an introductory history and theory of medicine, detailed remedies for 250 maladies, and a list of rules for maintaining good health. Though his therapies are worlds apart from modern medicine, they were compatible with the medical wisdom of the day. More important for our purposes, his medical theory and practice were based on a religious view of personal identity and human solidarity that is of enduring worth to all those concerned with health and medicine. In the words of Martin Marty, Wesley's medical nostrums, despite their quaintness, showed "a passionate regard for humans in their suffering, a warm concern for their bodies, and a sense that he and his workers must care and cure not only in the realm of soul-saving, their chosen sphere, but also in the search for temporal well-being" (Marty 1986:xi).

There certainly are no clear sanctions for self-chosen death in the Wesleyan tradition. Indeed, Wesley took a very hard line on suicide, which he called "self-murder." He recommended nothing less than hanging in public places the naked bodies of men and women who had killed themselves as a discouragement of such "madness" (Wesley 1958–59b:481). He even reckoned that Judas Iscariot's suicide was a more heinous sin than his betrayal of Christ. For Wesley, only the Lord gives life and only the Lord takes life away. In the Wesleyan tradition, however, we do find detailed discussions of freedom and responsibility, suffering and dying, justice and mercy, and healing and caring that may provide religious warrants for euthanasia under certain conditions of terminal illness or degenerative disease.

Freedom and Responsibility as Context

John Wesley's approach to health and medicine was rooted in his view of human nature. Against the eighteenth-century philosophers who celebrated humankind's rationality and dignity, he held to the orthodox Christian doctrine of original sin. But Wesley did not take the doctrine of the Fall to the extremes of the Reformed or Lutheran traditions. Rather, he maintained a lively sense of prevenient grace—that grace of God which is operative in the life of fallen humankind and which preserves human freedom and responsibility.

Wesley argued that human nature in its primitive integrity embodied a natural, political, and moral "image of God." The natural image of God denoted the ability to seek understanding, make choices, and act freely. The political image of God affirmed that human beings exercise dominion over the natural world and animal life. By the moral image of God, Wesley meant the capacity for love. The ideal of human behavior was loving concern for others. "Implicit in Wesley's depiction of the image of God was an ethic which prohibited the suppression of understanding, the shackling of choice, the subversion of proper dominion, and the denial of love" (Holifield 1986:112). By grounding this ethic in the doctrine of creation, Wesley assured these rights and assigned these duties to all persons, whether Christian or not. Moreover, his depiction of the image of God provided an ideal vision of human and social order without ignorance and want, without coercion and inequality, without pain and violence.

Of course, Wesley acknowledged that the natural, political, and moral image of God had been shattered by the Fall. But all human beings are beneficiaries of a prevenient grace that restores in part the capacities of their created nature. By his prevenient grace, God enlightens understanding, strengthens resolve, sustains liberty, encourages dominion, and restores love. Every person shares a general knowledge of good and evil and suffers the pangs of a good or bad conscience. Prevenient grace preserves both the capacity for moral freedom and the burden of moral responsibility. Prevenient grace "reinscribes" the moral law that was "engraved" in the heart at creation but lost in the Fall. Moreover, prevenient grace prepares the ground for that higher moral possibility that comes only from sanctifying grace—the freedom and responsibility of a life of love. That way of love is fully realized only by those who know the love and truth of God, but such love does not supervene or circumvent the moral law that God has planted and revived in every human mind and heart. For Wesley, law and love never stand in contradiction, though they do remain in tension.

Thus Wesley argued for a balance between freedom and responsibility. On the basis of his doctrine of the image of God, he could assume that certain moral claims are grounded in human nature and, as such, can be known and practiced quite apart from special religious sources and sanctions. He could appeal to philosophical and commonsense principles without assuming that persons were so mired in original sin that these appeals fell on deaf ears or stony hearts. Such rules were useful for Christians and non-Christians alike for restraining wickedness and encouraging righteousness. But these rational principles point beyond themselves to the loving relationships that they both intend and reflect. As such, every moral choice and action is ultimately answerable to the criterion of love for God, neighbor, and self.

Wesley's view of human nature clearly recognizes that human beings are capable of choosing to end their own lives, though they are accountable to the human community and to God for that fateful use of freedom. Herein the Wesleyan tradition differs from most contemporary advocates of patient rights who ground the right to die in individual autonomy and dignity. For them, human freedom and responsibility are finally illusory if individuals do not have radical control over their own minds and bodies. That line of thinking underlies the 1990 decision by the U.S. Supreme Court that some commentators have welcomed as constitutional protection for the right to die. In the Court's ruling on *Cruzan v. Missouri*, the majority held that a competent patient's right to refuse unwanted medical treatment is derived from our common-law traditions of bodily integrity and informed consent (*Nancy Beth Cruzan* 1990). To be sure, the Court also ruled that liberty interests must be balanced against relevant state interests and that the state of Missouri acted constitutionally in demanding "clear and convincing evidence" that the refusal of treatment expresses the true intent of a competent person. Moreover, the Court did not directly address the question of euthanasia, ruling only on the withholding or withdrawing of life-prolonging treatment. But the *Cruzan* decision does ground the right to die in human freedom. The choice to die is protected constitutionally for competent individuals, although the method of dying remains in question.

But there are strong counterarguments in our religious traditions and scientific theories against the idea of voluntary death as a fundamental right based on individual liberty. While recognizing that suicide can be a freely chosen act, both the Jewish and Christian traditions have for the most part condemned suicide as a radical misuse of freedom. Since human life belongs to God, we are not at liberty to take innocent life. Suicide, like murder, is a violation of divine and human law. Indeed, suicide is worse than murder because the very act excludes the possibility of repentance and forgiveness. For that reason, the religious and civil sanctions against suicide have traditionally been severe. In the past, suicides were routinely denied proper religious burial, and often their personal goods and property were forfeited to the state (Williams 1957:248–310). In England, the threat of suicide was taken so seriously that the penalty for *attempted* suicide was death! Suicide was seen as an act of rebellion against God and the state that must be suppressed at all costs. Aiding and abetting suicide was also treated as both a sin and a crime, though subject to less severe punishments.

Of course, both the church and state made exceptions for deranged people who took their own lives. Those who were driven by irrational or pathological conditions to commit suicide were not held accountable for self-murder. Not surprisingly, the horrific treatment of suicide victims evoked a reaction among compassionate authorities both secular and sacred who increasingly attributed suicide to insanity, thereby excusing the victim and freeing the family of the blame and shame of a relative's self-murder. John Wesley, like many other religious leaders of the day, condemned the wholesale exoneration of suicide by reason of insanity as "a vile abuse of the law" and an encouragement of "this execrable crime" (Wesley 1958–59b:481). But by the turn of the twentieth century, most of the horrific medieval laws were repealed in England, though attempted suicide was still a crime punishable by a fine or imprisonment and the successful suicide was denied funeral rites if he took his life while "of sound mind."

This "softer" view of suicide was buttressed by the findings of the social sciences, launched in the late nineteenth century by the work of Enrico Morselli and Emile Durkheim, who approached the phenomenon of suicide as a psychological and social problem rather than a religious and moral one (Droge and Tabor 1992:8–14). Using statistical analysis, Morselli attributed suicide to unconscious trauma rather than self-conscious choice. For Morselli, suicide and insanity were alternative pathological reactions to the individual's failure to compete successfully in the struggle for existence, which in the modern world had become increasingly an intellectual rather than a physical struggle. Durkheim located the cause of suicide in the pathology of the society rather than of the individual. Once again using statistics, Durkheim demonstrated that suicide can be correlated to distinctive patterns of social control in times of social or individual duress. The *altruistic* suicide occurs among those whose lives are viewed as secondary to the claims of the group. The *egoistic* suicide is common among individuals whose attachments to family, church, and community have broken down. The *anomic* suicide results from either the breakdown or the absence of social rules to guide individuals who find themselves in situations of social dislocation or unrest. Later social scientists have refined but continued these pioneering efforts to "medicalize" suicide. They attribute the cause of suicide not to individual choice but to psychological or sociological pathology. Thereby, they take accountability for suicide away from the individual.

For understandable reasons, both the secular society and the religious community welcomed these medicalized views of suicide. Suicide could thereby be decriminalized without accepting or encouraging suicide as the responsible act of a rational person. But the price to be paid for accepting this medical hegemony over suicide is greater than it first appears for those who care about our civil liberties and religious traditions. The act of suicide can be removed from the realm of moral and religious behavior only at the cost of further strengthening the hand of a medical care system that has already become too powerful and too intrusive in our lives. The militant proponents of the right to die may well be the protectors of informed consent and patient rights for all health care issues. Indeed, they may be the vanguard against a growing covert "duty to die" movement—the trend to take treatment decisions out of the hands of individuals and put them in the hands of governmental agencies and insurance carriers who will decide who lives and dies through the rationing of health care.

The carte-blanche acceptance of the medicalization of suicide poses an even greater threat to our religious traditions. Removing suicide from the realm of moral and religious behavior runs the risk of denying responsibility for all self-destructive behavior. However brutal their consequences, traditional religious strictures against suicide at least recognized the awesome reach of human freedom and depth of human responsibility. The Wesleyan tradition reminds us of a volatile world where human beings always retain some margin of moral choice and moral accountability. An even greater danger of removing suicide from the realm of moral and religious behavior is the risk of impugning the integrity of all self-sacrificial acts. Life voluntarily laid down for the sake of others falls under the same pathological cloud as life ended for selfish reasons, an equation that was clearly drawn in Durkheim's concept of altruistic suicide. The Wesleyan guidelines remind us of a vulnerable world where human beings always retain some capacity for moral sacrifice and moral heroism.

Of course, there are suicides that are irrational and pathological. Far too many people are driven to end their own lives by psychological despair or sociological desperation. But there are very good reasons for carving out a guarded space for voluntary death, especially for persons in extremis. Nonetheless, that space should not be conceived as a solitary or even autonomous space. Though our civil traditions speak more of individual rights than of civic duties, our religious traditions place the emphasis on radical freedom *and* responsibility. We are free to take our own lives, but we are accountable to God, country, and family for that decisive act of individual freedom. Whether such a voluntary death can be both rationally chosen *and* morally justified remains to be seen in the analysis that follows. What should be clear at this point is that the best of our civic and religious traditions allow for the possibility of a voluntary death rationally contemplated and freely chosen.

Suffering and Dying as Crisis

Like all theists, Wesley wrestled with the question of theodicy: Are suffering and dying a curse or a gift, an enemy or a friend? Should suffering and dying be fought or accepted? Do suffering and dying embody God's intention or contradict God's purposes? Wesley's response to these questions can be summarized in a simple way: suffering and dying are life crises, but they need not rob life of its meaning and purpose. The two sides of the formulation must be kept in balance. Wesley did not believe that we should simply accept suffering and dying as our inevitable lot in life. These are evils that need to be combated and resisted. But neither should we allow suffering and dying to destroy life's meaning and purpose. Indeed, suffering and dying rightly borne can lead to a happiness and holiness beyond all ordinary human expectation and understanding.

Wesley's deep concern over health and medicine was an outgrowth of his belief that the law of love compels Christians to battle against suffering, which includes both physical and emotional pain, both bodily and mental derangement (Holifield 1986:63–84). Wesley's medical tracts and dispensaries grew out of the same motivation that fueled his concern about slavery, poverty, prostitution, and alcoholism. The Christian's primary task when faced with suffering is to overcome it, for suffering is an enemy and not a friend. Yet even suffering as enemy can serve as an occasion for deepening holiness and happiness. Wesley's conviction that suffering could be purposeful reflected a deep conviction that the strength needed to bear the pain and loss of suffering would always be given. Suffering should be faced realistically, but it must be borne with patience. Christians need not deny their pain or mask their hope for deliverance. But they should not allow suffering to overpower or destroy them. For Wesley, that patient endurance "was the faith that pain bore a meaning beyond itself, that it created a pathway to holiness and hence, mysteriously, to happiness" (Holifield 1986:65).

The same dialectical tension found in Wesley's response to suffering is also evident in his vision of dying as both penalty and promise (Holifield 1986:85–105). This tension enabled him to avoid the sentimental illusion that death is unreal and the despairing conclusion that death is invincible. Wesley's view of death as a penalty was tied both to original sin and to actual sin. He insisted that death—physical and spiritual, temporal and eternal—must be viewed as a punishment for sin. Because of original sin, physical and temporal death is the inevitable fate of all human beings. Because of actual sin, spiritual and eternal death is the deserved lot of all human beings. By thus viewing death as

a penalty for sin, Wesley avoided all romantic notions of death as a natural completion of human growth or as a beautiful passage to the fuller
life. Death is neither merely a biological event nor a spiritual benefit.
Dying is an enemy to be feared and an event to be dreaded. But Wesley
also believed that dying contained a promise. He believed in the immortality of the soul and the resurrection of the body. Dying frees the faithful from the limitations of bodily existence and frees them for the con-
solations of eternal life. Therefore, while rightly dreading the prospect
of death, the Christian can faithfully embrace the process of dying, for
"to die is gain." Death is to be resisted stoutly but not fought indefinitely.

The Wesleyan tradition's linking of suffering and death on a continuum of loss is confirmed by a growing medical, philosophical, and
autobiographical literature on the experience of pain. As Elaine Scarry
has shown, pain has the power to "unmake" the world (Scarry 1985).
The experience of great pain lays bare the radical interdependence of
self and body. For persons in intractable pain, the body moves from the
background to the foreground of their experienced world. Their culturally instilled sense of transcendence of self over body collapses into
either radical identification or radical alienation. Pain can undercut a
person's capacity "to move out beyond the boundaries of his or her own
body into the external, sharable world" (Scarry 1985:13). The body can
virtually become one's world, as pain occupies more and more of one's
consciousness and crowds out awareness of anything else. Or unrelenting pain can have the opposite effect of destroying a person's familiarity with his or her own body. The body is then interposed between the
individual and reality. In that case, the body can become the *enemy*. The
body stands opposite to the self. Instead of serving, it demands service.
In either case, intense pain can destroy a person's self and world, "a
destruction experienced spatially as either the contraction of the universe down to the immediate vicinity of the body or as the body swelling
to fill the entire universe" (Scarry 1985:35).

Of course, physicians have a remarkable pharmacopoeia at hand to alleviate physical pain. Palliative care for the terminally ill who are in great pain has come a long way to overcome the slow and agonizing death. But what of that other kind of pain which is just as destructive of a person's life-world and selfhood? We tend to ignore or minimize mental pain as if it were somehow less real than physical pain. David B. Morris traces this separation to what he calls "the myth of two pains." Our culture divides physical and mental pain into two types "as different as land and sea. You feel physical pain if your arm breaks. You feel mental pain if your heart breaks. Between these two events we seem to imagine a gulf so wide and deep that it might as well be filled by a sea that is impossible to navigate" (Morris 1991:19). Like all cultural myths, this separation contains some serviceable truth. Yet in the long run, this nineteenth-century separation of pain into two radically different sources and valences has emptied physical pain of any meaning ("it's only a neuro-electric impulse") and deprived mental pain of any standing ("it's all in your head").

But numerous interdisciplinary pain studies and grief therapies are challenging this widespread myth. We are relearning scientifically and philosophically what all of us *know* for sure in the lived world of our own embodied existence. Put in simplest terms, when our hearts ache our bodies hurt, and when our bodies hurt our hearts ache. Pain and grief are the Siamese twins of all human suffering. Here the word *grief* denotes an overwhelming sense of loss and despair. Grief is a peculiar amalgam of such feelings as helplessness, rage, fear, guilt, doubt, shame, terror, anxiety, bewilderment, and hostility (Kliever 1995). Pain and grief are intertwined in such a way that it is impossible to experience them apart, however we may try to distinguish them in theory and in practice. Of course, short-term pain and grief create the illusion that they occur in logic-tight compartments because we can bring them under control before they synergize. This separation is reinforced by the management of pain and grief through a growing arsenal of medical analgesics. But the inseparability of pain and grief clearly emerges where there are no "magic bullets" to dissolve the compound of suffering that comes with chronic illness and degenerative disease.

Such suffering, born of unrelenting pain and unrelieved grief, can truly be a "suffering unto death." We are so accustomed to thinking of death as an event that we have forgotten that death is a process. Dying starts happening well before the moment of death arrives, as conventionally defined and medically determined. Psychiatrist E. Mansell Pattison describes this process as the "living-dying interval," that period of time when death is no longer the inevitable abstraction that it is when we are healthy, but a very real, time-bound condition (Pattison 1977:43–60). He further divides the living-dying interval into three clinical phases: (1) the *acute crisis phase* when serious illness or accident forcefully raises the existential prospect of death, (2) the *chronic living-dying phase* during which time the balance of the physical and psychological symptoms of a disease shifts from being under control to being in control, and (3) the *terminal phase* of physical deterioration and emotional disorganization that mark the onset of giving up and letting go of life itself. Finally, Pattison distinguishes the four types of death that occur during the terminal stage: (1) *sociological* death, where others withdraw and separate themselves from the patient, (2) *psychic* death, where the patient accepts death and withdraws into him- or herself, (3) *biological* death, where the mind-body organism as a self-conscious and self-sustaining whole breaks down, and (4) *physiological* death, where vital organs such as lungs, heart, and brain no longer function.

Distinguishing these four types of death is important because they can cause profound suffering when they occur out of phase with each other. A person may become socially dead long before the other aspects of death occur. Or the social denial of death may prolong a person's dying after psychic and biological death have already happened. Such confusions of the dying trajectory are due in large measure to advancements in medicine and breakdowns of tradition. Dying was once a process that one usually entered and left rather quickly according to well-known medical symptoms and ritual gestures. Today, the diagnosis and treatment of a terminal illness may extend over a period of months or even years before death. Of course, the lengthening of the dying period can allow the dying person extra time to reach closure on life in a satisfying manner. But the prolongation of the living-dying interval can also multiply suffering exponentially. Our customs have not kept pace with our medical technology; in a culture bereft of normative behaviors and social settings for dealing with prolonged dying, the dying are often left to wrestle with their own pain and grief without the support of others or the solace of rituals. Problems of social isolation, chronic pain, diminished capacity, emotional distress, and financial cost can become such crushing burdens that a person is doing more dying than living. For many in these straits, death would come as a welcome friend. Instead, the sick are suspended between barely living and not quite dying by a medical technology and a moral outlook that requires them to suffer their way to death.

Justice and Mercy as Norm

What do we owe those who are suffering their way to death, and what do they owe us? If we take the Wesleyan tradition seriously, this is a question of justice *and* mercy. We must always weigh what law requires and prohibits as well as what love allows and demands in such situations of extremity. Moreover, these questions must be addressed within a context that holds freedom and responsibility together in a moral balance. Both these interlocking norms and dimensions of human choice must be addressed if religious warrants for euthanasia are to be found.

Wesley spoke from time to time in his writings of justice and mercy, but law and love were his preferred categories for articulating these biblical norms of the righteous life. Certainly the demands of justice (giving to each according to his or her due) are enshrined in the laws of God. But the constraints of mercy (giving to each according to his or her need) are evoked by the love of God. Here again we encounter the same inner dialectic that characterized Wesley's fundamental approach to all theological and moral issues. The polarity of law and love creates a tension between the minimal requirements of equity and the maximal requirements of generosity. The duties of law establish the social order. The demands of love address the situational need. This polarity of law and love embodies the Wesleyan conviction that the moral life requires both structure and compassion.

Wesley believed that the will of God is expressed in and through four levels of law (Holifield 1986:114–16). The *eternal* law is identical with the divine reason that structured the world and as such is the supreme and unchangeable order that stands behind the world of finite things and visible appearances. The *moral* law is the model of truth and goodness written into the structure of human nature and as such is discernible to the faithful and faithless alike as the rule of conscience. The *revealed* law is the written law in the Old and New Testaments, which bring to light the moral law engraved in human nature. The revealed law includes the Decalogue and its exposition by the prophets and its intensification by Christ and the apostles. Finally, the *civil* law prescribes those duties that are "due to Caesar." While the Christian is obligated to honor the political leaders and laws of the land, civil laws are answerable to the higher levels of law and therefore may be challenged and changed for the sake of justice. While he believed that the laws of God lend themselves through church and state to precise formulation and clear obligation, Wesley reduced these several dimensions of the law to three general rules of conduct that he imposed on all members of his "societies." First, they were to do no harm. Second, they were to do good. Third, they were to attend to the ordinances of public worship and private devotion.[4]

This hierarchical ordering of the law implicitly recognizes an element of tension between the concrete expressions of law in society and Scripture and the timeless grounds of law in human nature and divine reason. This tension is further intensified by the Wesleyan polarity of law and love. Finally, love is the intention and fulfillment of the law (Marquardt 1992:103–18). Love alone is the indispensable condition for any deed to be called good. Through the operations of prevenient grace, such loving deeds are possible for all human beings. Of course, the loving deeds of those who have not yet received the love of God through sanctifying grace remain provisional and relative. Only a person prompted and shaped by the unlimited love of God can fulfill God's law with the full sensitivity and generosity of divine love. Thus believers and unbelievers alike live under a higher demand than mere justice—giving others what they deserve under the law. They are also constrained by the demands of mercy—giving others what they need in the name of love.

For Wesley, this tension between law and love does not destroy their essential continuity. Law is the instrument of love as surely as love is the intention of law. But maintaining the Wesleyan tension between law and love has several salutary moral implications for the care of the sick. For one, the tension between law and love makes "doing good" a matter of public policy as well as private virtue. The Wesleyan tradition has always sought to embody the works of love in social structures as well as in individual deeds. Moreover, the tension between law and love undercuts all simple utilitarian solutions to the ethical problems of medicine. The constraints of love always stand in judgment against the prudent calculations of distributive or retributive justice. Finally, the tension between law and love tempers all "universalizable" solutions to the ethical dilemmas of medicine. Despite the importance of fixed principles of moral reflection, no one set of rules can prescribe what love will always require in particular circumstances.

We can see something of this tension between law and love at work in the remarkable changes in medical treatment of the dying over the last twenty years. The concept of a right to withhold or withdraw extraordinary means of treatment is gaining wide acceptance as a matter of moral principle, legal right, and medical practice in most modern societies. Of course, the withdrawing or withholding of treatment is limited to the *terminally* ill, most often to patients in a comatose or permanently vegetative state. But less severely compromised individuals are beginning to exercise their rights as well to forgo life-extending and death-delaying treatments that they judge to be futile.

Religious sanctions for allowing people to die without heroic intervention have a long history. The traditional Roman Catholic distinction between ordinary and extraordinary means of preserving life arose four hundred years ago in a period of great medical and scientific advances (Bole 1990). New therapeutic and surgical procedures were both painful and costly, thereby raising questions about their desirability and necessity. The theological tradition isolated three factors that alone or in combination could render treatment to preserve life extraordinary and therefore non-obligatory. The first was hard-to-obtain means. The second factor was extraordinarily burdensome treatment, burdensome because it was financially excessive (requiring *sumptus extraordinarius*, inordinate cost, or *media pretiosa*, extravagant means), physically excessive (involving *quidam cruciatus*, considerable torture, or *ingens dolar*, immoderate grief), or psychologically excessive (producing *vehemens horror*, ardent repulsion, *summus labor*, laborious effort, or *nimia dura*, lasting indignity). The third factor was insufficient expectation of recovery, an assessment based on poor quality and meager quantity of life. Of course, these venerable guidelines were all but eclipsed by the rise of "heroic" medicine (which battles death to the bitter end) and the decline of "traditional" religion (which accepts death as a part of life). But, in recent years, both Jewish and Christian traditions have for the most part reached a consensus that extraordinary efforts to preserve life are not morally obligatory if the patient deems such medical procedures disproportionate to the expected result.

But permission to forgo extraordinary means to preserve the life for those who are overmastered by dying is limited to allowing to die, and that usually for physical suffering alone. Overt consideration is seldom given to the excessive psychological and financial burdens of the terminally ill. Moreover, active medical intervention to speed the dying process is not allowed, but only the withholding or withdrawing of treatments that artificially and fruitlessly prolong the dying process. An apparent exception is made for terminal cases where crushing physical pain cannot be controlled safely by analgesics. The elevated use of opioids to control severe pain may hasten death by repressing the central nervous system. But most bioethicists and physicians justify this treatment in terms of some "principle of double effect."[5] In such cases, death is not directly sought or intended, even if the strong likelihood of death is recognized. The intention is to relieve pain, although death is an unintended effect of such relief.

Justice may well be served by such allowing to die, but where is the mercy for those patients who are so disabled by bodily or mental impairments that existence is a constant psychological or physical torment? What possible benefit will they derive from the pain and shame of such a death? Wherein lies the real moral difference between *allowing* and *helping* those who are suffering their way to death to complete the process of dying? Of course, all manner of medical and moral distinctions can be drawn between allowing to die and euthanasia (Beauchamp and Childress 1989:134–54), but they all come down to a single fact. In allowing to die, the underlying pathology causes death, while the medical intervention causes death in euthanasia.[6] In either case, death is the express choice of the patient whether that intention is voiced through direct instruction or medical directive. Why then must the means of death be chosen only by others? Once safeguards are built in to protect against impulsive or irrational requests for help in dying, why should not those who are overmastered by physical or psychological suffering be free to get help in speeding the dying process? Why are they legally and morally free to choose to die lingering deaths by refusing treatment, disconnecting machines, or withholding nutrition, but

not free to choose a quick, painless death which their doctors could easily provide? Why must some underlying pathology rather than a caring
physician be "the old man's friend" who brings physical and psychological suffering to a merciful end?

Viewed in this light, existing moral and legal constraints against
active euthanasia seem more for the protection of others than for the
dying patient's good. Such constraints protect family and physicians
from the spiritual burdens and legal liabilities of *causing* the patient's
death. But opponents of euthanasia will object that these constraints
rest on the sanctity and solidarity of human life—principles that must
take precedence over the dying patient's autonomy and best interest.[7]
Those who want to cut their lives short because of their diminished
quality are breaking faith with the human community and doing violence to the sanctity of life. Deliberately ending a human life—our own
or another's—denies its social or its cosmic value. Finally, both the living and the dying are responsible to protect the sanctity and solidarity
of life, no matter what the physical, psychological, or financial cost to
those involved.

Viewed another way, however, the sanctity and solidarity of human
life can provide warrants that permit rather than proscribe euthanasia.
In the Wesleyan tradition, life's sanctity is based on prevenient grace
and eternal life. All life is valuable because every human being embodies the image of God and the promise of immortality. For those very
reasons, the sanctity of life has nothing to do with quantitative measures
of life's strength or length. Prolonging suffering or postponing dying
adds nothing to the intrinsic value of a person's life. Nor does evading
suffering or embracing death negate life's inherent worth. Death is neither an unmitigated tragedy nor an unavoidable discipline in the
Wesleyan view. Rather, death is both a threat to be fought with courage
and a promise to be met with gratitude.

Something of this same reverence for life and acceptance of death
can also be affirmed by those who do not believe in life after death. The

dying process can be seen as the seal of life rather than as the door to eternity. Ending life appropriately is as important as living life earnestly. "It is a platitude that we live our whole lives in the shadow of death; it is also true that we die in the shadow of our whole lives" (Dworkin 1993:199). This double-edged truth lies behind the emphasis we put on dying with *dignity*. The death we die should keep faith with the life we lived.

In other words, the sanctity of life is not some universal property, least of all some biological function. The sanctity of a person's life is rooted in the distinctive form of that person's life. Each person shapes his or her cultural inheritance into a distinctive life project. The sanctity of life is rooted in biography rather than biology, which is precisely why, given the choice, people will deal with dying in different ways. Some will battle death to the end, even through terrible pain or hopeless treatment, because they were fighters all their lives. Others will prefer death to a life of dependence and degradation because they lived an active and self-reliant life. Finally, these choices are matters not of taste but of character, matters not of autonomy but of sanctity. None of us wants to die out of character. We want our dying to be of a piece with our living.

But what of the claim that the person who chooses to die rather than live with intolerable physical or psychological pain is acting selfishly? Even if the choice were in character, would it not still be against the community? Does choosing immediate death rather than prolonged dying not represent a final negative judgment on the usefulness of the life taken and trustworthiness of the supporting fabric? At stake here is what the dying owe to the living in upholding the solidarity of human life. Can the decision to end a life wracked by suffering or submerged in unconsciousness ever be an affirmation rather than a betrayal of community? Put more dramatically, can there ever be a self-chosen death of the sickroom that enjoys the same honor as the martyrdom of the battlefield?

Of course, dying for the sake of others enjoys the highest moral approbation in both our secular and religious views of the commonweal. But these traditions typically draw a categorical line between martyrdom and suicide. The martyr's death is self-sacrifice; the suicide's death is self-murder. These distinctions, however, devolve on persuasive definitions. One person's martyrdom is another person's suicide (Droge and Tabor 1992:188). The decisive question is *why* a person chooses to die. Surely some critically or chronically ill persons have longed for death in order to evade social abandonment or escape chronic depression. But just as surely others have wished to die to free their loved ones from unhealable wounds of grief or extravagant means of care. Failing to mark the difference in attitude toward others in these different reasons for wanting to die is morally obtuse. Those who wish to die to avoid "being a burden to others" may be acting out of the deepest respect for life and commitment to others. To close the door to such charitable and courageous acts of euthanasia is both insensitive and uncaring.

In short, there are times when euthanasia *supports* the sanctity and solidarity of human life. But everything depends on what is consistent with the character and appropriate to the circumstance of the person involved. Seen in this light, we can understand why people differ so dramatically about how their lives should end. Whether our lives should end one way rather than another depends on what has sanctified and sustained our lives—the distinctive values we treasured, causes we served, people we loved, meanings we embraced. Thus we can also understand why the state should not impose some uniform way of dying but encourage people to make provision for their own way of dying or, lacking such individual or advanced directives, leave those decisions in the hands of people who had intimate knowledge of the patient and what he would want for himself (Dworkin 1993:213).

Healing and Care as Goal

Some commentators are willing to admit that hastening the death of those for whom life has become unbearable may be morally permissible under certain circumstances, but they remain dead set against any involvement of physicians in enabling such persons to end or to take their own lives. Their arguments are twofold. Physician-assisted suicide—and physician-performed euthanasia, even more—contradicts the goals and means of medicine. The age-old rule against mercy killing by a physician embedded in the Hippocratic oath has its roots in the very idea of the physician as healer. Turning the healing art into the killing art would pervert the practice of medicine and undermine the public's confidence in the profession (Kass 1985:157–223). Furthermore, any such medicalization of killing may be a first and fateful step toward euthanizing the mentally impaired, the socially unproductive, and eventually the ideologically unwanted (Lifton 1986). Authorizing the killing of suffering or insentient patients for their own benefit could open the door to killing those same patients for the social benefits their deaths would provide. Voluntary euthanasia could lead to involuntary euthanasia.

These are formidable dangers, but whether physician-supported euthanasia compromises the means of medicine depends on our definition of the ends of medicine. If the primary aims of medicine are death prevention and life prolongation, then euthanasia is inconsistent with the true practice of medicine. But this widely held view that preservation of life is the true goal of medicine is open to serious question. For the Wesleyan tradition, neither the prolongation of life nor the prevention of death is the end of medicine. Rather, healing and care are the true work of medicine. Moreover, these twin goals of medicine must take due regard for the physical and spiritual aspects of healthiness (Holifield 1986:160–80). Good health and well-being were never simply equated, though Wesley certainly affirmed bodily health as a desideratum of spiritual well-being and recognized the impact of spiritual well-being on bodily health. Human wholeness is ultimately a matter of the capacity to love and serve. Healthiness embraces both bodily and relational integrity. Thus healing and care were always held in dialectical tension. Healing involved caring for the physical and spiritual needs of the ill. Even when healing was impossible, caring for the ill and dying remained the physician's duty. For Wesley, medicine was always practiced within the tension between life's possibilities and life's limitations.

This Wesleyan view of medicine is remarkably consonant with a growing *humanistic* understanding of medicine. Against the popular idea that physicians battle death and prolong life, physician Leon R. Kass argues that the goals of medicine are restoring health and relieving suffering (Kass 1985:175–86). Of course, good health is a relative condition because it involves the "well-working" of the organism and the well-being of the person. Healthiness is always a matter of physical *and* human functioning. Medicine at its best attends to both the physical and the psychosocial dimensions of helping patients get well. For the acutely ill or seriously traumatized, the primary focus of medical care is the treatment of disease. But for the chronically ill or permanently disabled, the balance of medical treatment should shift from fighting disease to improving life functions and life situations.

What happens when physical pain and personal suffering are so burdensome that human well-being is simply crushed? Of course, easing pain is always a crucial goal of medical treatment, but relieving suffering becomes the *only* goal when medicine can no longer heal. Seen in this light, continuing medical interventions that are neither healing nor comforting is incommensurate with the twin goals of medicine—to restore health and to relieve suffering. But is it enough merely to withhold or withdraw therapeutic measures that increase or prolong physical pain and personal suffering? May not the physician be obligated by the very goals of medicine to assist the patient who wants to die rather than live a tortured and useless existence? What greater care could a physician show for patients who are suffering their way to death than to honor their resolute requests to speed their dying? Clearly, euthanasia is wrong if it does injury to someone or is contrary to the known preferences of someone. But helping terminate a person's life does no intrinsic violence to the goals of medicine when there is a rational and responsible request to speed the dying process.

Nor does the warning that physician-assisted euthanasia leads to involuntary euthanasia hold up under critical scrutiny. This "slippery slope" argument rests on the implicit assumption that euthanasia always undermines the sacredness and solidarity of human life. But, as argued above, there are times when euthanasia confirms the value of human life and affirms the bonds of human community. Indeed, the way of dying that cheapens human life and dissolves human community is our modern medicalization of death. Death is no longer a momentous event that takes place at the end of life in the company of trusted others. Death is a lonely process under the control of physicians in the company of strangers. We may have more to fear of the debasement of life and the routinization of death from "heroic" and "bureaucratic" medicine than from compassionate and controlled euthanasia.

But is such compassion and control possible, given the way medicine is practiced in this country (Battin 1991:302–3)? Here we reach what many believe is the most compelling argument against physician-performed euthanasia. The moral space and sanctions for euthanasia sketched above depend on the physician's knowing how a self-chosen death fits into the dying patient's life story and knowing that it represents the dying patient's best interests. But how often does such clear and convincing discussion between doctor and patient happen in modern medical practice? Medicine today is increasingly impersonal and technical. The dying patient is a collection of pathologies treated by different specialists. The attending physician *manages* the case rather than *cares* for the patient. Moreover, health care today is increasingly expensive and therefore rationed by the ability to pay. The financial aspects of dying are such that the "right to die" could become the "duty to die" in the face of mounting medical bills or limitations of coverage. How can we be sure that dying patients are not prompted or even coerced to end their lives as long as we lack a system of primary-care medicine and universal health insurance? Perhaps the American way of dying is bad enough without adding euthanasia to the mix.[8]

No one can deny that these are real weaknesses and dangers in our impersonal and inequitable medical care system. But there are two rejoinders to the argument that we must wait for a more personal and equitable health care system before approving euthanasia. The first is that, even in our current system, the comparatively few patients wanting to speed their dying could receive assistance if physicians were not so afraid of legal or professional reprisal (Brody 1993:A18). There are many sensitive and caring physicians who are willing to shorten the dying process, but their hands are tied by moral, legal, and professional constraints. Only the notorious or courageous few are willing to put their patients' rights and needs ahead of their own interests. Still, even in our flawed system, we are only a step away from providing medical assistance for those who are ready to die: withholding or withdrawing treatment is, in fact, a way of helping people to speed the dying process. The second objection, closely related to the first, is that the current American practice of withholding or withdrawing treatment in end-of-life situations is itself open to a wide range of abuses, precisely because such practices are not scrutinized as closely as more direct life-terminating practices would be. The comparative invisibility of withdrawing or withholding treatment invites the termination of curative care at the direction of insurance carriers or the discretion of physicians without due regard for the patient's autonomy or best interests. As things stand, the opportunities for depriving the dying of proper medical care are as great with our unstructured practices of letting people die as they might be with a properly administered system of helping people die.

Finally, all arguments for and against compassionate and controlled active euthanasia turn on how we understand the sanctity and solidarity of human life as well as the goals and means of medicine. Legal, moral, and medical professionals have reached a near consensus that these interests are best preserved and served by the practice of allowing to die only. But the fact remains that withholding or with-drawing treatment can negate these very principles. Many terminally ill or severely compromised patients are required to suffer their way to death over the extended downhill course of degenerative diseases that cause the majority of deaths in all advanced industrial democracies (Battin 1991:298). Of course, physicians try to control pain and mini-mize symptoms while withholding treatment, but these measures may disguise the fact that they are letting the disease kill the patient rather than bringing about death more directly. Moreover, the way such end-stage degenerative diseases as AIDS, Alzheimer's, or multiple sclerosis kill people is far more dehumanizing and agonizing than the way physi-cians might help terminate patients who are ready and willing to die.

How then are we to proceed in letting justice and mercy "flow down" to those who are unwillingly suffering their way to death? Given the way we practice and pay for medical care in this country, *legalizing* physician-administered euthanasia seems quite ill-advised even if morally permissible. Hoping that our legal system will follow the Dutch practice of protecting from prosecution those physicians who perform euthanasia is naive, given our polarized and litigious soci-ety. Physician-assisted suicide does, however, provide a way of giving physicians some control over the circumstances while leaving the fun-damental decision about ending life to the patients themselves (Quill et al. 1992:1380–83). Of course, physicians would supply the means for ending life to patients whose condition was hopeless and whose suffer-ing was intolerable. But whether to use those means would remain up to the patient and his or her moral and spiritual advisors. In this approach, "the physician is involved, but not directly; and it is the patient's choice, but the patient is not alone in making it" (Battin 1991:305). Moreover, all that would be required with respect to legalization of physician-assisted suicide would be the decriminalization of assisted suicide.

Because suicide is irreversible, this extraordinary treatment should be made available from the patient's primary physician only after other alternatives for a comfortable and dignified death have been exhausted. Moreover, such a course of action should meet carefully defined criteria to ensure that the patient is acting freely and in his or her own best interests. Timothy E. Quill, Christine K. Cassel, and Diane E. Meier have proposed that physician-assisted suicide meet seven clinical criteria (Quill et al. 1992:1381–82): (1) the patient must have a condition that is incurable and associated with severe, unrelenting suffering; (2) the physician must ensure that the patient's suffering and the request to die are not the result of inadequate comfort care; (3) the patient must clearly and repeatedly, of his or her own free will and initiative, request to die rather than continue suffering; (4) the physician must be sure that the patient's judgment is not distorted; (5) physician-assisted suicide should be carried out only in the context of a meaningful doctor-patient relationship; (6) consultation with another experienced physician is required to ensure that the patient's request is voluntary and rational, the diagnosis and prognosis accurate, and the exploration of comfort-oriented alternatives thorough; and (7) clear documentation to support each condition is required. Guided and guarded by such criteria as these, physician-assisted suicide does no violence to the sanctity and solidarity of human life or to the goals and means of medicine.

All moral decisions and policies are situational meldings of factual circumstances and value judgments. The Wesleyan tradition of health and medicine represents such a joining in the past. Of course, Wesley's guidelines for the care of the sick and dying were grounded in his theological convictions and empirical knowledge. For that reason, his views on freedom and responsibility, suffering and death, justice and mercy, and healing and care cannot be transposed uncriticized and unchanged into the contemporary debate over "choosing death in America." But these guidelines can furnish the framework for a fresh appraisal of the Christian tradition as it relates to the broad questions of allowing to die and euthanasia and to the narrower distinctions between physician-assisted suicide and physician-performed euthanasia.

Emulating the spirit of John Wesley, I have tried to bring together the spiritual and the physical, the religious and the ethical, the ancient and the modern, and the customary and the scientific in a fresh way of thinking about voluntary death. If the foregoing Socratic dialogue with myself has not fallen too far short of clarity and consistency, then a broadly defined religious case has been made for euthanasia under carefully controlled and properly administered conditions. Speaking in traditional terms, this religious case is based on *natural* rather than *revealed* theology. Put in a more contemporary framework, this case is grounded in civil religion rather than historic faith. What it offers is a clear alternative to both narrow philosophical defenses of euthanasia based on individual autonomy and dogmatic theological proscriptions of euthanasia based on the sanctity of life. In no sense have I argued that euthanasia is a religious or moral *duty*. But euthanasia can be a rational and responsible decision, fully consonant with religious and moral integrity.

Having claimed that for my argument, I must confess that I made up my mind about euthanasia in the process of researching and writing this paper. What began as an open question has ended in a firm conviction. But behind this change of mind based on careful study is a change of heart that I owe to ongoing conversations with my ninety-three-year-old mother. Amanda Kliever is a fiercely proud and independent woman who has lived virtually alone since my father died in 1949. She has enjoyed a lifetime of remarkably good health, but the last four years have forced her to concede that she is "finally getting old." In response to her hardening arteries and failing knees, she had to give up her beloved car and take up a despised cane.

Other less trivial events have cast the shadow of mortality over Amanda's life. The recent death of her oldest child, which breached an earlier vow that she would never bury another child, and grief over her older sister's long struggle with Alzheimer's disease have brought her own dying to mind. A woman of simple but profound piety, she speaks easily of dying "when her time comes." But she shrinks in horror at the thought of a lingering death filled with physical pain or enfeebled dependence. Indeed, she would happily die in her sleep, but she cannot bear the thought of someone finding her without her wig and her dentures in place. And so, like Nietzsche with whom she has nothing else in common, she wants to "die proudly when it is no longer possible to live proudly" (Nietzsche 1964:88).

Amanda has left no doubts about the way she wants to die. She most decidedly does *not* want to die hooked up to a machine or warehoused in a nursing home. For that reason and with my assistance, she has executed a directive to physicians and given me durable power of attorney for health care issues. Copies of both documents have been filed with her doctor, and other family members have been told of her wishes. Still she talks with me from time to time about her eventual dying, as if to reassure herself that I really do understand that she does not want to live out her days in pain or shame. The thought of agonizing pain is no more daunting to her than the thought of unrelenting shame. The prospect of losing control of bodily functions is no more acceptable to her than losing touch with reality. These conversations about end-of-life issues always end with my promising to honor her wish to die with some bodily integrity and personal dignity intact. Only now, I have a much better idea of how and why I will keep that promise.

NOTES

1. The term *voluntary death* includes both suicide and martyrdom as well as physician-assisted and physician-performed euthanasia. The moral distinctions between these forms of self-chosen death will be explored below.

2. Methodism is certainly not a creedal tradition. Methodist churches and church members are not bound by a shared confession or an official theology. But there is a discernible theological style in Methodism despite the rich variety of belief and practice within Methodist churches. This distinctive theological style is rooted in the four theological criteria to which Wesley appealed in his writings and teachings—Scripture, tradition, experience, and reason. See the chapter on "Wesley and His Tradition" in *Health and Medicine in the Methodist Tradition: Journey toward Wholeness* (Holifield 1986:3–27).

3. My appropriation of the Wesleyan heritage on health and medicine is heavily dependent on Holifield 1986 and Harold Y. Vanderpool 1986:317–53.

4. It is worth noting that the first two of Wesley's general rules of conduct are the same as the classical principles enshrined in the Hippocratic oath—non-maleficence and beneficence—and invoked in virtually every discussion of medical ethics. For example, see Beauchamp and Childress 1989:120–255.

5. The Roman Catholic tradition has given precise statement to the principle of double effect. When a desired effect and an undesired effect result from the same human act, the act is morally good on four conditions: (1) the object of the act must be morally good, (2) only the good results of the act must be intended, (3) the good effect must not result from the bad effect, and (4) there must be a proportionately good reason for allowing the bad effect to occur. See O'Rourke 1992:165–67.

6. James Rachels argues that there is no moral difference between acts of killing and allowing to die in voluntary euthanasia. The only morally significant question about how self-chosen death occurs is, Which method will minimize the person's suffering (Rachels 1975)?

7. Religious arguments against euthanasia usually stress the sanctity of life, while secular counterarguments typically emphasize the solidarity of life. But both the sanctity and solidarity of life can be defined and defended on either secular or religious grounds (Dworkin 1993:81–84, 194–96).

8. Opponents of euthanasia often point out the differences between our system and that of the Netherlands, where physician-performed euthanasia is permitted. In Holland, basic care is provided by the family doctor, who generally lives in the neighborhood, makes house calls, and remains the family's physician for years. In addition, Holland has a system of national health insurance that covers all aspects of health care from the cradle to the grave. Physician-assisted or physician-performed euthanasia is less vulnerable to abuse under these conditions than under the American health care system, although recent literature documents a surprising amount of euthanasia without the knowledge or consent of either the patient or the family of the patient.

REFERENCES

Battin, Margaret P. 1991. "Euthanasia: The Way We Do It, the Way They Do It." *Journal of Pain and Symptom Management* 6 (July): 298–305.

Beauchamp, Tom L., and James F. Childress. 1989. *Principles of Biomedical Ethics*, 3d ed. New York: Oxford University Press.

Bole, Thomas J., III. 1990. "Intensive Care Units (ICUs) and Ordinary Means: Turning Virtue into Vice." *Linacre Quarterly* 57 (February): 68–77.

Brody, Jane E. 1993. "Doctors Admit Ignoring Dying Patients' Wishes." *New York Times*, 14 January, A12.

Clemons, James T. 1990. *What Does the Bible Say about Suicide?* Minneapolis: Fortress Press.

Dax's Case. 1984. 16mm and VCR. Distributed by Film Makers Library, New York.

Droge, Arthur J., and James D. Tabor. 1992. *A Noble Death: Suicide and Martyrdom among Christians and Jews in Antiquity*. San Francisco: Harper.

Dworkin, Ronald. 1993. *Life's Dominion: An Argument about Abortion, Euthanasia, and Individual Freedom*. New York: Alfred A. Knopf.

Gadamer, Hans-Georg. 1975. *Truth and Method*. New York: Seabury Press.

Hauerwas, Stanley. 1977. "Memory, Community, and the Reasons for Living: Reflections on Suicide and Euthanasia." In *Truthfulness and Tragedy*, ed. Stanley Hauerwas, Richard Bondi, and David B. Burrell, 101–15. Notre Dame, Ind.: University of Notre Dame Press.

Holifield, E. Brooks. 1986. *Health and Medicine in the Methodist Tradition: Journey toward Wholeness*. New York: Crossroad.

Kass, Leon R. 1985. *Toward a More Natural Science: Biology and Human Affairs*. New York: Free Press.

Kliever, Lonnie D. 1995. "Rage and Grief: Another Look at *Dax's Case*." In *Chronic Illness: From Experience to Policy*, ed. S. Kay Toombs, David Barnard, and Ronald A. Carson. Bloomington: Indiana University Press.

———, ed. 1989. *Dax's Case: Essays in Medical Ethics and Human Meaning*. Dallas: SMU Press.

Laney, James T. 1969. "Ethics and Death." In *Perspectives on Death*, ed. Liston Mills, 231–52. Nashville: Abingdon Press.

Lifton, Robert Jay. 1986. *The Nazi Doctors: Medical Killing and the Psychology of Genocide*. New York: Basic Books.

Lowell, James Russell. 1939. "The Christian Life." In *The Methodist Hymnal*.

Marquardt, Manfred. 1992. *John Wesley's Social Ethics: Praxis and Principles*. Nashville: Abingdon Press.

Marty, Martin E. 1986. Foreword to *Health and Medicine in the Methodist Tradition* by E. Brooks Holifield. New York: Crossroad.

Morris, David B. 1991. *The Culture of Pain*. Berkeley and Los Angeles: University of California Press.

Nancy Beth Cruzan et al. v. Director, Missouri Department of Health, et al. 1990. *United States Law Week* 6:26–90, 58LW4916–4941.

Nietzsche, Friedrich. 1964. "The Twilight of the Idols." In vol. 16 of *The Complete Works of Friedrich Nietzsche*, trans. Anthony M. Ludovici. New York: Russell and Russell.

O'Rourke, Kevin. 1992. "Pain Relief: Ethical Issues and Catholic Teaching." In *Birth, Suffering, and Death: Catholic Perspectives on the Edges of Life*, ed. Kevin Wm. Wildes, Francesc Abel, and John C. Harvey, 157–70. Dordrecht: Kluwer Academic Publishers.

Pattison, E. Mansell. 1977. *The Experience of Dying*. Englewood Cliffs, N.J.: Prentice-Hall.

Quill, Timothy E., Christine K. Cassel, and Diane E. Meier. 1992. "Care of the Hopelessly Ill: Proposed Clinical Criteria for Physician-Assisted Suicide." *New England Journal of Medicine* 327 (November): 1380–84.

Rachels, James. 1975. "Active and Passive Euthanasia." *New England Journal of Medicine* 292 (9 January): 78–80.

Ramsey, Paul. 1970. *The Patient as Person*. New Haven: Yale University Press.

Scarry, Elaine. 1985. *The Body in Pain: The Making and Unmaking of the World*. New York: Oxford University Press.

Vanderpool, Harold Y. 1986. "The Wesleyan-Methodist Tradition." In *Caring and Curing: Health and Medicine in the Western Religious Traditions*, ed. Ronald L. Numbers and Darrel W. Amundsen, 317–53. New York: Macmillan.

Wesley, John. 1958–59a. "Thoughts on Slavery." In *The Works of John Wesley* 11:59–79. Grand Rapids, Mich.: Zondervan.

———. 1958–59b. "Thoughts on Suicide." In *The Works of John Wesley* 13:481. Grand Rapids, Mich.: Zondervan.

Williams, Glanville. 1957. *The Sanctity of Life and the Criminal Law*. New York: Alfred A. Knopf.

CHAPTER 12

Euthanasia and Physician-Assisted Suicide: A Believers' Church Perspective

Daniel B. McGee

J. Robert Oppenheimer described the reaction that he and others felt as they watched the multicolored splendor of the first atomic blast over the White Plains Missile Range: "A few people laughed, a few cried, most people were silent. . . . There floated through my mind a line from the Bhagavada-Gita in which Krishna is trying to persuade the Prince that he should do his duty: 'I am become Death, the shatterer of worlds'" (Goodchild 1981:161). As head of the Manhattan Project that had brought the power of the atom to this unveiling, Oppenheimer understood the awesome potential now in human hands. Today as we sense our newfound medical powers to control both death and life and the attendant choices regarding euthanasia, sometimes we laugh, sometimes we cry, and sometimes we are silent.

A recurring theme of the twentieth-century story is the way in which we humans, through ingenious schemes and persistent effort, have grasped new powers to ourselves only to have the triumphant yell of victory catch in our throats as we realize the awful (awe-filled) potential of our new capacities. This emotion is nowhere more evident than in the story of medical advances. From our control of reproduction to our control of the dying process, we seem to hold ourselves and our destinies in our own hands in ways that had been the stuff of fantasies. We have new powers of death and life, with all the exhilaration, confusion, and terror that go with these responsibilities.

One struggle attending these new capacities concerns voluntary euthanasia and physician-assisted suicide.[1] The increased complexity of some of these issues inclines us to despair because it seems that there are no clear traditions to guide us. What may at first seem to be a rather clear-cut decision about whether we are going to cause death or allow suffering becomes much more complicated. Who should die and who should live? Who should suffer and why and for how long? Who is to decide? What images, stories, or rules control our decisions? What consequences do we pursue? How much are we willing to pay for our decisions, and who is to bear the financial, emotional, and other costs of those decisions? I contend here that, even though it seems that our new powers have created radically new dilemmas for us, there are ancient stories, values, and images from the Judeo-Christian tradition that help clarify our experiences and choices.

I am a Baptist and come to the questions about voluntary euthanasia and physician-assisted suicide from the perspective of the Believers' Church tradition. Baptists comprise the largest number in this tradition that is often referred to as the radical reformation. It is marked by emphasis on voluntary church membership, the congregational form of church government, religious freedom, and a clear distinction between believers and the world.[2] Several features of the Believers' Church tradition are evident in this chapter. One is the frequent appeal to biblical themes, images, and stories. Another is the development of three theological and ethical motifs: the priesthood of believers, stewardship, and vocation. (Though shared with the larger Christian community, these motifs have been especially important to the people of the Believers' Church tradition.) We turn now to the four themes that provide structure for our consideration of euthanasia: freedom and responsibility; suffering and dying; mercy and justice; and healing and caring.

Freedom and Responsibility

Freedom and responsibility—we tend to embrace the first and avoid the second. Can we get away with that? Should we view one as more important than the other? Should we think of these two moral imperatives as alternatives between which we can choose? What is the relationship, if any, between freedom and responsibility?

The Believers' Church tradition of the priesthood of all believers gets at the heart of the question of human freedom and responsibility.[3] Central to the claim that all believers, not just a special class within the church, are priests is the view that humans are created and called by God to a high level of competence and responsibility.

This view stands in contrast to an emphasis upon the sovereignty of God that denies any genuine or meaningful human freedom and responsibility. The Believers' Church has resisted hierarchical religious and political systems that allow little responsibility and freedom for the ordinary believer or citizen. At times, adherents of the Believers' Church have espoused extreme views on individualism and egalitarianism (Bloom 1992:200–233), advocating freedom from limitations and from others. In its fullest and most authentic expressions, however, this tradition has embraced a communal sense of the human experience (as in the congregational form of church government). Priests view their access to the power and presence of God as a responsibility to serve the community, not as a privilege for personal benefit. In this case, it is not freedom *from* something but rather freedom *for* one's own relationship with God. Freedom has responsibility as its Siamese twin.

This understanding of the human experience encourages us to view the dramatic advances in modern medicine as presenting us with these interlocked realities of freedom and responsibility. As with Siamese twins, we cannot satisfy the demands of one without meeting the needs of the other. No longer can we play one against the other, nor can we collapse or reduce either one into the other. We must satisfy both together.

Just a few decades ago the common sickbed scene involved a patient and one physician with a small black bag containing every medical instrument that he knew how to use. After limited ministrations to the sick the physician stepped back and said, "Well, it's in God's hands now." There was little freedom of choice and correspondingly limited responsibility. Today the scene is very different. A never-ending line of physicians passes by the sickbed. Each is a specialist, trained to use innumerable techniques and technologies. Should any one of them exhaust his or her bag of treatments, another specialist can be called in. The problem remains in our human hands because it appears that there is always something that can be done. Increased freedom of choice means increased human responsibility.

There are two common responses to these new realities. One I call the *humble stance*. This response resists the impulse to take into our hands new responsibilities: it leaves them in God's hands or lets nature take its course. Questioning human wisdom and fearing technology, those who embrace this view warn us that the most basic human sin is pride. Eating from the tree of knowledge (Genesis 3:3–7) and building towers into God's face (Genesis 11:1–9) stand as the defining stories of human sin and its consequent confusion and decline. In contrast, the *heroic stance* promotes the virtue of courage and calls for bold and adventurous action. Its defining biblical image pictures God giving humans dominion and responsibility over all of creation (Genesis 1:26–31). This heroic impulse is often translated into the modern commandment to do everything that can be done.

The biblical story of the faithful steward may suggest a more helpful response to these new responsibilities than the humble or the heroic models described above. The stories about the faithful steward (for example, Isaiah 22:15–25; Luke 12:41–48) have a common structure and theme. There are three characters—the master who owns the household, the steward who has been given the freedom and responsibility to manage the household, and the members of the household who are dependent upon the ministry of the master and steward. The steward can fail and be unfaithful in two ways. The steward may reject the invitation to accept the assigned responsibilities, in which case the sin parallels that of the one who buries his or her talent (Matthew 25:14–29). Or the steward may turn the opportunity into a time of self-indulgence. In either case the master's will and purpose are thwarted, and the needs of the household are not met. The unfaithful steward fails both the master and the household.

In this story freedom and responsibility are intense experiences in the steward's life. He feels exhilaration in realizing the immense freedom and power that go with being in charge. The master is away, and the steward has been given the opportunity to run the show. At the same time this freedom to act brings great responsibility. The household is waiting for its needs to be met, and the master will return for an accounting.

With our new powers to control life and death, we are forced to ask what it means to be a steward of the life that God has given us (Ashley 1992). We have in our hands unaccustomed powers. We can reject these powers and the attendant responsibilities, or we can grasp these powers as an occasion for arrogant self-serving. The stewardship model suggests the different strategy of accepting the new and intimidating responsibility with a sense of sober hope that in using our new freedoms we can serve the people who share our time and place in history.

The Humble Stance: Abandoning Responsibility

There are many ways in which we can abandon responsibility concerning euthanasia and physician-assisted suicide. We can continue to leave the decision about who lives and dies to a health care system that does not meet the needs of many within the household. U.S. health care expenditures have risen from $12 billion in 1950 (4.5 percent of the Gross National Product) to $942.5 billion in 1993 (over 14 percent of the GNP), and yet millions of Americans do not receive even minimal health care (U.S. Department of Commerce 1994: sec. 42, p. 1). While we claim that we dare not decide who lives or dies, we allow an unjust system to make that decision for us. Many within our household are constrained by severe financial limitations in making their decisions about life or death. Elderly patients decide against continued treatment because they do not want their mates to be left bankrupt (McCormick 1991:1134). It is illusory for us to imagine that we have no responsibility for these decisions that are coerced by our social, economic, and health care system. It is the height of irresponsibility to turn these decisions over to systems that take actions we cannot condone.

A faithful steward who had been given the most advanced medical resources in the world cannot tolerate the neglect of vast numbers of those within the household. The first step toward responsible decisions about euthanasia must be the creation of a health care system that neither wastes resources on useless efforts nor discriminates unfairly against the very poorest of our neighbors. We cannot view ourselves as fully responsible until we create a health care system that is far more just.

Another way to avoid responsibility is to turn over the tough decisions of life and death to what has been called the "technological imperative" (Callahan 1973:256). The impulse here is to use every technology available. This reaction grows out of our modern fascination with and confidence in technology and out of our tendency to put the machine between ourselves and the decision (Annas 1991). We just do all that we can do, with little weighing of the costs or consequences. With little or no discrimination, every effort is made to prevent death or control life. The result can be a useless expenditure of resources or prolonged suffering for the patient. Ultimately this can be an abdication, a shifting of responsibility to our technological capacity, which allows us to avoid troubling choices.

A third way to shirk responsibility is to turn the decisions and actions over to health care professionals. Much of the talk about physician-assisted suicide seems to be driven by this inclination. Clearly the specialized training of health care professionals warrants granting them certain responsibilities and authority; however, we must not attribute to any one person or group a God-like authority to make life and death decisions. The inclination of patients or families to allow professionals to make these decisions is often a refusal to accept responsibility for their own lives.

A final way we can evade responsible stewardship is to design a rigid set of rules, either religious or legal, that will make the decisions for us. Such escapism produces decision making that is strangely void of the real blood and guts of human pathos and struggle (Wolf 1992:31). A moral life is imagined in which there is a fixed pattern of behavior that can be objectified and put into a precise set of rules. Much of the contemporary effort to write laws quickly that cover the questions raised about controlling life and death seems to be driven by a desire to eliminate the struggle of choosing. Once this system is in place, we believe, we can avoid moral complexity and ambiguity. All we have to do is obey the rules because they make the decisions for us. Yet no matter how helpful such rules may be as guidelines, they are not likely to cover adequately all situations. The faithful steward will still have real decisions to make and actions to take. Furthermore, the steward must be prepared to accept full responsibility for those actions.

Many shrink from such heavy responsibility because it appears dangerous to entrust important decisions about life and death to an uncertain future. We are warned about stepping out on a slippery slope with the inevitable slide into moral oblivion (Brock 1992:19–21). The truth is that the tougher decisions of life are always made on slippery slopes. There are no broad plains of moral certainty to which we can flee. Like St. Paul we always see through a glass darkly (1 Corinthians 13:12). Realization that we are on a slippery slope does not lead, however, to ad hoc decision making with no consistent moral perspective. Indeed, realization of the dangers should prompt the most careful attention to where we step and the consequences of those steps. The person on the slippery slope will be very much in need of clear moral traditions for help along this dangerous journey, but the number of variables makes it impossible to set out a fixed path across the slope.

The Heroic Stance: Presumptuous Arrogance

At the other end of the spectrum from abandoning responsibility is the mistake of presumptuous arrogance. We are tempted to claim an absolute freedom that recognizes no limits or need for others. Again the story of the steward reminds us that we act within the context of a community with God and neighbor.

American values concerning decisions of life and death are influenced by the frontier mentality that pictures the individual in sole possession of his or her life. This sentiment has been promoted by the well-known drama *Whose Life Is It Anyway?* The implication is that we can do with our own lives whatever we like. This radical individualism stands in sharp contrast to the biblical image of the steward, whose life is intertwined with all the household and who holds his or her life and all its resources as a trust from God. The apostle Paul described the symbiotic relationships of human existence with the image of the body composed of multiple and diverse organs (1 Corinthians 12:12–31). He portrays the folly of the eye's claiming that it is the whole body or that it does not need the other parts of the body. It is a serious mistake for anyone to claim that no one else has a legitimate interest in his or her life, so that each individual faces decisions regarding death and suffering alone.

Another expression of arrogance is to deny the growing reality that we have limited resources. The heady belief that our new technologies allow us to do anything we want to do has run up against the hard facts of our limited financial resources and our mortality. It is beyond our capacity to avoid either suffering or death. Both are part of the human experience, and any dream of escaping them is an arrogant delusion.

The faithful and wise steward takes a realistic inventory of what can be done and what resources are available to do it. At this point we cannot do everything that we are technologically capable of doing because, as individuals and as a nation, we simply cannot afford it. Our decisions about life and death must be made within the context of this sobering realization.

Our freedom of action should be controlled also by the realization of our limited wisdom. Medical knowledge is limited. This is reflected by the frequent changes in the accepted wisdom of the day. Diagnoses are never absolutely certain. Though we cannot use this as an excuse to hold out for some miracle, a certain modesty should mark our considerations. One result of this modesty will be to acknowledge that we can never have all the information that we might want, nor can we be absolutely certain of the results of our actions. We must be prepared to live with that uncertainty.

A final limitation within which we live and act is our sinfulness. Our moral insights and inclinations are distorted by this human reality. One way we protect ourselves from our limited virtue is to subject ourselves to certain restraints. For example, we should constantly test our moral judgments against those of others within our community (Schmidt 1989:476). We should also recognize the place of rules and limitations in protecting us from the most blatant mistakes, even though the process of formulating rules is complicated by our living within pluralistic communities and by the difficulty of balancing the needs for enough structure to maintain order and enough flexibility to protect freedom (Brock 1992:14–21; Minogue 1990; Gula 1990). Finally, Christians should recognize the need for serious and regular participation in worship, reflection, and meditation as a way to correct and renew our moral selves.

In the face of difficult decisions about controlling life and death, we find that freedom and responsibility come to us as companion friends, not as competing values. We are created free so that we might be responsible. Our call is not to use our freedom to declare independence from God and others. Our search should be for communities of sharing and action in which we can pool our resources to make the tough decisions that have come with our new powers and freedoms. We must shun all the subtle ways in which we avoid, delay, and transfer our questions and obligations to others. We need to seek ways to embrace our personal responsibilities even as we learn to share our burdens and victories with others.

Suffering and Dying

The experiences that precipitate our decisions about euthanasia and physician-assisted suicide are suffering and dying. These scourges of human existence gnaw away at our being and threaten the meaning of our lives. Many of the strategies of living, both those sophisticated ones of philosophy and theology and those informal ones of our mores, are designed to make sense of suffering and death. Unfortunately, in our current medical environment many look to the swirl of suffering and death and believe that we must choose between the two. Some view death as so destructive that they must endure any suffering to avoid it. Others fear suffering to the extent that they embrace death as a quick and easy solution to suffering (May 1983:69–73). My view is that neither response reflects an adequate grasp of either the Christian understanding of suffering and death or our current experience of them.

Suffering and Death in the Christian Story

At the heart of the Christian story of life is the crucifixion and resurrection of Christ. It has seemed strange to many that a religious faith that claimed to bring good news and hope to humanity would choose the cross, a symbol of suffering and death, as its most prominent visual representation. This bold, even scandalous (Galatians 4:11) claim was possible because the resurrection was the twin component.

In this Christian story we see an acceptance that the terrifying experiences of suffering and death are an inevitable part of the human experience. No human can escape them—not even God when in human flesh. Furthermore, although much of Christian art has made the crucifixion seem antiseptic and inoffensive, in reality it was not a pretty scene. It was the picture of human sin and failure in all its destructive terror, embracing physical pain, fear, abandonment, hatred, duplicity, despair, and death.

Within this central event of the Christian drama, suffering and death are inseparably joined. Much discussion of these two experiences has treated them as if they are qualitatively different. Obviously there are differences, but both threaten the meaning of human experience, both assault the very core of our being. Christ's suffering is not secondary, not just a prelude to the really grand threat of death in the crucifixion event. His suffering took him to the very depths of human annihilation as he felt himself abandoned by everyone, including God (Matthew 27:46). The story offers no justification for viewing death as the real threat to human existence and suffering as only a minor trial. Suffering threatens our identity and the meaning of our existence (Smith 1987:259).

The central claim of the crucifixion-resurrection faith is that, although life is threatened by both suffering and death, the resurrection of Christ affirms the power of God to overcome both for us. Christ faced both boldly and did not flee finally from the terror of either. The good news of the Christian story is that though suffering and death are inescapable dimensions of our human experience, neither of them destroys our meaning or value. The task of the Christian is to deal with both death and suffering in such a way that life is enriched and affirmed. We are not to flee either of them as if they have the power to destroy the meaning and purpose of our lives, nor are we to romanticize them as hidden goods. In truth, both suffering and death are human tragedies that are overcome in the power of a loving God (Simmons 1977:151–57).

In the context of the present discussion, such an understanding of the Christian story resists any language or activity that treats life—to use Barth's term—as a "second God." The phrases "sanctity of life" or "reverence for life" should be used cautiously or replaced by an expression like "profound respect for life." The long and noble history of Christian martyrdom and Christ's own persistent march to his cross proclaim the truth that there are times when death is voluntarily chosen over life (Clark 1986).

Suffering and Death in Modern Medicine

The term *euthanasia* has an extended and circuitous history (Fye 1978; Anderson 1987:208–15). The first evidence of its usage dates from 1646. Its meaning of "good death" or "easy death" referred to the efforts to keep terminal patients free from pain. Then it came, in the late 1800s, to refer to the choice of death in cases where terminal patients were experiencing intense and intractable pain. From the beginning until now the term has pointed to experiences of suffering and death and their relationship within the medical setting. In practice distinctions have arisen among *passive euthanasia* (allowing to die), *double-effect euthanasia* (a potentially lethal act with the primary intent to relieve suffering), and *active euthanasia* (causing to die) (Vaux 1989:20). My focus here is limited to active euthanasia, specifically active euthanasia in which the terminal patient participates in the decision and freely chooses to die.

Until the middle of the twentieth century the definition of death as the cessation of heartbeat and respiration had been standard. New advances in medical technology make it possible for patients to recover from conditions that match this traditional definition of death. Furthermore, our new powers allow us to maintain heartbeat and respiration in an increasing number of patients (or are they cadavers?) when there is no realistic hope of any further self-sustained activity. This capacity forces a reassessment of the traditional definition and leads to such formulations as the Harvard criteria, which focus upon brain function (Ad Hoc Committee 1968). Debate regarding the adequacy of this definition of death continues, along with efforts to clarify and interpret its meaning and usage ("An Appraisal" 1977; Veatch 1975; Jonas 1974). Today we continue to describe and distinguish among a number of medical conditions that some associate with death, including persistent vegetative state, coma, dementia, irreversible coma, chronic and reversible coma, neocortical death, and locked-in syndrome (Cranford 1988). The dispute continues concerning what should count as death.

It is instructive to note that within modern medicine more attention has been given to defining and preventing death than to identifying and preventing suffering. Some charge that "medicine tends to ignore suffering" (Gunderman 1990:18). This relative neglect of the suffering dimension of the medical experience is anomalous when we remember that the term *patient* literally means "the one who suffers." It is encouraging that discussion about pain and suffering has increased recently within the medical setting (Cassell 1991). Some limit its meaning to physical pain, while others claim that any experience of dehumanization is suffering (Schneiderman 1990). The inexpressibility of something so real and intimate as pain has made it difficult to describe and identify suffering (Scarry 1985). Yet while we struggle to define it, we see the reality of suffering on the modern medical scene. Indeed, advances in medicine, while providing new methods to control suffering, have also generated new ways of creating and extending it. Our heroic efforts to prevent death often take the shape of torturous suffering. Ironically, much suffering today is so destructive of human meaning and value that it is difficult to distinguish it from death. It is time to face that fact and see from the perspective of the crucifixion that both are bound up together as destructive enemies of human life, even as we see from the resurrection that neither is finally destructive of our meaning and purpose.

The Christian understanding of crucifixion-resurrection teaches us that both suffering and death are tragic, but neither is an ultimate tragedy. We should avoid romanticizing or demonizing either. Neither can solve the problem of the other. Our preoccupation with the threat of death has led us to prolong life as long as technically possible without recognizing that the suffering thereby created is often as destructive of life as the death we seek to escape (Landau and Gustafson 1984). Conversely, our compulsion to seek the perfect life of comfort, free from suffering, has led some to rush to death as the quick solution to suffering. Neither response is faithful to human experience or to Christian truth as reflected in the crucifixion and resurrection.

Mercy and Justice

The prophet Micah put it succinctly: "He has showed you, O man, what is good; and what does the Lord require of you but to do justice, and to love kindness, and to walk humbly with your God?" (Micah 6:8, Revised Standard Version; all subsequent biblical references are to the RSV). Mercy and justice (along with peace) are the most dominant of the ethical images or standards promoted in the Judeo-Christian tradition. Though they are sometimes portrayed as two different sides of God's character, I view mercy and justice as two complementary and defining features of God that become moral standards by which the people of faith live.

Mercy and Justice in the Scriptural Setting

Chesed (in Hebrew Scriptures) and *agape* (in Christian Scriptures) are the terms most often translated into English as love, mercy, or compassion. One difficulty of using the terms *love* and *mercy* is that they have become so common and all-encompassing that their meaning is fuzzy and unclear. They mean everything and therefore nothing. It is important to recapture a clear meaning of mercy.[4]

Mercy is born in the recognition of God's love for us, and it is our proper response to that love. "Beloved, if God so loved us, we also ought to love one another" (1 John 4:11). We love because God first loved us. One of the first things we notice about God's love is that it always takes concrete form (Molin 1987:113). It becomes incarnate. The mercy we are called to emulate is not just a mystical feeling or sentiment. Though planted deep in our inner being, such impulses of mercy are real only when they take on hands and feet and action. It is not a Platonic pity but a robust commitment of action.

When one is empathetically committed to the other, one is prepared to sacrifice. There is an extravagance in this mercy that is full of surprises—surprises regarding both who is loved and what is done. It involves an abandonment that defies logic and the established rules, similar to Jesus' "rule" that one should be willing to forgive "seventy times seven" (Matthew 18:22). A feature of this "beyond logic" loving is a steadfastness that patiently waits and endures beyond reasonableness. The core feature of love is its goal of reconciliation. Its empathy reaches out and identifies with the other, the unlikely other, for the purpose of bringing healing to broken and alienated humanity.

As with mercy, the norm of justice is defined by the character of God.[5] The acts of God are both the motive and model of justice. "You shall not pervert the justice due to the sojourner or to the fatherless, or take a widow's garment in pledge: but you shall remember that you were a slave in Egypt and the Lord your God redeemed you from there; therefore I command you to do this" (Deuteronomy 24:17). The people of faith do justice because it was first done to them. We are driven not by fear or guilt but by gratitude for the acts of God on our behalf.

These acts of God then define justice. It is action that favors those whom life has neglected. It responds to others not on the basis of their merit or worth but on the basis of their need. The recurring formula is, "You do justice to the widow, the orphan, and the stranger within your gate" (Deuteronomy 10:17–18; Isaiah 1:17; Exodus 22:21). The Jewish tradition of the jubilee year, a time of restoration, is based upon this understanding of justice. The reign of God is characterized by favored treatment for those who have been disenfranchised by life.

This jubilee dream for justice became the hallmark of Christ's ministry as he defined it at the beginning. "The Spirit of the Lord is upon me, because he has anointed me to preach good news to the poor. He has sent me to proclaim release to the captives and recovering of sight to the blind, to set at liberty those who are oppressed, to proclaim the acceptable year of the Lord" (Luke 4:18). This was the ministry that was marked by the scandalous behavior of eating with sinners, talking with women, and befriending Samaritans and other untouchables. This is a justice whose agenda is determined by who is hurting the most and has the fewest resources to heal the hurt.

Mercy and Justice in the Medical Setting

How do these qualities of mercy and justice speak to our questions about voluntary euthanasia and physician-assisted suicide? Within the history of medicine, the normative ideal of beneficence and the rule of "do no harm" reflect the spirit of mercy. In our own time the compassionate impulse of mercy should find ready identification with those who suffer. It is this impulse that through the centuries has drawn Christians to the health care scene as professionals and as volunteer caregivers. It is the antithesis of the tendency in modern medicine, and indeed in many modern professional contexts, to deal with people in abstract or impersonal terms, to identify patients as "the coronary," "the Downs," or "the amputee." Human beings are reduced to their condition or their disease, and in the process we lose sight of their humanity. Mercy abandons such categories and touches the real hurt of real people. Compassion rejects all efforts to romanticize suffering or to take comfort in some hidden blessing that lies concealed within the torment of unrelenting pain and suffering.

Mercy not only reaches across our conventional professional distance but also draws us into doing the unexpected. The spirit of mercy works to establish orderly structures and systems that serve human needs; however, when structures and systems become contributing factors to human misery, mercy does not hesitate to break the rules. Mercy impels us to take risks, to go the second mile, to do the surprising and extravagant deed in pursuit of healing. In this pursuit, professional protocols, hospital rules, and even societal laws are subject to serious challenge.

Mercy also pushes beyond our fascination with technical wizardry and proficiency. We can be hypnotized by the miracles of technology and fail to see that we often become captives of the machines that promised to be our saviors. The eyes of mercy are not blinded by the bright lights and technological glitz of modern medicine. These eyes remain fixed on the patients and their plight.

The norm of justice is more orderly and structured than mercy, but it seeks a certain kind of order. It seeks an ordering of life that shows preference for those who are the neediest. Today justice inclines us toward a reordering of a health care system that leaves millions of citizens of the world's richest land without even minimal medical attention. This sense of justice will cry out against social, economic, and professional structures that drive people to reach for death prematurely because to continue living will bankrupt their families. Concern for the outcast will identify and oppose those tendencies to disvalue some and to coerce them into agreeing that their lives are no longer worth living (Teno and Lynn 1991:297). The elderly, the handicapped, the despised, those with costly illnesses will find a friend in justice who affirms their value and allows them to face their suffering and death with the same sense of value as the most fortunate among us.

Healing and Caring

At the heart of the Reformation faith is the recovery of a sense of divine calling for all the faithful. This understanding of Christian vocation, which brings daily work and divine mission together, has been especially important for the Believers' Church. Not only is every Christian to view her or his work as a calling from God, but also the work of the church is shared by the laity and the clergy. There are no moral distinctions among the various tasks that are done at God's behest. There is no hierarchy among these vocations, but rather all legitimate work is viewed as a part of God's work and therefore worthy of being viewed as a vocation from God.

Of course, some kinds of human activity cannot be viewed as a Christian vocation because they produce that which is clearly destructive or useless and therefore not God's calling. Three characteristics have traditionally been attributed to a Christian vocation: "(1) a systematic and persistent doing of *needful work;* (2) a putting forth and development of *an individual's own constituent powers;* (3) a willing *contributive share* in the world's work and *the common life*" (Calhoun 1935:53–72, emphasis mine). The vocations of healing and caring should be marked by these three features. The value or needfulness of both activities is obvious. We should also engage in healing and caring in such a way that our individual humanity is enriched and developed in the process. Our unique gifts should inform and be shaped by these works. Finally, we should always recognize that we share these tasks with others, that some aspects of the work are best done by others who have different talents and skills. No one of us can do the work alone.

The terms *healing* and *caring* describe activities that have a rich history in the Christian tradition and that are worthy of being considered a Christian's calling. Here I use the term *healing* to describe the "making whole" that we usually associate with the practice of health care. The term *caring* is used in a more inclusive sense to describe a wide range of services designed to take care of a human being. Our task here is to identify as precisely as we can what is involved in the Christian vocations of healing and caring for those who are suffering and dying.

Christ himself set the example of healing as a legitimate vocation. Out of this has grown a substantial involvement of the church in the work of healing. The church as an institution has included health care activities as a part of its ministry. These activities have ranged from healing services to the financial support of hospitals and clinics.

There can be no question about the legitimacy of healing as a Christian vocation. What is in dispute is how the purpose and extent of this work is defined (Nagi et al. 1981). One tradition views the defining purpose of medicine as the prevention of death; this view is reflected in the use of the human skull as a symbol of the enemy that medicine fights. This has fostered the development of military imagery and language within the medical community (May 1983:63–86). The focus upon death prevention as the basic purpose of medicine finds support from those values that identify death as the ultimate human tragedy. The technocratic mind-set also promotes this definition of purpose, which allows practitioners to measure results objectively and precisely—death lends itself more easily to such measurements than does the more elusive reality of suffering.

This narrowly defined purpose of the medical vocation has contributed to the relative neglect of pain reduction among the medical skills. There is a tendency to conclude that if death cannot be prevented, then there is little that medicine can do. Defining medical purpose in this way has also meant that those medical specialties that focus on preventing death receive the greatest acclaim and rewards.

A needed corrective is the recovery of a strong sense of caring as a vocation. The essence of caring is the simple but often demanding ministry of presence (Campbell 1984:27–28, 111–12). It is the kind of tenacious presence that stays close during the most difficult time of life. A broader definition of the physician's calling includes not only the reduction of pain and suffering but also an affirming, reassuring presence.

This understanding is found in that part of the medical tradition which stresses the standard of "do no harm" and the virtue of beneficence. Some suggest a compromise that assigns the "hard science" side of health care to the physician and the more compassionate caring to the nursing profession, yet such a breakdown of tasks may stem from gender stereotyping rather than a reasoned and fair division of labor (Campbell 1984:34–39).

In defining our callings a division of labor *is* necessary. Our calling is "a willing contributive share of the world's work and the common life" (Calhoun 1935:59). No one of us does all of God's work. We have different talents, opportunities, and vocations. It is a serious mistake to fail to recognize that most of the physician's work is very specialized and beyond the capacity of most of us. It is an irresponsible sentimentalism to imagine that the call of the physician is just to be present. The physician's vocation requires special skills to meet the special needs of the sick (May 1975:37). We must understand that fulfilling the unique role of physician does not allow doctors the time to be present to most patients most of the time. Furthermore, we should confess that sometimes our complaint that physicians need to be more caring is really an attempt to pass on the caring responsibility to someone else. We turn over the tough decisions to the professionals and avoid the risk of making mistakes for which we feel responsible. We want someone else to take on the demanding task of holding the hand of those who are suffering and dying. This abandonment is part of a modern tendency to professionalize as many human services as possible. We turn over to the experts our problems and tasks as a way to flee those obligations, and then we often project our sense of guilt by criticizing physicians for not caring. We have been especially derelict in fulfilling our call to care because it takes so much emotional and physical energy. While we can properly ask physicians to be more caring, the major responsibility in caring for the suffering and dying belongs to families and other intimate communities. The primary, though not exclusive, responsibility for healing belongs to the physician and other health care professionals.

An even more critical question for our discussion here is whether the vocation of caring includes the responsibility to kill in order to be compassionate. If there is ever an occasion when euthanasia is appropriate, does that task fall within the realm of the medical profession's responsibility (Gaylin et al. 1988; Brock 1992:16–17; Pellegrino 1992)?

Euthanasia and Physician-Assisted Suicide

With increasing frequency the options of euthanasia and physician-assisted suicide are being considered as solutions to the dilemmas of intense suffering, especially that suffering associated with prolonged dying. We turn too readily, I believe, to active euthanasia as the solution to our problems. A number of preliminary steps would dramatically reduce the frequency with which people seek euthanasia. One such step is to establish a more just health care delivery system. The threat of financial disaster from the cost of extended health care drives many to the cheaper option of a quick death. We should not invest an inordinate amount of resources in delaying an inevitable death, nor should we sanction the injustice of a health care system that provides exorbitant, extraordinary treatment to some, while others cannot afford even modest measures to protect life and relieve suffering.

A second step we should take is to make the forgoing of life-sustaining treatment more readily available to those who face terminal conditions (Kass 1990:41). The evidence is clear that many want the option of euthanasia because they fear being captured in a network of medical and legal procedures that will not let them die, whatever the circumstances. We should abandon our obsessive fear of death that compels us to practice curative medicine even when there is no meaningful hope for a cure.

A third step is to establish concrete programs to provide genuine and substantial care for people who are facing death and its attendant suffering. Many times euthanasia appears the only option for those who have been abandoned to pain and neglect. The only way out of their loneliness appears to be death. A genuine caring ministry will rescue these people from their desperate plight and limited choice. Our care should be wide-ranging in its dimensions and its providers. Caring is not the exclusive or even the primary responsibility of the physician. Families, friends, and especially faith communities should overcome their uneasiness in the presence of death and suffering so that they can provide the caring presence that will witness to the truth that life can be worth living.

This brings us to the question of whether there are times when life is not worth living. Can we ever approve positive action to cause death? I believe that some extreme and rare circumstances do justify euthanasia. As stewards of the Master's resources we are called to use our God-given capacities to serve human needs, and those needs might include escape from a life that is worse than death. Nonetheless, I believe that it is a mistake at this time in history to establish a public policy condoning active euthanasia.

If there are occasions when death is better than life, why not institutionalize this option in public policy? A primary reason is that all moral responsibility cannot and should not be established in rules and laws. Moral values find existence in virtues and goals as well. Rules of behavior are crucial elements in the life of the moral person, but so are the freedom and responsibility to go beyond the requirements of law. We should be more trusting of the discernment that grows out of moral character (Smedes 1987:17–18). The attempt to establish laws to cover every eventuality in the complex issues before us here reflects a lack of faith in God's leadership and in our capacity to respond to that leadership as faithful stewards.

The inadequacy of laws to comprise the entire moral life does not mean that they are unimportant. If we establish a policy that allows for euthanasia, we will formalize mechanisms for what should be carefully deliberated decisions in uncommon circumstances. With established policy and procedures we may turn too easily to killing as a quick and cheap solution to suffering. Our society already sanctions too much killing for me to be comfortable with yet another officially approved taking of life.

There is the further danger that the public sanctioning of euthanasia will be interpreted by the weak and disvalued as a coercive move that points them in the direction in which society wants them to go. Those who are disfavored in society already see clear evidence that society does not want them anymore. Our public policies should be marked by the kind of justice discussed above, a justice that takes special note of the needs of the outcast and seeks to bring them into the community of caring.

I do not favor a public policy endorsing euthanasia, and yet I recognize that in rare circumstances moral responsibility will move us beyond the bounds of law to euthanasia. Physicians should be free to participate; in fact, there is good reason for them to do so. There is wisdom in placing euthanasia within the context of a competent and caring community. This brings a knowledgeable judgment and responsibility to the decision and protects against malevolent or careless killing. The medical profession's commitment to defend life will also act as a deterrent, a check on the decision-making process. The inclusion of physicians in this decision and perhaps the act itself also recognizes that preventing death is not the only purpose of medicine.

Even though physicians may have an important role to play in decisions concerning euthanasia, I do not favor a physician-*administered* euthanasia, because this places all the burden and responsibility upon the medical community. All of us should share this responsibility and risk. It is important to protect physicians and others who participate in the rare euthanasia from punitive legal sanctions, or even the threat of sanctions, unless there is clear evidence of malicious intent.

I also do not favor establishing a specialty within the medical profession to do this work. This assumes a far wider practice of euthanasia than I envision, and it yields to our penchant for specializing every task. The physician who is most needed in this intimate and caring community is the one who is closest to the patient and family, not a specialist brought in just to do this task.

In conclusion, let us consider an ancient story of healing.

> After this there was a feast of Jews, and Jesus went up to Jerusalem. Now there is in Jerusalem by the Sheep Gate a pool, in Hebrew called Bethzatha, which has five porticoes. In these lay a multitude of invalids, blind, lame, paralyzed. One man was there, who had been ill for thirty-eight years. When Jesus saw him and knew that he had been lying there a long time, he said to him, "Do you want to be healed?" The sick man answered him, "Sir, I have no man to put me into the pool when the water is troubled, and while I am going another steps down before me." Jesus said to him, "Rise, take up your pallet, and walk." And at once the man was healed, and took up his bed and walked. (John 5:1–9)

In this story we see a profile of the one whom Christians have called "the Great Physician." On a feast day when every prominent religious leader was at the temple, Jesus is found in a place where society's castaways are gathered. These are the ones whose only hope is in a rare and miraculous moving of the waters. Furthermore, Jesus turns his healing care to the one who has waited for years and who has no one to help him get to his only hope. It is the most neglected and the most desperate one whom Jesus heals. The story continues by describing the reaction to this healing by the officials of Jesus' day. They were distressed because he healed on the sabbath, thus breaking an important law—a law that Jesus acknowledged as important. Jesus gave preference to the forgotten and suffering one over the law, and so the officials "sought all the more to kill him, because he not only broke the sabbath but also called God his own Father, making himself equal with God" (John 5:18).

We experience equal suffering by many who are forgotten and neglected on the sickbeds of our day. The Believers' Church tradition, with its emphasis on individual responsibility, rejects all the ways in which this responsibility to care for the suffering is abandoned. The call is for us to go to the forgotten sufferers and to do the unexpected. We do this even if we are accused, on occasion, of "playing God." We view ourselves as those who are called by God to share divine or "priestly" power and responsibility. We accept this call not arrogantly but with the awe-filled sense of one who has been given a power that must be used responsibly. As those who first felt the power of nuclear energy, sometimes we laugh, sometimes we cry, sometimes we remain silent.

NOTES

1. For two helpful bibliographies and summaries of issues see Hamel 1991 and McCarrick 1992.
2. A thorough treatment of the Believers' Church tradition is found in Garrett 1969.
3. The most complete account of the doctrine of the priesthood of believers in the Judeo-Christian tradition is found in two volumes by Cyril Eastwood: Eastwood 1963 covers the period from the biblical material to the Reformation, and Eastwood 1962 covers the period from the Reformation to the modern era. Treatments of this doctrine within the Believers' Church tradition can be found in Garrett 1969, Pitts 1988, and Marney 1974.
4. For helpful discussions of the meaning of love and mercy in the Judeo-Christian tradition, see Williams 1968 and Furnish 1972.
5. For helpful discussions of the meaning of justice in the Judeo-Christian tradition, see Berkovits 1969; Gallardo 1983; Haughey 1977; and Yoder 1972.

REFERENCES

Ad Hoc Committee. 1968. "A Definition of Irreversible Coma." *Journal of the American Medical Association* 205 (5 August): 337–40.

"An Appraisal of the Criteria of Cerebral Death." 1977. *Journal of the American Medical Association* 237 (7 March): 982–86.

Anderson, J. Kerby. 1987. "Euthanasia: A Biblical Appraisal." *Bibliotheca Sacra*, April–June, 208–17.

Annas, George J. 1991. "Killing Machines." *Hastings Center Report* 21 (March–April): 33–35.

Ashley, Benedict M. 1992. "Dominion or Stewardship? Theological Reflections." In *Birth, Suffering, and Death*, ed. Kevin Wm. Wildes, Francesc Abel, and John C. Harvey, 85–106. Boston: Kluwer Academic Publishers.

Berkovits, Eliezer. 1969. *Man and God: Studies in Biblical Theology*. Detroit: Wayne State University Press.

Bloom, Harold. 1992. *The American Religion*. New York: Simon and Schuster.

Brock, Dan W. 1992. "Voluntary Active Euthanasia." *Hastings Center Report* 22 (March–April): 10–22.

Calhoun, Robert L. 1935. *God and the Common Life*. Hamden, Conn.: Shoe String Press.

Callahan, Daniel. 1973. *The Tyranny of Survival and Other Pathologies of Civilized Life*. New York: Macmillan.

Campbell, Alastair V. 1984. *Professional Care*. Philadelphia: Fortress Press.

Cassell, Eric J. 1991. *The Nature of Suffering and the Goals of Medicine*. New York: Oxford University Press.

Clark, W. Royce. 1986. "The Example of Christ and Voluntary Active Euthanasia." *Journal of Religion and Health* 25 (winter): 264–77.

Cranford, Ronald C. 1988. "The Persistent Vegetative State: The Medical Reality." *Hastings Center Report* 18 (February–March): 27–32.

Eastwood, Cyril. 1962. *The Priesthood of All Believers*. Minneapolis: Augsburg Publishing.

————. 1963. *The Royal Priesthood of the Faithful*. Minneapolis: Augsburg Publishing.

Furnish, Victor Paul. 1972. *The Love Commandment in the New Testament*. Nashville: Abingdon Press.

Fye, W. Bruce. 1978. "Active Euthanasia: An Historical Survey of Its Conceptual Origins and Introduction into Medical Thought." *Bulletin of the History of Medicine* 52 (winter): 492–502.

Gallardo, Jose Cortes. 1983. *The Way of Biblical Justice*. Scottdale, Pa.: Herald Press.

Garrett, James Leo, Jr. 1969. *The Concept of the Believers Church*. Scottdale, Pa.: Herald Press.

Gaylin, Willard, Leon Kass, Edmund Pellegrino, and Mark Siegler. 1988. "Doctors Must Not Kill." *Journal of the American Medical Association* 259 (8 April): 2139–40.

Goodchild, Peter. 1981. *J. Robert Oppenheimer: Shatterer of Worlds*. Boston: Houghton Mifflin.

Gula, Richard M. 1990. "Moral Principles Shaping Public Policy on Euthanasia." *Second Opinion* 14 (July): 73–83.

Gunderman, Richard B. 1990. "Medicine and the Question of Suffering." *Second Opinion* 14 (July): 15–25.

Hamel, Ron, ed. 1991. *Choosing Death: Active Euthanasia, Religion, and the Public Debate*. Philadelphia: Trinity Press International.

Haughey, John C. 1977. *The Faith That Does Justice*. New York: Paulist Press.

Jonas, Hans. 1974. *Philosophical Essays: From Ancient Creed to Technological Man*. Englewood Cliffs, N.J.: Prentice-Hall.

Kass, Leon R. 1990. "Death with Dignity and the Sanctity of Life." *Commentary* 89 (March): 33–43.

Landau, Richard L., and James M. Gustafson. 1984. "Death Is Not the Enemy." *Journal of the American Medical Association* 252 (2 November): 2458.

McCarrick, Pat Milmoe. 1992. "Active Euthanasia and Assisted Suicide." *Kennedy Institute of Ethics Journal* 2 (March): 79–99.

McCormick, Richard A. 1991. "Physician-Assisted Suicide: Flight from Compassion." *Christian Century* 108 (4 December): 1132–34.

Marney, Carlyle. 1974. *Priest to Each Other*. Valley Forge, Pa.: Judson Press.

May, William F. 1975. "Code, Covenant, Contract, or Philanthropy." *Hastings Center Report* 5 (December): 29–38.

————. 1983. *The Physician's Covenant*. Philadelphia: Westminster Press.

Minogue, Brendan P. 1990. "The Exclusion of Theology from Public Policy: The Case of Euthanasia." *Second Opinion* 14 (July): 84–93.

Molin, Lennart. 1987. "Christian Ethics and Human Life." *Covenant Quarterly* 44 (August): 113–24.

Nagi, Mostafa H., Neil G. Lazerine, and Meredith D. Pugh. 1981. "Euthanasia, the Terminal Patient, and the Physician's Role." *Journal of Religion and Health* 20 (fall): 186–200.

Pellegrino, Edmund D. 1992. "A Doctor Must Not Kill." *Journal of Clinical Ethics* 3 (summer): 95–102.

Pitts, William L., Jr. 1988. "The Priesthood of All Christians in the Baptist Heritage." *Southwestern Journal of Theology* 30 (spring): 34–45.

Scarry, Elaine. 1985. *The Body in Pain*. New York: Oxford University Press.

Schmidt, Stephen. 1989. "Living with Chronic Illness: Why Should I Go On?" *Christian Century* 106 (3 May): 475–79.

Schneiderman, Lawrence J. 1990. "Exile and PVS." *Hastings Center Report* 20 (May–June): 5.

Simmons, Paul D. 1977. "Death with Dignity: Christians Confront Euthanasia." *Perspectives in Religious Studies* 4 (summer): 141–59.

Smedes, Lewis B. 1987. "On Reverence for Life and Discernment of Reality." *Reformed Journal* 37 (June): 15–20.

Smith, David H. 1987. "Suffering, Medicine, and Christian Theology." In *On Moral Medicine: Theological Perspectives in Medical Ethics*, ed. Stephen E. Lammers and Allen Verhey, 255–61. Grand Rapids, Mich.: Wm. B. Eerdmans.

Teno, Joan, and Joanne Lynn. 1991. "Voluntary Active Euthanasia: The Individual Case and Public Policy." *Journal of the American Geriatrics Society* 39 (August): 296–99.

Theological Dictionary of the New Testament, s.v. "love." 1964. Ed. Gerhard Kittel. Grand Rapids, Mich.: Wm. B. Eerdmans.

U.S. Department of Commerce. 1994. *U.S. Industrial Outlook 1994*. Washington, D.C.: U.S. Government Printing Office.

Vaux, Kenneth L. 1989. "The Theologic Ethics of Euthanasia." *Hastings Center Report* 19 (January–February): 19–22.

Veatch, Robert M. 1975. "The Whole-Brain-Oriented Concept of Death: An Outmoded Philosophical Formulation." *Journal of Thanatology* 3, no. 1: 13–30.

Williams, Daniel Day. 1968. *The Spirit and Forms of Love*. New York: Harper and Row.

Wolf, Susan M. 1992. "Final Exit: The End of Argument." *Hastings Center Report* 22 (January–February): 30–33.

Yoder, John Howard. 1972. *The Politics of Jesus*. Grands Rapids, Mich.: Wm. B. Eerdmans.

EPILOGUE

Martin E. Marty

When our children were young, they were given a game or a testing device that, I am told, had some features in common with the Ouija board. It consisted of a chart made up of circles; it looked like a target. On the left was the word "Yes" and on the right the word "No." The other item of equipment was a stick with a string at the end and a steel ball at the end of the string.

The player was to hold the stick in the hand of an outstretched and thus unsupported but still relaxed arm. Someone would ask her or him a question: "Would you rather play Little League than go camping with the family?" Or: "Do you love Ellie?" If the player was relaxed and thus cooperative, it was thought that in a few seconds the conscious mind that had tried to hide the information or the unconscious and previously unconsulted mind would give impulse to the arm until it made subtle gestures and led the stick-holder toward "yes" or "no" answers.

I have no idea whether any kind of science undergirded the theories of mind, arm, and hand to which this game was devoted. I do recall that we had a good time embarrassing each other or positively revealing our secrets and outlooks. But now and then a round of the game ended when the ball either stayed on dead center, at the figurative target's bullseye, or swung wildly from pole to pole.

While reading these chapters I often felt the way I did when I was the holder of the wand in that game. When the questions concerning active voluntary euthanasia and physician-assisted suicide came up, I would be moved by the theology or logical rationale of the writer. "Yes!" would come easily from my unconscious; but it would be canceled by the equally firm "No!" that resulted from convictions formed as I read the next article in the sequence. One thing did not happen: my figurative arm and wand never stayed still over the center. The essays here forced a responsive attitude and sometimes moved me emotionally; they were all convincing and compelling, as I imagine they were for other readers of this book.

So what good is an argument or a conversation about religious beliefs and practices in respect to "choosing death" if the result is indecisiveness and a new awareness of complexity? Much, in many ways; one of the delights of this book is to watch authors convincing themselves. One is quite explicit: it was *during* the writing of his chapter that he found which way he'd been leaning all along. But others were more ready to resort to the language of continued and perhaps permanent ambiguity and paradox in religious discourse on this subject. The chapters are designed to show the minds of experts in action and to help readers, who may or may not have given as much thought to the subject, to make up their minds.

What one is most likely to take from the cumulated chapters is not a definitive answer to the rightness or wrongness question. Instead, one will have a larger repertory of options, a more reasoned support for many of them, a more sympathetic approach, greater understanding of troubled people who go in a direction different from one's own chosen path, and some awareness of how religious and theological thinkers discuss a subject.

That many of these religious thinkers live with ambiguity and paradox is important to note, for many ethical decisions are made by people who are sure, too sure, of themselves and can see only their option as credible. Believers on the left and the right regularly criticize each other for being too ideologically pure and forceful. Yet most of the thoughtful ones are hesitant to mount a pulpit or pose as a prophet. The scriptures and traditions that they expound do not give clear guidance on this subject, at least not in the new settings that confront people who must make moral choices today.

Also noteworthy is the mode of discourse that many of the religious thinkers choose. However ready they may be to marshal evidence and argue the claims of autonomy or justice in philosophical terms, somewhere along the way most of them turn to narrative. They tell stories about someone near to them or about their own experiences. I do not trace this tendency to the current fashionableness of "narrative theology"; it seems to spring more from the fact that, however reducible to dogma and canon many religions are, they rise from event-centered accounts of how God or the gods became entangled with the affairs of humans. Such religions state their case chiefly through stories, in this case, stories of suffering and dying, stories of how people coped with the experience of their end. Retelling stories of the agonized who are near death but cannot die allows the religious and theological thinker to adduce many relevant and revealing aspects of a case that might otherwise be overlooked. The physician, religious or not, who goes by the book is using the book of law, prescription, or oath. For the religious person when not in the physician's role, going by the book likely means going by a scriptural narrative which "complexifies" or, I would prefer to say, "thickens" the case. It thus allows for many more factors to be taken into consideration than otherwise would be, and a certain humanization results.

A narrative of my own will identify me with the "yes" and "no" thickeners of discourse. While reading these chapters, I remained aware of the currently most vivid case in my orbit. A church leader of great consecration, learning, and skill, and with as impressive a record as he had a circle of friends, was dying of AIDS. Evidently—and stories like these always need such qualifiers—he responded to both his experience of suffering and his impulse to be generous. Rather than watching his savings be depleted to pay for medical treatment, he set up a scholarship at his alma mater, a place that means much to me, and then, evidently intentionally, let his car engine run in a closed garage so that he died of carbon monoxide poisoning.

My "yes" side joined with the many friends who, having prayed for him all along, now celebrated: how sensible and thoughtful was his act. "I probably would have done the same thing, if I had the wit and grace." My "no" side joined with the others who, having prayed for him all along, were now uneasy: should not someone like our friend have set an example by the way he faced suffering and let nature and history take their course? Such a response would have done justice to many religious norms in support of life. I do not know whether he did right, or whether the authors in this book who would have understood his action, if not celebrated it, are right. But reading these essays has helped me "thicken" my discourse with myself.

Most of those who have reservations about voluntary active euthanasia write about a "slippery slope": if we allow this, will we not be on a course to really and clearly bad things? Watching the religious thinkers worry about the slippery slope leads me to mention another tendency of theological discourse in our time: the general message is "slow down" or "go slow." (There are flamboyant exceptions, of course, people who say "hurry up" or "go further," but none is in the company of authors in this book.) In other words, the religious community has interests in seeing to it that the scientific community takes time to reckon with issues that go far beyond the technical or the pragmatic. During the past four centuries scientific pioneers from Galileo through Darwin had to oppose religious leadership in order to win freedom to pursue their inquiries; in their eyes, issues of human dignity were at stake. Now the religious thinkers sometimes have to oppose scientists, or those who use science, in order to change ethical understandings and do their own protecting of human dignity. If I am an individual sufferer who cannot legally participate in the taking of my own life, my pain will lead me to say that going slow is a luxury. If I am concerned about what a culture and a society value and what the religious in them consider to be a proper response to God, the counsel to go slow (or go not at all) may commit me to taking one side in debates that demand appraisal of many sides on urgent issues affecting human dignity. So one must proceed deliberately at such a moment.

Religion is cultural, but it also seeks to be countercultural. One of the authors in this book is both somewhat dismissive and quite accurate when she observes that the culture has shaped religion more than religion has shaped the culture. What is surprising is that religion has done as much shaping as it has and that it is quite possibly doing more than it did for some decades in the recent past. We are hearing some quickened, informed, and helpful religious voices where for some time only secular rationality prevailed in medical ethics.

In this book some authors use the prefix "de-" rather generously, as in *deinstitutionalizing*, *detechnicalizing*, and *demedicalizing* death. In a similar vein, religion scholar José Casanova has recently written about the *deprivatization* of religion. Religion has reentered the public arena, in no small measure because of rapid developments in medical technology and societal expectations. So this book has reminded us again that while religion, like death, may be "a private affair," it has public dimensions. Add another element to be deduced from the presence of the religious here: religious thinkers tend to see death in the context of community, and attitudes toward it as telling much about culture and society—much more, indeed, than can be embodied in laws about euthanasia.

The Spanish philosopher José Ortega y Gasset has written that history is made less often by war, famine, and earthquake than when the "sensitive crown of the human heart" tilts ever so slightly in cultural shifts. He cites the motion from optimism to pessimism, or from despair to hope, as examples. That sensitive crown has tilted rather recently and rather rapidly toward an ever readier acceptance of euthanasias—I use the plural advisedly, since many forms are in this book—and these authors give some accountings why. Part 1, "A Cultural Analysis," is supposed to be about that subject; but Part 2, "Theological Responses," finds the religious thinkers also preoccupied with the cultural context.

Their responses point to many factors that induce change in the tilt of the sensitive crown of the human heart in our time. But the main element seems to be an attempt to minimize, avoid, and even eliminate suffering. While one or two of the religious thinkers are somewhat moved to turn sympathy for the suffering into positive support for active euthanasia, most of them work hard to see value in suffering. They may advocate better treatment of pain, but they have not bought the softer side of the therapeutic revolution in its suggestion that suffering can disappear; nor are they politically ready to extend the notion of entitlement further than it can be stretched —in this case, to the point of saying that we are all entitled to avoid suffering and to take easy, or at least easier, ways out when it comes. Buddhism, Judaism, and Christianity, and maybe *all* religions, address themselves in some way to suffering. Few of them picture human life exempt from it. How to deal with it is a part of religion and of the religious thought of the "pro-ambiguity" thinkers, those cautioning us to "go slow," who predominate in this volume.

It no longer works to say that science is based on reason and religion on emotion. Too many philosophers of science have shown how reason is based in the affective life of the people who employ it, and too many theologians have employed reason too forcefully to permit such a line to go unchallenged. Nevertheless, most of the religious thinkers here want to be sure that in a culture where "rationality" pervades bureaucracy, government, and medical systems, the voice of experience is heeded. That voice impels one to listen not only to the one who wishes to die but also to those she will leave behind, to the experience of the community and the tradition. And the experience of a life-in-context can no more be reduced to "may I help kill this person" than be reduced to "I must do everything to keep him alive." Attention to experience brings many factors to bear that no legislature can anticipate as it drafts laws and that no physicians' or hospitals' codes can reduce to canon.

It would embarrass the six authors, chosen from several Western theological traditions, if this afterword suggested that they were "know-it-alls" because they kept religious questions vivid, as they were asked to do. They might not even be thought of as people who "know more than," or who would place themselves above the medical specialists or purely secular-minded ethicists. Most of the way, they reveal themselves to be people who "know the same as," which means that those with a secular agenda are alert to religious concerns and those with a religious preoccupation are at home in the environment where secular discourse prevails. The overlap between the two parts of this book illustrates this. But more than any of these, scholars with religious interests "know other than." That is, while religion is being deprivatized, they want to be sure that the theological voice is also rendered public. It will raise questions that demand address where there cannot be answer. This religious voice will "thicken" the answers to questions that demanded more immediate answers. It will listen to intuition and experience, tradition and community, memory and hope, as well as affectivity and affection. Those who do the uttering will not close their ears to the voice of humane and humanistic thinkers, who have much to say, some of them in this book. In sum: the two parts overlap and are fused. Maybe the good "slippery slope" is the one that has ethicists and physicians sliding into theological discourse patterns and theologians sliding to show their familiarity with what is going on in the world around them, where belief and nonbelief are jumbled together. The authors in both halves want to be sure that human dignity continues to be reckoned with, and for that intention, one that I believe they fulfill, they have left us in their debt.

Now we can get out the children's board game one more time, hold the wand, outstretch the arm, and see whether the pull is more toward the "yes" or the "no" in respect to active euthanasia. Deciding will be as hard as ever. Living with the decisions, however, may be pursued with better conscience and certainly with more information and insight than before.

INDEX

abating treatment. *See* treatment (forgoing life-sustaining)

Abel (biblical figure), 231

abortion, 269

    Supreme Court decision on, 51, 72–76, 78

Abraham (biblical figure), 157, 231

absolutism (in bioethics), 103–4, 108

active euthanasia. *See* euthanasia

Adam (biblical figure), 154, 158, 231

Adkins, Janet, 127–28, 134

Admiraal, Dr. Peter, 61

adultery, 162

advanced directives, 7, 27–28, 123, 299

afterlife (resurrection)

    Baptists on, 312–13, 315–16

    Jews on, 155–57, 162

    Lutherans on, 205, 208, 223

    nonbelievers in, 289–90

    Reformed tradition on, 247–48

    Roman Catholics on, 180

    Wesleyans on, 281, 289

agape, 316

Ahithophel (biblical figure), 162, 164

AIDS, 68, 165, 296

    patients with, 25, 30, 32, 121–23, 126, 130, 333–34

air hunger, 125, 130–31

Akiba (rabbi), 155

allowing to die. *See* treatment (forgoing life-sustaining)

altruistic suicide, 277, 279

Alzheimer's disease, 93, 128, 134, 192, 296, 299

American Bar Association, 35

American Medical Association, 35

American Society of Internal Medicine, 135

American value(s)

    association between morality and legality in, 78

    autonomy as, 7, 28, 34, 107, 126–27, 200–201, 260

    and support for euthanasia, 16, 28, 34, 37

amyotrophic lateral sclerosis, 97–98

anesthesia, 99n.6, 125, 126

Angell, Marcia, 92–93

anomic suicide, 278

anti-authoritarianism, 17, 19, 28, 34, 37

anti-Semitism, 228–29

Ariès, Philippe, 126, 127

Aristotle, 45

Arizona Supreme Court, 79n.5

Asher, Rabbenu, 163–64

assisted suicide, 141

    in absence of terminal illness, 198–225, 266–302

    books on, 29

339

RONALD P. HAMEL, director of the Department of Clinical Ethics at Lutheran General Hospital–Advocate Health Care in Park Ridge, Illinois, co-edited *Choosing Death: Active Euthanasia, Religion, and the Public Debate.*

EDWIN R. DUBOSE, a clinical ethics consultant at the Park Ridge Center for the Study of Health, Faith, and Ethics in Chicago, is the author of *The Illusion of Trust: Toward a Medical Theological Ethics in the Postmodern Age.*